Dark Medicine

BIOETHICS AND THE HUMANITIES
Eric M. Meslin and Richard B. Miller, editors

EDITED BY
WILLIAM R. LAFLEUR,
GERNOT BÖHME,
AND
SUSUMU SHIMAZONO

Dark Medicine

Rationalizing Unethical Medical Research

INDIANA UNIVERSITY PRESS
Bloomington and Indianapolis

This book is a publication of

Indiana University Press
601 North Morton Street
Bloomington, IN 47404-3797 USA

http://iupress.indiana.edu

Telephone orders   800-842-6796
Fax orders   812-855-7931
Orders by e-mail   iuporder@indiana.edu

The paper used in this publication meets the minimum requirements of American National Standard for Information Sciences—Permanence of Paper for Printed Library Materials, ANSI Z39.48-1984.

Manufactured in the United States of America

Library of Congress Cataloging-in-Publication Data

Dark medicine : rationalizing unethical medical research / edited by William R. LaFleur, Gernot Böhme, and Susumu Shimazono.
    p. ; cm. — (Bioethics and the humanities)
  Includes bibliographical references and index.
  ISBN 978-0-253-34872-2 (cloth : alk. paper) 1. Human experimentation in medicine—Moral and ethical aspects. 2. Medicine—Research—Moral and ethical aspects. 3. Medical ethics—History. I. LaFleur, William R. II. Böhme, Gernot. III. Shimazono, Susumu, date IV. Series.
  [DNLM: 1. Human Experimentation—ethics. 2. Human Experimentation—history. 3. Bioethical Issues. 4. History, 20th Century. W 20.55.H9 D219 2007]
  R853.H8D3776 2007
  174.2'8—dc22

                                                                                          2007000635

1 2 3 4 5   12 11 10 09 08 07

Americans were kept in the dark about the effects of what was being done to them . . . for these experiments were kept secret.

President Bill Clinton, on October 3, 1995, concerning the Report of the Advisory Committee on Human Radiation Experiments

Contents

PART TWO

THE CONFLICTED PRESENT AND THE WORRISOME FUTURE

Preface

Nations involved today in international competition in biotech research often behave like drivers in an old-fashioned stock-car race. Each is constantly aware of others in the race and uses anxiety about relative "position" to rationalize stepping harder on the accelerator and taking ever-greater risks.

In fact, a kind of raw fear can grip the so-called advanced nations if there seems to be some evidence, perhaps real but possibly only fabricated, that nations deemed just a few years ago to be underdeveloped in science and biomedicine have not only already caught up but have been sighted as now *in the passing lane*. This perception then gets infused into debates about bioethics. For instance, although one can construct a cogent moral argument on behalf of federal funding of therapeutic stem-cell research, a sizable portion of the "case" for this, as presented both to the American general public and to the U.S. Congress in 2006, depended on conjuring images of an America no longer able to be first among nations in these domains. Although this is utterly dubious as an *ethical* argument to justify any program in medicine, in today's world blatant appeals to scientific nationalism get imported into politics . . . and even into bioethics.

Asian societies, taken as monolithic, get cited by speed-enthralled Americans as now poised to cop the really big prizes of biotech hard-driving. And the putative reason for this, we are told, is that Asians have no inhibitions in this domain. No limit-obsessed God, no heavy-handed church, no sentiment about life's sanctity will, we are told, stand in the way of Asians' rushing ahead of the West in the domain of what Renée Fox has—tellingly—called "frontier medicine."

This is a half-truth. It has, if you look, already resulted in some recent wreckage on the scene; Korea's Dr. Woo Suk Hwang, prior to the horrendous 2005 crash of his fraudulent cell nuclear transfer project, had been touting his "Buddhism" as the reason, at least for him, human cloning posed no ethical problems whatsoever. And, until his big crash, some American scientists and ethicists publicly expressed envy of Hwang's perceived advantage.

More fundamentally, however, the problem with the version of an uninhibited Asia cherished today by some Western scientists is naïve—at least when it is not craftily manipulating blissful ignorance (plus the "findings" of quickie junkets to Asia) to rationalize acceleration at home.

This book, at times through studies of the past that may prove downright painful to some readers, is intended by its editors to put the lie to such naïveté. For instance, the Japan examined here will not fit easily into any facile sketch of an "uninhibited Asia." While Japan is probably the world's most advanced nation in robotics and some other technologies, many Japanese—including many bioethicists and a surprising number of physicians—are deeply skeptical vis-à-vis biotechnology's getting shoved onto the fast lane. As essays here will show, for many Japanese some notion of a limit-demanding God need not be part of things in order to have good bases for exercising caution. Other reasons show themselves quite readily. And among these surely it is *history*—a deeply troubling "been there/done that" kind of mid-war history—that makes many Japanese skittish today.

In this the Japanese resemble the Germans, also a people deeply and continuously sobered by knowledge of having in the past gone far too far into the dark side of medical research. We should probably not be surprised to see that many of today's Japanese and Germans are considerably more skeptical than their Anglo-American counterparts when faced with intellectually greased trajectories into what is called "liberal" eugenics.

That modern medicine has provided our societies with innumerable good benefits is beyond doubt. This volume, by looking hard at how and through what rationalizations medical research did—and still can—slip into its dark mode, will, we hope, help it retain its earned reputation as one of humankind's goods.

Acknowledgments

This book had its origins in conversations, both in person and in cyberspace, among its three editors. We agreed on the urgency of raising the questions asked in these chapters—and decided to assemble world authorities on both the historical cases and the contemporary issues investigated here. Unwilling to imply that unethical medical research is a problem only of the past, we sought to explore how the rationalization mechanism operates today as well.

The persons we pinpointed for this project gathered for a conference at the University of Pennsylvania April 28 to May 1, 2004. We convened in Philadelphia under the rubric "Going Too Far: Rationalizing Unethical Medical Research in Japan, Germany, and the United States." We enjoyed strong support from two research units at Penn—the Center for East Asian Studies, under the direction of G. Cameron Hurst III, and the Center for Bioethics, directed by Arthur F. Caplan. Financial support was provided by a grant to the CEAS from the U.S. Department of Education. Generous additional support was received from the US–Japan Friendship Commission through its director, Eric Gangloff; Penn's School of Medicine and its dean, Arthur H. Rubinstein; the special fund of the Dean of the School of Arts and Sciences; the Penn Humanities Forum; the Penn Lauder CIBER; the E. Dale Saunders Council; individual departments at Penn; and the discretionary fund of the Director-General of the International Research Center for Japanese Studies.

Sadly, one of our colleague-contributors, Rolf Winau of Berlin, died very suddenly while this volume was in preparation. In addition to being a physician, he had been a leading authority on the history of the research use of human subjects. We are very grateful to his colleague, Volker Hess of Berlin's Center for Humanities and Health Sciences, Charité, for checking the final proofs of Winau's essay here.

Paula Roberts, the Assistant Director of Penn's Center for East Asian Studies, skillfully and unflappably coordinated our funding, travel, and conference logistics. Max Dionisio was an absolutely reliable coordinator of all on-the-ground details; he made the conference flow with ease. Since we decided early on to reach out for quality of expertise not necessarily complemented by a scholar's ability to write and lecture in English, translators and interpreters would, we knew, be required. During what were often lively conference interchanges, Alexander Bennett and Frank Chance adroitly sent comments in Japanese into English and vice versa. The team of persons who, in advance and often within terribly compressed time-frames, had skillfully translated most of the papers was composed of Nona Carter, Adrian Daub, Denis Gainty, Jeffrey Graves, William Hammell, Sari Kawana, Stephen Miller, Robin Orlansky, Rika

Saito, and Jonathan Siegel. Also assisting with logistics were Jennifer McCaskie and Kenji Saito. Cheri Love designed a stunning poster for the conference and Nicole Riley assisted later in handling manuscripts and proofs.

The collaboration of Penn colleagues was invaluable. Those who contributed greatly by giving prepared responses to the conference papers were Ronald Granieri, Nien-hê Hsieh, Rahul Kumar, Luigi Mastroiani, and Paul Root Wolpe. Linda Chance, Jennifer Conway, Ruth Cowan, Sherrill Davis, Margaret Guinan, Richard Herring, Lynn Lees, Irene Lukoff, Cecilia Segawa Seigle, Wendy Steiner, and Liliane Weisberg helped us greatly. Ongoing discussions with colleagues in Penn's Faculty Seminar on Ethics in the Professions were also a stimulus for completing this work. Ann Mongoven, on the faculty of Indiana University, not only attended but also contributed a comment on one of the papers. Attendees came not only from within the United States but from Japan as well.

During the summer and fall of 2003, Kyoto's International Research Center for Japanese Studies provided funds and a venue for William LaFleur to explore the possibility and shape of this project. Its director at the time, Tetsuo Yamaori, was supportive from the outset.

Persons at Indiana University Press deserving mention in gratitude are Robert Sloan and Jane Quinet. Carol Kennedy was a careful and always helpful copyeditor. Thanks for helpful comments go also to anonymous readers of the original manuscript.

Dark Medicine

Introduction: The Knowledge Tree and Its Double Fruit

William R. LaFleur

Nearly two thousand years ago Marcus Aurelius articulated a standard that, if applied to the professions, held that all their members should "*be* upright, not be *kept* upright." But this high ideal, we know by bitter experience, is unrealistic. The professions, including those of medicine, today enjoy the general public's confidence in part because mechanisms have been put in place in order to *keep* their actions "upright."

One of these mechanisms consists of making public those actions—in both the past and the present—that violate generally agreed upon ethical standards. This was made strikingly, even shockingly, clear by what had been reported concerning some physicians serving with the American military in Iraq's Abu Ghraib prison. *The Lancet*, Britain's premier medical journal, performed a service by pointing out, "Government documents show that the U.S. military medical system failed to protect detainees' human rights, sometimes collaborated with interrogators or abusive guards, and failed to properly report injuries or deaths caused by beatings" (Miles 2004, 725; now also Miles 2006).

We no longer dare excuse gross lapses in professional ethics by appealing to "wartime conditions"—as if these are statistically so rare or so unusual that when they occur, ordinary standards may simply be waived. In fact, what we might wish were a sharp, clear difference between "seasons of war" and "seasons of peace" has, especially in recent centuries, been blunted by something in between, namely, seasons of rumored, anticipated, or planned-for wars. The years of what we call "the Cold War" were precisely such a season, one lasting for half a century and generating its own "culture" (Whitfield 1991).

And medicine was caught up in the dilemma the Cold War posed—from that war's very outset in 1945. The horrendous level of radiation poured onto two Japanese cities, we are at last beginning to see, produced a subsidiary "value" in addition to accelerating the end of World War II. And that "value" was realized because a portion of America's medical establishment was drawn into the research producing it. While we have no direct evidence that the production of data relating to radiation and its effects was an explicit motive in dropping the bombs, the huge amount of human energy exerted by the United States into the collection, preservation, and study of *data* recoverable on the ground and from the bodies and body parts in Hiroshima and Nagasaki, presents us with something deeply disturbing. Even if only a "windfall" benefit, this hoarding of data was part of an evolving research project, one subsequently carried out by the Atomic Energy Casualty Commission but very quickly seen by many Japanese as one that had used the noncombatant citizens of Hiroshima and Nagasaki as "guinea-pigs" in a radiation test.

That project's motives seemed especially sullied when the AECC adopted a "no treatment" policy with respect to the *hibakusha*, persons radiated but still alive, who were suffering and desperately in need of care. Official American policy required that even American physicians in the bombed cities were expected to gather data and, correspondingly, to refuse to administer anything that would smack of therapy (Lindee 1994, 124–42). Since it is an acknowledged fact that raw data will necessarily be "contaminated" once the bodies providing such data are medicated in any way, and since the Americans were obsessed with collecting data as pure as possible, the burden of proof surely lies on those who might wish to explain away the suspicion that many, even if not all, American physicians in Hiroshima and Nagasaki let their deepest professional obligations be sidelined by the "needs" of research.

Importantly, the war propelling this abrogation of professional ethics was *not* the war just concluded but, rather, a war then merely envisioned as occurring in the future. As Lindee notes: "The American medical teams [arriving in Japan in late September 1945] were expected to develop plans for atomic triage in a future war" (Lindee 1998, 382). And such plans required, it seems, that the data be brought home for easy access and close study. Thus, the AECC transported at least "twenty-thousand items, including photographs, autopsy records, clothing, and four thousand pieces of human remains" half a world away to Washington, D.C., where they were to remain as objects of research until being returned—on Japanese insistence—to Japan in May 1973 (Lindee 1998).[1]

Rationalizations initially masquerade as reasons. It is often only in hindsight that they are seen for what they had really been. Under construction, rationalizations have as a central component some kind of appeal to "special" or "extraordinary" conditions. Of course, wars, whether in process or only anticipated, can hardly be outdone in terms of providing "conditions" useful to rationalize practices that go far beyond what is usually deemed ethical in medicine.

However, some of us now wonder whether the scientific competition prized in our day does not itself take the form of "research wars" and, as such, jack up the impression that "unusual conditions" justify running research agendas down the fast lane. Ironically, very advanced biotechnical research can now be done in the laboratories of nations still undergoing "development" in many other domains. Some of the more economically advanced nations—such as the three that come into focus in this volume—have at times made attempts to put regulations in place. But a deep fear, one projected out to the public in an image of national scientists in a state of panic, has its uses. A fear of losing out in the competition and even of being scientifically "outclassed" by others pervades. "If *we* don't do it, *X* will" becomes the reiterated base rationale for researchers and enterprises demanding that regulations be lifted.[2]

Gross risk and great opportunity are the Janus-faces of "crisis." The ethics of research can be relativized either by the atmospherics of war or by the blandishments of opportunity. And when the public is being massaged into acceptance of an extraordinary breakthrough in the offing, the reasons given for going forward with research immediately are, virtually without exception, noble and unobjectionable: forms of therapy, cure, and prevention heretofore scarcely imagined—a new level of medical "miracle." If located, it is argued, such therapies will benefit far more people, far more quickly, and far more efficiently. What is presented as "extraordinary" in such cases is the *opportunity*—to do good.[3]

The fruits that heal and the fruits that kill all too often hang on the same knowledge tree. And persons trying to pick only the former can hardly avoid knocking some of the latter into their baskets. In the context of research, the altruism of healing can scarcely avoid getting mixed up with the natural egotism of persons or groups doing things that may bring fame or elicit the praise and support of those who govern. And the alternative to collaboration often presents itself as a future of professional isolation, even obscurity—as well as the professionally miserable state of going unfunded. Motives come mixed.

Germany in the epoch of the Third Reich presents us with such a graphic, if horrifying, example of all of the above, that its materials, we feel, need to be continuously kept in view and analyzed for what they tell us about the process of rationalization. Given the present volume's readiness to juxtapose and compare unethical medical research in three different twentieth-century nations, some readers may feel that we have implicitly taken sides in the intense debate that took place in Germany during the 1980s concerning what some within that debate, Jürgen Habermas especially, insisted was the *singularity* [Einzigartigkeit] of the Holocaust and the crimes of the Third Reich (Knowlton and Cates 1993). Such is not the case. This book does not relativize the demonic depths of Germany's policies and practices during that epoch. Specifically, we recognize the specific genocidal motive in the Holocaust and do not find evidence of such a dimension in either the Japanese or American medical programs examined in this volume.

This is not to suggest that the results of their programs were not horrendous. Unit 731 was the now infamous medical unit of the Japanese army that operated under a government mandate and carried out murderous research in China and Manchuria. The number of persons killed in such medical experiments seems to rise with each new effort to calculate it and may have been, as Chinese writings claim, in the thousands. And the United States is not without its own version of dark medicine. With the passage of the Freedom of Information Act and due to dogged research into files long kept secret, it has become clear that, according to Eileen Welsome, within the United States after 1945 "thousands of human radiation experiments, many of them unethical and without therapeutic benefit, were funded by the Atomic Energy Commission over the next three decades of the Cold War" (Welsome 1999, 193).

Historical "accidents" can blunt memory. Welsome (469–70) notes that President Bill Clinton's October 3, 1995, public apology to the victims of American medico-military research and his startling declaration that "Americans had been kept in the dark" concerning that research was lost on that same public, one easily captivated two hours after Clinton's statement by news of the courtroom verdict in the sensational murder trial of O. J. Simpson in Los Angeles.

Or, is it not more likely that nations, like individuals, often *prefer* to remain "in the dark" about times and ways in which some of the medical research sponsored and conducted by their own governments had gotten dark—both because it was ethically compromised and because it operated most "efficiently" when kept concealed? We do not like being disabused of our belief that only one kind of fruit, the healing variety that we so much prize, hangs from the tree of medical research.

The impulse to forget or even to repress such knowledge is not unique to certain nations or peoples. As Frederick Dickinson's contribution to this book makes clear, references, largely in Western media, to a peculiarly Japanese national "amnesia" concerning the crimes of Unit 731 are overblown. Dickinson's data and analysis fit my own discovery in Japanese materials that I had been reading about bioethics there. Inured as I was to the usual rhetoric here about a pervasive Japanese unwillingness even to mention the medical crimes of Unit 731, I was surprised in the late 1990s to find multiple references to its atrocities in what I was reading. Japan's so-called amnesia was far from total; I had stumbled across historians and bioethicists in Japan who were candid about this history and were ready to explore how it might be instructive concerning the need to deal ethically with research programs that, if not downright dark, had in them enough shadow to give reason to pause, ponder, and possibly move forward only with the greatest of caution.[4] My discovery of these materials was a catalyst for the project that produced this book.

The focus of this volume may be clarified by a comparison. Much recent Chinese research and publication on Japan's wartime medical research seems to be mired in the politics of the present, specifically the repeated Chinese demand that Japanese living in 2006 pay reparations for crimes against the Chinese committed during the first half of the last century. Also, in the absence of proof of a specific genocidal intent, Chinese references today to Japan's medical experiments as an "Auschwitz" in Asia seem misdirected. Moreover, the ascription of the crimes of that era to a "militarism" assumed to be a continuing idiopathology of the Japanese blunts the chance of seeing the more universal problem, the one we have been intent on investigating in this book. The problem of rationalizing unethical medical research is, we would be best to assume, not one to which China has successfully immunized itself.

The focus of this volume, then, is not so much on the history of the episodes of dark medical research in three nations considered as it is on how such research was rationalized—precisely because the patterns of rationalization are more likely to show up again in our own time than are the specifics of past actions. Chapters by Böhme, Winau, Müller-Hill, Frewer, and Caplan focus on such patterns within Germany. Programs involving "man's inhumanity to man" were made to seem justifiable by the theorizing of Viktor von Weizsäcker, arguably one of the twentieth century's finest researchers in psychiatric medicine and someone whose international image in the postwar period has not been like that of the gruesomely ruthless Dr. Josef Mengele. Gernot Böhme's groundbreaking essay is the first in any language to demonstrate the process of rationalization in von Weizsäcker. Böhme subjects these materials to a philosophical analysis and suggests that, contrary to our fond wishes, we do not yet have in place safeguards that would keep us from slippage into a similar ethical debasement.

Andreas Frewer gives us the core of a book he wrote in German, one demonstrating the slide of *Ethik,* German's premier journal on ethics, into an embrace of what was patently contrary to everything ethical. Frewer's is a classic example of a sobering account, tracing how, step by step, both medical practice and a complicit ethics moved from prioritizing the health of the patient as the highest law (*suprema lex*) in medicine to a focus, instead, on what was taken to be the "health" of the general public. He describes how such a subversion of intellectual integrity occurred and may do so again.

Rolf Winau's research reaches back into times well before the Nazi era, showing us something easily overlooked in studies, namely, that there is nothing new in touting "medical progress" when setting out to use humans in experiments. His discussion also shows the clear affirmation of informed consent reached already in Germany of 1930—that is, prior to the epoch of its most egregious violation there. The code's articulation and its basest violation occurred at almost the same time. "Guidelines" had been articulated but, tragically, had no effect on practice.

Benno Müller-Hill is a scientist who insists that scientists not ignore or paper over scientific crimes of the past—some of which he himself unearthed. His own work (Müller-Hill 1984) forced open this issue within Germany. In his chapter he builds a strong case against permitting researchers and scholars to keep silent about patently unethical agendas. His own personal experiences dealing with the ploys by others, members of the German scientific community, to deny or conceal evidence makes for a compelling account.

The chapter by Arthur L. Caplan is both a vivid reminder of the kinds of things that, in the wake of the Holocaust, should have been much more thoroughly investigated and a critique of explanations—in terms of incompetence, madness, and coercion—that will not wash. Caplan 1992 is one of the earliest works to connect Third Reich–era medical experiments with contemporary bioethics. In the present volume his essay puts forward evidence to show that, perhaps because some of the rationalizations of the Nazi doctors find resonance within contemporary thinking about medicine, bioethics as a discipline still tends to resist truly *serious* grappling with what went on in the Third Reich.

What is presented here concerning Japan will quite likely be relatively new to many readers in the English-speaking world. American society's ignorance of horrendous wartime crimes in the name of medical research sponsored by

Japan's rulers is an ignorance that, as shown also by Hurst here, was brought about by design, not by default. It was part of the American government's policy during the Cold War, a point reinforced by the extensive materials presented in Welsome 1999. War, even if "cold" and still only potential, rationalized American officials' decision in the immediate postwar era to procure the "results" of Japan's wartime research and, as a consequence, to refrain from including such persons, in spite of their clear criminality, as defendants in the "Tokyo War Crimes Trials" conducted between 1946 and 1948.[5]

Here a discussion of Japan's wartime research is the primary focus of essays by Tsuneishi and Dickinson, although attention to that sordid history is also part of the articles by Yamaori, Shimazono, and Komatsu. Kei-ichi Tsuneishi, who in 1981 published the first extensive exposure of this material and is widely regarded as the world's premier authority on the history of Unit 731's gruesome deeds,[6] emphasizes in his chapter that it was the *medical profession*, not the military per se, that sought to benefit—both in terms of new research findings and in terms of making a demonstrable contribution to nationalist goals—from subjecting unwitting human subjects to excruciating pain and death. Tsuneishi finds shocking also the degree to which, even in the postwar context, Japan's community of physicians, while generally aware of how Unit 731's findings had been procured, has tended to behave as if there had been nothing barbaric in science of that sort.

As noted above, Frederick R. Dickinson's research directly challenges the assumption that a peculiar kind of national "amnesia" keeps Japanese awareness of Unit 731's crimes from surfacing. He presents rich detail to show that, in fact, the political polarization within Japan during the Cold War was a catalyst for Japan's Left to force a substantive public exposure there of the biological warfare research carried out prior to 1945. By contrast, Dickinson contends, within the United States there has been, again for political reasons, nothing comparable in terms of a political situation forcing a revelation to the public here of American efforts to put a cover over the facts of Unit 731 and virtually no "appetite" for revealing the history of America's own biological warfare research.

Books, like experiments, run risks. And one of the risks accepted from the outset by this project has been that of being criticized, especially within the United States, for drawing any parallel between American research and that of Germany and Japan. Therefore, it bears reiterating here that we are not suggesting anything parallel in scale or intensity. There is a difference too in a program that is aimed specifically at genocide and one that, begun for other reasons, shows the features of blatant racism as choices are made along the way concerning who receives therapy and who does not. America's government-sponsored "Tuskegee syphilis experiment," in which African American men were deemed too valuable as research subjects to be given the penicillin that would have healed them, is an infamous and egregious case (Brandt 1978; Jones 1981).

G. Cameron Hurst III's historical study facilitates this volume's linkage between Japan and the United States in the employment of unethical research programs. By examining long-standing claims that Americans used biological weapons during the Korean War, Hurst suggests that we ought not dismiss such charges out of hand. He provides a concrete case of how the political ethos of the Cold War—which, of course, got very *hot* on the Korean peninsula!—not only quite likely served as "cover" for Americans' military usage of Japan's mid-war research but also reaches down into the present. Accusations today that it is only America's terrorist enemies who would even *conceive* of using biological agents to kill are, at least in terms of things discussed by Hurst, worthy of being met with considerable skepticism.

M. Susan Lindee's chapter forcefully demonstrates why American research absolutely may not be exempted from very close scrutiny both by historians and by scholars concerned with the ethics of medicine. The details of American ballistics research during the Cold War are excruciating. And perhaps because so routinely described by researchers in the quantifying language of "normal science," the bodies subjected to "experimental wounding" poignantly illustrate the nature and depth of our problem, a transnational one.

And evidence that the history of the discipline we call "bioethics" needs rewriting is presented by Jonathan D. Moreno here. He examines specific instances of gaps, sometimes resulting in deaths to research subjects, between the official American adoption of the norm of "informed consent" and government-sponsored research. He uses in-practice violations of the "informed consent" norm adopted by the American government to force a reconceptualization of some of our key terms. Moreno challenges us to go beyond our standard account of the "origins" of bioethics and suggests that doing so will help us more adequately deal with present and future arguments in favor of using human experiments for the sake of national security.

The second half of this volume, "The Conflicted Present and the Worrisome Future," while less focused on history than the book's first half, more directly addresses certain contemporary—and probably future—questions and dilemmas in the field of bioethics.

In her chapter, Renée C. Fox calls our attention to something very troubling but generally overlooked, namely, iatrogenesis as harm intrinsic to all forms of medical care. Fox's demonstration of this important point, one we emotionally and institutionally resist, accentuates the presence of a kind of "dark knowledge" within the thickened plot of this volume. After scrutinizing harm caused within gene therapy trials, Fox offers here a tantalizing "counter-intuitive hypothesis"—namely, that physicians more easily admit that they have committed an "error" than that some kinds of harm are inherent in medicine itself and beyond their control. Thickening this book's plot, she shows how certain kids of discomforting knowledge even today routinely get pushed into the dark.

Fox's essay also resonates well with that of Tetsuo Yamaori in this aspect. Yamaori is a Japanese scholar with the status of a "public intellectual" there—someone widely quoted. Although, as here, he faces what is repulsive in Japan's militarism in the early twentieth century, Yamaori also often draws upon Japan's Buddhist traditions to note why Japan need not follow the West in any knee-jerk fashion. Looking here at the implications of the history of Unit 731 and the wider implications of cadaveric organ transplantation, Yamaori sees us as needing to move beyond employing a simplistic "survival theory" to rationalize some of our medical procedures, including organ transplantation. His chapter has deep theoretical and practical implications, and his personal account of how he himself hopes to be able to die presents a vivid and sharp contrast to what Renée Fox and Judith Swazey describe as an American transplantation ethos that embraces a "bellicose, 'death is the enemy' perspective" (Fox and Swazey 1992, 199).

This is closely connected to the major theme of Yoshiko Komatsu's strong and informed critique of concepts that rationalize what he calls a continuing "barbarism" in whole areas of medical ethics today. With Unit 731 and Nazi era atrocities in view, he here presents in English the core of what in Japan has received attention and praise as Komatsu's ethically sensitive concept of "reverberating death." Here he draws out its implications across a range of bioethical issues and problems.

Susumu Shimazono's informative and important essay uses history and religious difference to explain something that is often a conundrum to persons viewing Japan from abroad—namely, that society's toleration of easy access to abortion but deep reservations about the ethics of cadaveric organ transplantation and current forms of regenerative medicine, recombinant stem cell use in particular. His explanation of why the recombinant stem cell use but *not* abortion may, at least in the eyes of many Japanese, constitute ethically problematic practice implicitly challenges the notion, widely held at least in North America, that only abortion-opposed, "right-to-life" proponents will resist far-reaching biotechnology and a "progressive" bioethics. Shimazono's perspective illustrates why attitudes in bioethics around the globe cannot, and probably, should not, be as uniform as some wish to make them.

Miho Ogino points out that Japan's early legalization of abortion in 1948 had its own dark underside, inasmuch as it was linked to eugenics both in name and in practice. Her research shows why an invoking of language about "rights" does not assuage the concerns of persons with disabilities, nor does it remove the ethical dilemma even of feminists in Japan. The element of "choice" in new reproductive technologies does not mean the "new eugenics" comes free of deep problems.[7] Public language about the "right to choose" exercised by infertile women and couples, she writes, contributes to the way in which the hasty application of new reproductive technologies gets rationalized.

In this book's final chapter I indicate why some of our current dilemmas result, at least in part, from themes and rhetoric that were part of European philosophy as it tried to modernize itself. Apologists for what today is called the new, "liberal eugenics" tell us there is absolutely no similarity between it and the "old" eugenics that was touted as advanced medicine not only in the Third Reich but also in America and elsewhere prior to World War II. But the utopianism near the surface of their claims and their argument against any possible historical parallels should occasion, instead, suspicion and caution. I also assert that we need to see the nexus between Hans Jonas's experience in the Holocaust and his insistence upon rigorous caution in the development of certain kinds of biotechnologies.

* * *

Historical research tends to be sobering. There is probably a subtle linkage between, on the one hand, the fact that the authors in this volume refuse to close the books on past episodes of repulsive medical research and, on the other, the fact that all or most of these same writers will wish to inject substantive calls for caution when deliberating the ethics of innovative or groundbreaking new research. In some of the essays that linkage is made explicit.

Having noted that, we consider it important to state clearly that it would be a mistake to view this volume as "anti-modern" or even "anti-science." Scientists themselves must, we feel, acknowledge that their reputation has in our time been tarnished in part by a growing awareness that "the largest part of the expenditures for scientific-technological manpower has hitherto been invested in the military sector" (Böhme 1992, 9). Nevertheless, although this project involves a study of the processes of rationalization, these authors do not take a reductionist approach to elucidating that process. That is, they stay clear of insisting, for instance, that it is *only* the "bottom line" of corporate profits that, when all is said and done, offers the true explanation for certain research agendas or, alternatively, that *only* envisioned praise and prizes motivated medical researchers' cooperation with their governments in projects we now see as dangerous, even nefarious.

In part because it is, in fact, the more *difficult* route, our preference is to avoid being reductionist. These chapters demonstrate that it is possible to exercise what Paul Ricoeur called "the hermeneutics of suspicion," but, precisely because the motivations of human beings are far too complex to be rendered down into one or more *base* (in both senses of that word) factors, that very complexity must, we hold, be honored within our own research (Ricoeur 1970, 32–36; Ricoeur 1986, 95–100).

If, as noted, historical research is sobering, we need to keep continuously active the question whether a truly responsible bioethics may avoid taking history into account. Gernot Böhme holds, contrary to many of his fellow philosophers, that it absolutely may not avoid history. Considering, for instance, the question of physician-assisted suicide, he insists that one cannot decide such a matter simply by weighing the Hippocratic code against what, through modern medicine, becomes an artificially protracted lifespan and "a humanly degraded form of existence." History may not be left out of the picture. "It is quite impossible to decide on this question today without seeing it against the background of a misuse of the idea of euthanasia—if the practice of the Third Reich can be described as that. What is at issue here, therefore, is not only basic values but our society's historical understanding of itself" (Böhme 2001, 11). The conclusion, then, seems clear. If history, especially that of the twentieth century, is sobering, we ought not expect that the ethics of our medical research and our bioethics will be other than themselves sobered by attention to it. A bioethics trained to detect times and ways in which dark motives for doing certain kinds of research are present will be a bioethics more able to tell the scientist and physician which fruit to grasp and which ones to leave unpicked.

Notes

1. Hogle 1999 also brilliantly analyses how body parts and body tissue were related to ways in which Germans attempted to deal with the history of the Holocaust.

2. In her study of human experimentation in the United States in the first half of the twentieth century, Susan D. Lederer points out that the "martyrdom" of not a few medical researchers who did initial trials on themselves, sometimes resulting in death, did much to abate public criticism and suspicions (Lederer 1995, 137). That mode of gaining public confidence is not, for various reasons, of course, in use today.

3. Sermons advocating eugenics in America during the 1920s and 1930s employed the notion of "crisis" in both senses: dire inasmuch as the human gene pool was depicted as rapidly deteriorating but, on the other hand, extremely hopeful in that eugenics, if applied quickly and extensively, would materialize on earth what the Scriptures had called "the Kingdom of God." See Rosen 2004.

4. Representative, even if far from exhaustive, references in Japanese to Unit 731 atrocities in the context of discussions of bioethics (in order of their appearance) are: Akimoto 1983; Kimura 1987, 267–68; Yamaguchi 1995, 70; Komatsu 1996, 48–49; Kondō 1996; Tsuneishi 1998; Abe 2000, 43; Kanamori and Nakajima 2002, 69.

5. Although Harris 1994 is the best-known exposé of this policy of concealment in an English-language publication, a reader for Indiana University Press pointed out to me that Harris was preceded by Powell 1981 and by Williams and Wallace 1989.

6. Surely facts about Unit 731 were brought to a wide Japanese reading public through Ienaga 1968, and, although via fiction, facts about the vivisection of downed American pilots were revealed in a spectacular manner in a novel, widely read in Japan, by Shūsaku Endō (Endō 1958).

7. Insisting on the concerns of persons with disabilities has been an especially strong motif in Japanese bioethics. An important writer on this has been Masahiro Morioka. See, for instance, Morioka 2003.

References

Abe, Tomoko. 2000. Bunka toshite no shi no kaitai to ningen kaitai o maneku "Nōshi, zōki ishoku." In *Watakushi wa zōki o teikyō shinai,* ed. Kondō Makoto et al., 26–56. Tokyo: Yōsensha.

Akimoto, Sueo. 1983. *I no rinri o tou: Dai 731 butai de no taiken kara.* Tokyo: Keisō shobō.

Böhme, Gernot. 1992. *Coping with Science.* Boulder, Colo.: Westview.

———. 2001. *Ethics in Context: The Art of Dealing with Serious Questions.* Cambridge, U.K.: Polity Press.

Brandt, Allan M. 1978. Racism and Research: The Case of the Tuskegee Syphilis Study. *Hastings Center Report* 8: 21–29.

Caplan, Arthur L., ed. 1992. *When Medicine Went Mad: Bioethics and the Holocaust.* Totowa, N.J.: Humana Press.

Endō, Shūsaku. 1958. *Umi to dokuyaku.* Tokyo: Bungei shunjū.

———. 1973. *The Sea and Poison.* Trans. of *Umi to dokuyaku* by Michael Gallagher. Tokyo: Charles E. Tuttle.

Fox, Renée C., and Judith P. Swazey. 1992. *Spare Parts: Organ Replacement in American Society.* New York: Oxford University Press.

Harris, Sheldon H. 1994. *Factories of Death: Japanese Biological Warfare, 1932–45, and the American Cover-up.* New York: Routledge.

Hogle, Linda F. 1999. *Recovering the Nation's Body: Cultural Memory, Medicine, and the Politics of Redemption.* New Brunswick, N.J.: Rutgers University Press.

Ienaga, Saburō. 1968. *Taiheiyō sensō.* Tokyo: Iwanami shoten.

———. 1978. *The Pacific War, 1931–1945: A Critical Perspective on Japan's Role in World War II.* Trans. of *Taiheiyō sensō* by Frank Baldwin. New York: Pantheon Books.

Jones, James Howard. 1981. *Bad Blood: The Tuskegee Syphilis Experiment.* New York: Free Press.

Kanamori, Osamu, and Hideto Nakajima. 2002. *Kagakuron no genzai.* Tokyo: Keisō shobō.

Kimura, Rihito. 1987. *Inochi o kangaeru: Baioshikkusu no susume.* Tokyo: Nihon hyōronsha.

Komatsu, Yoshihiko. 1996. *Shi wa kyōmei suru: Nōshi, zōki ishoku no fukami e.* Tokyo: Keisō shobō.

Knowlton, James, and Truett Cates, trans. 1993. [No original editor] *Forever in the Shadow of Hitler? Original Documents of the Historikerstreit, the Controversy Concerning the Singularity of the Holocaust.* Atlantic Highlands, N.J.: Humanities Press.

Kondō, Makoto. 1996. *Kanja yo, Gan to tatakau na.* Tokyo: Bungei shunjū.

Lederer, Susan E. 1995. *Subjected to Science: Human Experimentation in America Before the Second World War.* Baltimore: Johns Hopkins Press.

Lindee, M. Susan. 1994. *Suffering Made Real: American Science and the Survivors at Hiroshima.* Chicago: University of Chicago Press.

———. 1998. The Repatriation of Atomic Bomb Victim Body Parts to Japan: Natural Objects and Diplomacy. *Osiris* 13: 376–409.

Miles, Steven H. 2004. Abu Ghraib: Its Legacy for Military Medicine. *The Lancet* 364 (Aug. 21): 725–29.

———. 2006. *Oath Betrayed: Torture, Medical Complicity, and the War on Terror.* New York: Random House.

Morioka, Masahiro. 2003. *Mutsū bunmeiron.* Tokyo: Toransubyū.

Müller-Hill, Benno. 1984. *Tödliche Wissenschaft.* Reinbek bei Hamburg: Rohwalt Taschenbuch Verlag.

Powell, John W. 1981. Japan's Biological Weapons: 1930–1945, A Hidden Chapter in History. *Bulletin of the Atomic Scientists* (Oct.): 41–45.

Ricoeur, Paul. 1970. *Freud and Philosophy: An Essay on Interpretation.* Trans. Denis Savage. New Haven, Conn.: Yale University Press.

———. 1986. *Lectures on Ideology and Utopia.* Ed. George H. Taylor. New York: Columbia University Press.

Rosen, Christine. 2004. *Preaching Eugenics: Religious Leaders and the American Eugenics Movement.* Oxford: Oxford University Press.

Tsuneishi, Kei-ichi. 1994. *Igaku to sensō: Nihon to doitsu.* Tokyo: Ochanomizu shobō.

——. 1998. Igaku to sensō: Ima, igakkai ni towarete iru koto. In *Seimei rinrigaku kōgi: Igaku, iryō ni nani ga towarete iru ka,* ed. Kōyama Arifumi, 187–216. Tokyo: Nihon hyōronsha.

Welsome, Eileen. 1999. *The Plutonium Files.* New York: Random House.

Whitfield, Stephen J. 1991. *The Culture of the Cold War.* Baltimore: Johns Hopkins University Press.

Williams, Peter, and David Wallace. 1989. *Unit 731: Japan's Secret Biological Warfare in World War II.* New York: Free Press.

Yamaguchi, Kei'ichirō. 1995. *Seimei o moteasobu: Gendai no iryō.* Tokyo: Shakai hyōronsha.

Part One: The Gruesome Past
                    and Lessons
              Not Yet Learned

1 Rationalizing Unethical Medical Research: Taking Seriously the Case of Viktor von Weizsäcker

Gernot Böhme

An anthology on bioethics recently published in Germany claimed in its preface that "the reception of many topics of bioethics occurred in Germany in light of what had taken place during the Third Reich. . . . It was the medical tests performed in the concentration camps, the Nazis' euthanasia programs and the programs of racial purification that formed the background for the reception of modern medicine."

The sentence sounds plausible enough, and what it claims is not wrong per se. When one reads the book mentioned, however, doubts arise: Germany's experience under the Nazis is not really discussed there. The book does not even ask in what way ethics would have to take that experience into account. But we, if we are to discuss the topic of "rationalizations for unethical medical research," *do* have to answer that question. Formulating our topic like this means coming to two realizations:

First, there were, during World War II, in Germany as well as in Japan and the U.S., types of medical research we must today regard as unethical.

Second, the legitimizing of these kinds of research took place during the time they were performed and, in some cases, even after the fact.

These two statements in combination contain the explosive notion that not only were these actions and programs reprehensible but, moreover, there may be in ethics itself or in its development something deeply problematic. We have to ask ourselves the following questions.

First, what were our experiences of the Nazi era? The point here is not to simply call to mind the atrocities committed by the Nazis, but rather to read these atrocities as events relevant for the development of morality.

Second, what would it mean for ethical theory to take these experiences seriously? Since arguments based on ethics were indeed given in defense of Nazi barbarities, some sort of transformation has to occur within ethics itself. This is required by our topic.

Third, what does it mean for praxis, be it in life research or in medicine today, that such crimes against humanity are in our history? Why was the context at the time (that is, the Hippocratic oath, humanistic ethics, European civilization) not strong enough to prevent the individual doctor and researcher from participating in these criminal programs? Is what Adorno says true, namely that "Auschwitz irrefutably proved the failure of culture"? If this is so, the question is that of a self-cultivation, of an ethical development such that individuals would become able to stand firm in comparable situations.

Morality between *Askesis* and Rhetoric

The terms "ethics" and "morality" are often used synonymously. However, some, Hegel for example, place importance on their distinction. I do not want to provide here an account of the different uses of these terms, but rather posit for the purposes of our discussion the point that ethics denotes the comprehensive area of normative regulations of human behavior, while morality denotes only a subset thereof. It is of prime importance for ethics that there be a wide range of modes of behavior that are unproblematic because they are based on custom. That is not to say that these are not normative regulations, but just that they have become norms to which we are habituated. There are situations, however, in which such habituation no longer provides sufficient grounds for orientation. This can occur

- because certain habituations conflict with one another,
- because they become problematic under certain points of view, or
- because challenges have to be met, and these require going beyond the habitual.

In these situations, then, things get serious. I define a moral question as a serious question. In so doing I distinguish between questions that are serious for the individual and questions that are serious for society as a whole. A question poses itself *seriously* for the individual when the making of a decision concerning it involves showing what kind of person one is, or how one is to be a person. A question poses itself *seriously* for society when the decision concerning it involves asking what kind of society we live in, or what we together regard as a humane life.[1]

In what follows I want to focus on those questions of serious importance for society. I am not going to try to answer the third question raised in the first section, namely the question of what enables an individual to remain steadfast in his or her convictions. An answer would involve, in my opinion, some sort of *askesis*, that is, practices by which one acquires character, as well as an ability to make decisions and a readiness to suffer.

What concerns me is instead the framework by which the kind of society we live in is determined, as well as what that society regards as humane living. Questions of this kind have to be decided on the basis of moral argumentation and in processes of public decision making. These can then lead to the establishment of new customs, but also of laws, of professional codes, and of administrative regulations.

What is decisive is that moral arguments are rhetorical in character. Rationality in ethics is not scientific. Rather, these arguments, because they are put forward in public, always depend on what the public being addressed already believes to be correct. That which one in each case believes and approves I will call, with Aristotle in mind, a *topos*. Aristotle wrote a book entitled *Topics*. It deals with the question of what people take for granted when ethical questions are at stake. To him the human good is not eternally given but must be found through consensus formation in public argumentations. What can be referred to in these argumentations as commonly accepted is called a topos, the whole context of them the *topics*, or belief system. This is the way I use the terms "*topos*," plural "*topoi*," "*topics*," and "belief system."

In order to analyze a moral discourse we have to get an idea of the *topoi* that discourse presupposes; in other words we have to describe a *topics*. Moreover, emotions will always play a role in moral discourses, since these revolve fundamentally around what one approves of and what one rejects. Rhetorical argumentation does not address simply the understanding, but the emotions as well.

So when do moral arguments come into play? We usually assign them a legitimating role. But that would mean they become necessary only after the fact, when we need to justify our action before some sort of authority, be it our parents or a court of law. But they have a role before the fact as well, namely when we rationalize an action or its context in order to justify taking that action. This will be the case when we need to justify it vis-à-vis inner doubts or what we call the stirrings of conscience. Here as well, the justification is addressed before the public, even if only a virtual public. Finally, all moral arguments become necessary in forming anew a field of actions, that is, in the establishment of new customs, laws, and regulations.

In what follows I would like to use an example from the Nazi era to draw out—as a paradigmatic case—the moral arguments that were used to justify crimes in the medical field (or at least were made to appear to justify them) and that perhaps provided the ideological background to make them possible in the first place. In so doing, I intend not to give concrete recommendations for solutions, but rather to provide a lead-in to the core problematic to which this volume is devoted. My example is the case of the well-known physician and neurologist Viktor von Weizsäcker.

Viktor von Weizsäcker

In choosing Viktor von Weizsäcker as my case study, I consciously took a person who was not a criminal—such as Dr. Mengele—or an outright sadist—such as Dr. Rascher[2]—but someone who is an important scientist and continues to be well regarded to the present day.

Viktor von Weizsäcker lived from 1886 to 1957 and had already participated in World War I as a troop and field doctor. Beginning in 1919, he was an assistant at Heidelberg Medical School. During World War II, in 1941, he became professor of neurology in Breslau and also director of the Institute of Neurological Research. He fled Breslau to escape the oncoming Russian army. At the end of the war he was a colonel in the medical corps of the Wehrmacht. In 1946 he became professor of clinical medicine at Heidelberg University Hospital, a position he held until retirement.

Von Weizsäcker was critical of medicine that is methodologically limited to pure, natural science. It has been said that he introduced consideration of the subject into medicine. He is regarded as one of the originators of psychosomatics and social medicine. These achievements secured for him an important and continuing position in the history of medicine. But in pushing a new medicine he often resorted to arguments and referred to *topoi* that led to his "being viewed not unsympathetically by the National Socialists" (Begegnungen und Entscheidungen [Encounters and Decisions] in von Weizsäcker 1986–2005, 1:280).[3] That this feeling was mutual is demonstrated by a talk he gave in 1933 at the invitation of the rector of the University of Freiburg, Martin Heidegger, as well as by his 1933 lectures entitled "Ärztliche Fragen. Vorlesungen über allgemeine Therapie" (Questions for Physicians: Lectures on General Therapy, 2nd ed. 1935, von Weizsäcker 1986–2005, 5:328). We will find that he developed in these and similar writings a mode of thought that could be used to legitimate crimes against humanity. Von Weizsäcker never actually committed such crimes himself, although he shares some responsibility for at least one. At the Institute for Neurological Research in Breslau, of which he was the director, the brains of children and adolescents murdered at the hospital of adolescent psychiatry in Loben-Lubliniec were used for neuropathological research. In this process, von Weizsäcker actually gave written instructions to the hospital in Loben-Lubliniec on how to prepare the brains and spinal cords (see Penselin 1994, 123–37).

I will now examine von Weizsäcker's discourse with special attention to his use of bioethical *topoi*. The center of von Weizsäcker's effort to transform medicine is the concept *Rentenneurose*—which we can perhaps translate, even if somewhat awkwardly, as a neurosis connected to compensation for a disability. Von Weizsäcker's other terms for the same pathology are: insurance neurosis, accident neurosis, juristic neurosis, and claims neurosis. In each case we are dealing with a pathology in which the somatic symptoms, upon an analysis based on a consultation between the doctor and patient, point to a *conversion* that has taken place. That is, a condition of social emergency such as being in dire straits, experiencing a personal humiliation, or having some great failure in life has been converted into a physical illness, and that, in turn, creates a patient who is making a legal claim on the social security system. Von Weizsäcker sees this pathology as indicating the necessity to open the medical field to the psychological dimension on one hand and the social on the other. In so doing, however, he introduces his particular view of the phenomena as well as certain bioethical *topoi*. He wrote: "Many of the[se] people were not sick at all. They had simply failed. For that reason they sought to nurse in themselves some sort of ailment, in order to base a legal claim on it. Illness became a legal claim and being ill a means to subsistence. Many had neuroses; but in most cases this was no longer real neurosis, but rather a general evacuation, a failure and collapse of one's way of life" (Begegnungen und Entscheidungen, von Weizsäcker 1986–2005, 1:267).

These so-called pension neuroses have been correctly associated with the war neuroses (shell shock) so common among the soldiers of the First World War. This connection also tells us something about von Weizsäcker's professional attitude toward the patient who has the pension neurosis. The subject that von Weizsäcker introduces into medicine here is not an autonomous subject but, rather, one in need of *guidance* by the doctor. Moreover, since von Weizsäcker became acquainted with such cases in his capacity as an expert or professional authority in the context of pension claim procedures, he compares the relationship between doctor and patient to that between a judge and a defendant. In keeping with this, the healing process is envisioned as a pedagogic measure, namely the denial of the pension in the one and work therapy in the other case. In both cases the patient is treated as somebody lacking discipline and self-responsibility.

We have thus identified an initial *topos* of von Weizsäcker's bioethical argument: he presupposes a fixed order of social hierarchies, an ordering of leaders and subordinates. But not only that. He also sets up an order in which human beings have more and less value. I quote: "From the physician's point of view it is clear that a healthy life has more value than a sick one" (Euthanasie und Menschenversuche [Euthanasia and human experimentation], von Weizsäcker 1986–2005, 7:99). But this hierarchical ordering of human beings does not stop with the physician; rather, above the doctor's responsibility is to be found that of the political. The doctor must therefore align his behavior with whatever the political leaders deem to be right. This system culminates and attains closure in the figure of the supreme leader, the Führer Adolf Hitler. It is in this spirit that in his 1933 Freiburg lecture von Weizsäcker grounds his proposals for dealing with the pension neuroses explicitly in the will of the Führer. And in his postwar 1947 essay, "Euthanasie und Menschenversuche," in which he deals with the actions of doctors during the Third Reich, he sees their legitimization—at the time—as having derived in the final analysis from Hitler himself: "When a physician believed Hitler to embody the greatest solidarity in himself, then he was, from his standpoint, justified in his actions" (Euthanasie und Menschenversuche, von Weizsäcker 1986–2005, 7:110–11).

To understand the whole meaning of this sentence, it must be noted that von Weizsäcker uses the term *solidarity*—as a sociologist such as Durkheim does—in the sense of *the unity of society.*

If you push this system, in which authorities are not in competitive relationships, but rather are ordered hierarchically, to its logical conclusion—as von Weizsäcker did—then it follows that the highest political authority must also sublate all particular expertise in himself: "For it is true that Hitler does not simply hold supreme political command, he is also the first physician" (Euthanasie und Menschenversuche, von Weizsäcker 1986–2005, 7:111).

In what we have noted thus far, the distinction between expert knowledge and political authority remains intact. But von Weizsäcker thinks that this distinction cannot hold. Perhaps more accurately, his experience was that a doctor can and will be forced to act politically, for instance as an expert who has to deal with insurance matters. In this role, the doctor not only decides about the monetary aspects of society, but affirms the existing order, namely the order of the social security system (Ärztliche Fragen: Vorlesungen über allgemeine Therapie [Questions for physicians: Lectures on general therapy], von Weizsäcker 1986–2005, 5:328). This order, however, is, according to him, precisely the habitat in which the pension neurosis flourishes. Therapy must therefore become social therapy, and the doctor must become a *politicized doctor* (Ärztliche Fragen, von Weizsäcker 1986–2005, 5:328).

It is certainly right to worry about social relations when it is realized that they themselves make people ill. But it is obvious that von Weizsäcker's arguments for the expansion of medicine address very particular circles, with which he feels himself in agreement, and that they address them by referencing very particular *topoi*. Von Weizsäcker expresses this unequivocally when he declares himself a "conservative revolutionary" (Begegnungen und Entscheidungen, von Weizsäcker 1986–2005, 1:227) and thereby positions himself more or less consciously close to Nazism. Looked at in greater detail, that position really entails two things: On the one hand, von Weizsäcker regards the activity necessary in the social domain as a form of therapy, and thus regards politics as therapy. In this he follows the age-old Platonic pastoral notion of politics: the rulers are seen as the leaders of the flock, the people, those who have been entrusted to them. The social totality is thereby regarded as analogous to an organism, and as such it allows the transference of the concept of sickness into the social arena. Social sickness then comes to mean the sickness of the people, as a single organism, the political body.[4]

On the other hand, von Weizsäcker does not regard the actual condition of social relations, the unequal distribution of wealth, or the means of production as radical social problems. Rather he explicitly defines his own position in direct opposition to the politics of social democracy. Social democracy was based on the idea that people had rights, rights *to* something. Even in 1945 von Weizsäcker wrote,

> The legal neurosis was thus not the illness of an individual human being, but that of a society, an institution, a state, perhaps even a nation. The reasons lay in a certain political mentality, the education of the working class in ideas of social democracy, which constantly informed its adherents of their rights. I tended to look upon this overestimation of the legal process as old liberalism's gift to socialism. One could say that its even earlier ancestors were the "human rights" of the French Revolution, things that revolution bequeathed to liberalism. (Begegnungen und Entscheidungen, von Weizsäcker 1986–2005, 1:279)

In contradistinction to social democracy, which had pursued social policies, there should now, he held, be social national policies (Ärztliche Fragen, von Weizsäcker 1986–2005, 5:322).

What should such policies consist of, according to von Weizsäcker? They were to lead to an insurance reform, even to a complete abolition of the system of social security. For the existing system had, according to him, merely provided monetary compensation for accidents suffered, for damage in war, or for the destitution due to unemployment. And this system of compensation gave a kind of permanence to damage, illness, or poverty. What mattered was, according to von Weizsäcker, to reintegrate affected individuals into society, depending on their fitness for work. He commented retrospectively in 1945: "What I was imagining was a gradual cutback in the possibility of juridical cases [that is, of the possibility of making legal claims to insurance benefits—GB] and in this way a prophylaxis and compulsory assignment of labor by manipulating the so-called job-market" (Begegnungen und Entscheidungen, von Weizsäcker 1986–2005, 1:279).[5]

And he added: "This is the path national socialism surely seemed to be heading down for a while" (Begegnungen und Entscheidungen, von Weizsäcker 1986–2005, 1:279).

It was clear to von Weizsäcker that this path would necessarily go hand-in-hand with a limitation of civil liberties and the right to privacy, and, at least from 1933 onward, it did in fact go along with such limitations: "The new forms of life entail multiple and relentless limitations of the private sphere" (Soziologische Bedeutung der nervösen Krankheiten und der Psychotherapie [Sociological significance of nervous diseases and psychotherapy], von Weizsäcker 1986–2005, 8:167).

We have thus arrived at another *topos* of von Weizsäcker's argument, the *Weltanschauung*, or the conception of the state held within political conservatism: The polity does not take shape as a civil society, but rather as a community —to borrow the terminology of Tönnies.[6] The integration, or, as von Weizsäcker puts it, the *solidification* of the individual happens not by way of the market or the justice system but, rather, by an organic integration, one that makes the individual useful for the whole, or, as von Weizsäcker puts it in old military jargon, *usable* (Ärztliche Fragen, von Weizsäcker 1986–2005, 5:275). National social policy—that is, what both von Weizsäcker and the Nazis wanted—would be the creation of the people's solidarity by means of work and war.[7]

In order to demonstrate the terrifying consequences, which von Weizsäcker developed on the basis of the *topoi* just discussed, we have to identify another *topos* and, more precisely, a mode of ethical rationalization. I call this mode the principle of ethical consistency—meaning that different principles or standards of measurement may not be used, as in "situation ethics," in differing cases. *When one has endorsed A, one has to grant B as well. Since one has already accepted A, . . .* In recent times, this principle has played a role in Germany in the debate over the uses of nuclear energy. The argument ran as follows: If one in fact accepts a technology such as that of motor vehicles, a technology that causes seven thousand deaths per year, one must, in the interest of consistency, also accept the risks connected with nuclear power plants. Von Weizsäcker's argument ran accordingly: The profession of a doctor is not limited to healing and care, but also entails destruction and killing. After all, a doctor may have to perform an amputation[8] or an abortion. For von Weizsäcker it follows quite generally that traditional medicine—that is, medicine based on the Hippocratic oath—that was entirely dedicated to the preservation of life, and that, as he puts it, treated destruction as a *pudendum*—that is, as something one would be ashamed of doing—was in need of expansion. "There was not and there still is not today any comprehensive doctrine of destruction as a supplement to medical science's traditional presentation of itself as a pure doctrine of preservation" (Ärztliche Aufgaben [Physicians' tasks], von Weizsäcker 1986–2005, 5:151).

This doctrine of destruction as having a role in medicine would have disastrous consequences once it was taken in combination with the concept of the nation as an organism. For in that case it may fall to a physician to have to excise the pathogenic elements of a social body. As early as 1933, von Weizsäcker had emphatically welcomed the law for the prevention of hereditary illness, which allowed for compulsory sterilizations (Ärztliche Aufgaben, von Weizsäcker 1986–2005, 5:15). But in this passage he went even further: "As physicians, too, we hold responsibility to play a role in the sacrifice of individuals for the common good. It would be illusory and, indeed, it would not even be fair if the German doctor believed himself above playing his responsible role in this emergency policy of destruction" (Ärztliche Fragen, von Weizsäcker 1986–2005, 5:323).

Von Weizsäcker attempted to give this policy of destruction added legitimacy through the notion of the sacrifice. In 1947, having already been informed via Mitscherlich about the atrocities uncovered in the Nuremberg Doctors' trial, he isolates "sacrifice" as the only possible justification for "euthanasia" in the sense of *the destruction of unfit life:* "It is only the notion of sacrifice by virtue of which an action so similar to murder can actually come about. In the notion of sacrifice alone inheres the particular dialectic, which can turn the mere motive into a law, an ought, a duty, an inescapable compulsion, a moral action [*sittliche Handlung*]" (Euthanasie und Menschenversuche, von Weizsäcker 1986–2005, 7:102).

Von Weizsäcker is quite aware that what he is invoking here is a religious *topos,* and he refers specifically to "the notion of sacrifice [as] an amalgam of killing and redemption" (Euthanasie und Menschenversuche, von Weizsäcker 1986–2005, 7:103). We will therefore have to devote ourselves to this aspect of von Weizsäcker's thought in more detail.

Like many others, von Weizsäcker returned from the First World War with a profound sense of the dissolution of all values and a readiness for radical change. He even shared the popular sentiment that the solution had to lie in a return to religion—an idea common, in fact, among those of his contemporaries who were not socialists. This "religious excitement" (Begegnungen und Entscheidungen, von Weizsäcker 1986–2005, 1:93), however, did not lead him, as it did Karl Barth, to a newly concretized Christianity. Nor did it bring about a turn to the church but, instead, to a sort of metaphysical existentialism. By this I mean a *topos* that combines a complex of generalized belief in transcendence, an ontology of essence or spirit,[9] and the concept of human freedom. He speaks, for example, of the essence of being a physician, of the destiny of humans, and of the idea of the "Volk" (people). This means that these concepts—humans, the physicians, and the people—are more than they appear to be empirically. But this "more" is open, is what is at issue, and has to be established in existence. This combination of nihilism and transcendentalism places von Weizsäcker in proximity to his contemporary existentialists. Sartre's "existence precedes essence" in particular would probably have been a term he would have found agreeable.[10] We have seen the same attitude in his discussion of the doctor's profession: a doctor's "being" has an essence, but it is this essence that is at issue. He puts this in the starkest terms in his jeering denunciations of the Hippocratic oath: "We *cannot* denounce a transgression of 'the' medical ethics, as if there unquestionably were such a thing in our time. There is no such thing. The Hippocratic oath does not concern us" (Euthanasie und Menschenversuche, von Weizsäcker 1986–2005, 7:121).[11]

Von Weizsäcker thought himself living at a time in which a radically new determination of the *essence* of being a physician was necessary. This demanded steps that he regarded on the one hand as heroic[12] and on the other as quite clearly transgressive of existing laws: "In dealing with letting-live and killing, the question was not in the least what medicine *is*, but rather how it *ought* to be. People employing medicine as well as people doing medicine were aware of this situation, at least partially. They both sensed the great new turn, and they drew from this the strength that allowed them to pursue, in the long run, very dangerous things" (Euthanasie und Menschenversuche, von Weizsäcker 1986–2005, 7:108).

With regard to the people (*Volk*) it is important to note that von Weizsäcker does not talk about the *Volk* per se but about the *idea of this Volk,* with the implication that the idea of a people is in each case historically determinable. I will quote the relevant passage so that we can note the consequence drawn from it: "A deficiency is after all only a deficiency in the context of a Volk, when it is in contradiction to the idea of that Volk. Whether there indeed is such a contradiction cannot be decided by medical biology; rather, it is the person who is leading bearer of this idea [of the Volk] who, in the pure passion of his sense of responsibility, has the last word in this matter" (Ärztliche Fragen, von Weizsäcker 1986–2005, 5:329).

It should become obvious what this means in plain language. The *leading bearer of the idea of the Volk,* the one who had in mind the notion of a racially pure *Volk,* was Adolf Hitler.

Concerning the individual human being, von Weizsäcker's viewpoint was strongly influenced by his experience, paradigmatic for him, of dealing with pension neuroses. With these experiences as his point of departure, he came to regard every disease as a failure to achieve a person's true destiny as a human, and disease itself was taken as a mode of inauthenticity. He claimed that "there lies in every sick person a resistance to convalescence" (Ärztliche Fragen, von Weizsäcker 1986–2005, 5:307). And, by the same logic, he concluded that "good health has to do with the authenticity [*Wahrhaftigkeit*] of a human being" (Ärztliche Fragen, von Weizsäcker 1986–2005, 5:285). This view easily leads to allotting to the physician the role of the custodian (the Führer!) of an incompetent. It remains unclear in von Weizsäcker—as it does in existentialism more generally—what is meant by "a person's true destiny as a human." Generally speaking, von Weizsäcker locates this end in transcendence—with the terminus *transcendence* essentially describing something beyond itself. But by one interpretation that can mean that the individual reaches his or her destiny vis-à-vis certain *eternal entities,* but by another it can mean that this destiny fulfills itself within the framework of *Volk* solidarity, in which case transcendence will come to mean something like *usefulness* or perhaps even *usability.*

I wish to explicate the significance of this point of view by looking at the conclusions, ones with dire consequences, von Weizsäcker draws with respect to the question of the legitimacy of annihilating unworthy human lives: "If the physician presupposes there to be *worth* in a given worldly and temporal life, but one void of eternal value, then that merely temporal worth can be so low that the life in question deserves annihilation. Put differently, any definition of life which sees its meaning, purpose or worth as other than transcendent, possesses no inner guardrail against the notion of a biologically worthless life" (Euthanasie und Menschenversuche, von Weizsäcker 1986–2005, 7:100).

In retrospective, then, von Weizsäcker regards a religious destiny for humans as the only protection against a ruthless calculus of utilization[13] and annihilation. His post–World War II opinion thus mirrors his post–World War I opinion: the true reason for the catastrophes he witnessed in both contexts is the turn away from religion. This is the only point at which von Weizsäcker, who otherwise suffered from the all too common delusion of being blameless,[14] something he himself had diagnosed in others, seems to have had a genuine inkling of the extent of his own guilt. He speaks of the "fate of the religious question" in his life between 1918 and 1933: "It was an attempted spiritual accomplishment, which started out as religious but was then segued into a seemingly unreligious research program, that ended without success. And it eventually attained an entirely new meaning in the context of the total catastrophe of total war. That is the framework within which I hope to explicate the decline of morality in the inner life of a single individual" (Begegnungen und Entscheidungen, von Weizsäcker 1986–2005, 1:232).

I have thus arrived at the end of this part of my elucidations, a case study in the role of *topoi* in bioethical argumentation. To summarize, von Weizsäcker's discourse makes reference to the *topoi* of:

- hierarchies within both society and values
- political conservatism (the *Volk* as an organism, a community instead of civil society)
- the demand for ethical consistency
- a metaphysical existentialism.

These *topoi* are, we need to recall, not mere principles von Weizsäcker followed, but rather points of reference to which he could make an appeal in his listeners and readers—at least those he deemed relevant at the time. We have to come to terms with the core ambivalence here. On the one hand these *topoi* were obviously fitted out to provide the ideological framework for Nazi crimes in the medical field, and on the other, these same observations led Viktor von Weizsäcker to expand medicine into the domains of the psychosomatic and the social.

Conclusion: Consequences for Bioethics Today

By way of a conclusion we have to ask ourselves what consequences arise from our analysis of a case such as von Weizsäcker's—or, more generally speaking, that of the experience of the Third Reich? What are the consequences for how we discuss and do bioethics? When we do that we have to stress first of all that, according to this analysis, the formulation of the title for this volume, namely *Rationalizing Unethical Medical Research,* falls somewhat short of what we need. After all, we are here dealing with *bioethical* rationalizations of a certain manner of dealing with human beings, a manner that at that time was not recognized as unethical by the physicians and scientists in question. The most unsettling aspect of their actions precisely is this: These physicians and scientists, by and large, had no sense of perpetrating injustices. And yet, the factual result of their behavior, notwithstanding their rationalizations, is so patently inhuman and criminal that the formulation "unethical research" appears in fact quite adequate. The first consequence we have to draw from the above is therefore that the moral intuitions, which allow the events in the Third Reich to appear as criminal, need to be taken seriously.

I need to state something more about "moral intuitions." The case of von Weizsäcker helps us to see that "moral intuitions" must be allowed a role as a *topos* in bioethics. It is not moral *principles* alone that have a role to play in bioethics. Also to be factored in are the feelings we harbor toward other human beings—and in particular feelings toward human beings who are ill, weak, and in need of help. The Nazi rulers were aware of these intuitions. This is the reason their euthanasia programs, the experiments they performed on the incarcerated, and so forth, were undertaken in extreme secrecy, and without explicit legal legitimation. The physicians and researchers who were involved used their bioethical rationalizations to suppress and subdue their moral intuitions.[15]

Since 1945 we have seen something of a reversal—namely the extension of these moral intuitions themselves into principles within the field of philosophical ethics. Above all Hans Jonas and Emmanuel Levinas come to mind as thinkers who did that. Hans Jonas articulated what he called the *principle of responsibility* (*das Prinzip Verantwortung*) based on a model of parent-child relations, and thus made clear that there is an asymmetrical relationship. Children are the needy ones with respect to their parents. And in this responsibility toward the needy Jonas located the prototype of ethical behavior. Similarly Levinas, who makes the experience of the face—that is, the sight of another human being in all its vulnerability—the basis of the ethical attitude. Moreover, we need to recall that the Allied Control Council in 1947 in ad hoc fashion established the "crime against humanity"[16] as a punishable criminal offense. This was in order to codify the intuitive realization that medicine of the Nazi type is criminal.

What is most important in these developments is the insight that a condemnation of the crimes of the Nazis is insufficient and that from these things certain consequences must be drawn for bioethics itself. Yet recognition of these fundamental consequences can easily be deflected and denied by assuming that such crimes were possible only within the context of a totalitarian regime. This volume, it is hoped, will cure us of taking that route of evasion; even in democracies comparable crimes are possible. Moreover, we see today that democracies become quite ready to suspend civil rights for jingoistic reasons or for policies of security. We have lost the Kantian hope for a condition of eternal peace. Kant's claim that states a republican form of government would not start wars has been falsified empirically (Kant 1996, 323–27 [8:350–53]). These considerations force us to refuse to rely on having a certain form of sociopolitical arrangement take care of these things automatically for us. Rather we must demand that things be set up in such a way that crimes against humanity in the area of medicine and research on human beings become no longer possible. And this brings us to one more *topos* within the bioethical discourse of our time— namely, the simple fact that in the twentieth century, such crimes have indeed taken place. This making of historical fact a point of reference in moral discourse will entail a fundamental transformation of the topic of bioethics. The philosopher Theodor Adorno expressed the same thought in the form of a paradox: "By means of Hitler human beings in their state of unfreedom have been forced to recognize a new categorical imperative—namely, so to transform their thought and actions that Auschwitz can never be repeated and that nothing comparable may ever happen" (Adorno 1996, 356).

In opening I claimed that such a taking of historical events as truly serious for doing bioethics has not come to realization. Much to the contrary, we can observe a certain flight from such facts, and it is a flight into principles. The recourse to *principles* is understandable in light of the consequences of the bioethical *topoi*, for instance in von Weizsäcker. The desire is precisely for a detachment from such historical, class-based, or even politically factionalized kinds of rationale. This desire leads to postconventional (in the sense of Kohlberg and Habermas) and universalistic concepts of ethics, but it leads us to ignore that general principles have their use only as foundations for arguments and not as the motivational directives of particular actions. For this reason even Kant was forced to look for something that would serve as a motor for his categorical imperative, in order to ensure that it would be followed. Universal principles can possess motivational efficacy only in cultures that are inheritors of European Enlightenment, and even in those places probably only amongst a small subset of the people.[17] Moreover, universalistic principles, precisely because they are meant to be valid irrespective of culture, religion, and class-identity, can lead only to the most minimalist form of ethics. And that, in turn, may lead to their granted allowance to modes of behavior that we *intuitively* know to be unethical. This applies for instance to the utilitarian principle of the greatest happiness for the greatest number of people: in such a framework the sacrifice of the few can appear quite justified. It applies as well to the concept of *informed consent* as a barrier against wrong actions by doctors and researchers. Here, those individuals incapable of becoming adequately informed about risks or incapable of giving their consent may be denied bioethical protection.

We are thus, as one perhaps should be at the beginning of an inquiry, in a bit of a quandary: We cannot eschew a topics (*Topik*) approach in bioethical discourse altogether, but we also want to avoid the particularity and dependence on the cultural and historical situation that necessarily comes along with it. Perhaps one might settle, in our world, which has turned multicultural already within the particular states, on general rules, yet on general rules that are founded on different *topoi*, depending on ethnicity, religion, and cultural background.

Notes

1. For further development of my conception of ethics published in English, see Böhme 2001.

2. S. Rascher purposely killed test subjects in vacuum chambers at the behest of the Luftwaffe. See also Mitscherlich and Mielke 1960, in particular p. 62. For the English translation, see *Doctors of Infamy: The Story of the Nazi Medical Crimes,* trans. Heinz Norden.

3. *Nota bene:* All references to the writings of Viktor von Weiszäcker are to the individual articles reprinted in his collected works, *Viktor von Weizsäcker: Gesammelte Schriften,* 1986–2005. Translations of titles into English will be provided only the first time each appears.

4. For example, as late as 1947, in his essay "Euthanasie und Menschenversuche," in which he explicitly rejects von Uexkull's demand for a limitation of the concept of therapy to the individual alone: "Such that 'sick' in this case can mean not just individuals, but also a solitary community, a collective, a people, or humankind itself" (von Weizsäcker 1986–2005, 7:102).

5. In his article "Soziologische Bedeutung der nervösen Krankheiten und der Psychotherapie," probably first published in 1935, he makes even more explicit reference to the institutions of National Socialism: "We all know how much of a shortening of the way [in therapy—GB] is entailed once the state invests itself in the establishment of organizations poised to fight against unemployment, such as work programs or the military, instead of resorting to therapeutic patchwork" (von Weizsäcker 1986–2005, 8:167).

6. Von Weizsäcker, incidentally, wrote in 1945 that he had never read Tönnies (Begegnungen und Entscheidungen, von Weizsäcker 1986–2005, 1:281).

7. Von Weizsäcker experienced the feeling of popular unity firsthand during his first days as a soldier in World War I: "In the weeks at Diedenhofen, before the first

battles, it wasn't really the war that excited me, but rather the supernatural identification [*Einswerden*] of a people [*Volk*] at this particular point in time" (Begegnungen und Entscheidungen, von Weizsäcker 1986–2005, 1:265).

8. Thus explicitly in "Euthanasie und Menschenversuche," von Weizsäcker 1986–2005, 7:102.

9. Von Weizsäcker does not seem to have had any relations with his colleague in Heidelberg, Karl Jaspers. This is noteworthy, because Jaspers, a doctor turned philosopher, would have made a perfect correspondent for von Weizsäcker, also a physician deeply interested in philosophy.

10. Years before the German translation of Sartre's *L'Etre et le néant* (Being and nothingness), von Weizsäcker had already written a long essay on it, an essay full of sympathetic passion, as he himself notes, von Weizsäcker 1986–2005, 1:424–34. Strangely enough, he does not touch the critical point mentioned above, although he even quotes Sartre's *L'Existentialisme est un humanisme* (Existentialism is a humanism).

11. Von Weizsäcker states explicitly that this statement should not be taken out of context. But then, the context is the paragraph titled "The licit use of violence in Medicine."

12. A true existentialist, von Weizsäcker interprets his situation as a tragic entanglement in guilt: "It follows that the choice between two kinds of guilt is a duty [*Aufgabe*] of the masculine kind" (Euthanasie und Menschenversuche, von Weizsäcker 1986–2005, 7:132).

13. This sharpening of the term "*Verwendbarkeit*" (usefulness) can be found in "Ärztliche Aufgaben: Vorlesungen über allgemeine Therapie": "We are powerless once hereditary disease takes hold where causal therapy cannot reach and where integration and usability run afoul of the severity of the deficiency" (von Weizsäcker 1986–2005, 8:151).

14. "We are talking here about a person who incurs guilt, but whose conscience is not roused by it. This too is a kind of delusion" (Begegnungen und Entscheidungen, von Weizsäcker 1986–2005, 1:336).

15. I interpret this as a fight against unconscious guilt with the help of such reassurances (i.e., "questions addressed to superiors or to the Führer") and other means such as alcohol, "idealism," "patriotism," and "obedience to duty" (von Weizsäcker 1986–2005, 7:123, trans. Dr. Edgar Taschdjian, 1949).

16. Law No. 10 of the Allied Control Council. Regarding the juridical problematic arising from the application of this law, see Mitscherlich and Mielke 1960, 277, 291.

17. See my talk at the Department of Philosophy at the University of Pennsylvania on April 27, 2004, on the topic of "Kant's Universalism and the Family of Man."

References

Adorno, Theodor W. 1966. *Negative Dialektik*. Frankfurt: Suhrkamp. (Reprinted as *Negative Dialectics*, London: Continuum Int. Publ. Group, 1983.)

Böhme, Gernot. 2001. *Ethics in Context: The Art of Dealing with Serious Questions*. Cambridge, U.K.: Polity.

Kant, Immanuel. 1996. Toward Perpetual Peace (Zum ewigen Frieden [1795]). In *Prac-*

tical Philosophy, ed. Mary J. Gregor and Allen Wood, 323–27 (8: 350–53). Cambridge, U.K.: Cambridge University Press.

Mitscherlich, Alexander, and Fred Mielke, eds. 1960. *Medizin ohne Menschlichkeit. Dokumente des Nürnberger Ärzteprozesses.* Frankfurt/M.: Fischer. Originally published under the title *Wissenschaft ohne Menschlichkeit* in 1948 by the West German Association of Physicians. For the English translation, see *Doctors of Infamy: The Story of the Nazi Medical Crimes,* trans. Heinz Norden (New York: H. Schumann, 1949).

Penselin, Cora. 1994. Bemerkungen zu den Vorwürfen, Viktor von Weizsäcker sei in die nationalsozialistische Vernichtungspolitik verstrickt gewesen. In *Anthropologische Medizin und Sozialmedizin im Werk Viktor von Weizsäcker,* ed. Udo Benzenhöfer, 123–37. Frankfurt am Main: Peter Lang.

von Weizsäcker, Viktor. 1986–2005. *Viktor von Weizsäcker. Gesammelte Schriften.* 10 vols. Frankfurt am Main: Suhrkamp.

2 Medical Research, Morality, and History: The German Journal *Ethik* and the Limits of Human Experimentation

Andreas Frewer

[T]he ethical problems arising from human experimentation have become one of the cardinal issues of our time.

—M. Pappworth, 1967

Human Experimentation in Twentieth-Century Medicine

The issues surrounding the subject of human experimentation are among the most intractable ethical dilemmas in medicine for persons attempting to strike a balance between research interests and the well being of individuals. The twentieth century witnessed great advances in medicine, but also severe crimes in the name of science. More than fifty years after the end of the Nuremberg Doctors' Trial the decisive factors and the full repercussions of a "medicine without humanity" (Mitscherlich and Mielke 1947 and 1960) can finally be grasped. The development of moral theory that was used to underpin the medical ethos of that time drew on numerous and complex sources during the period leading to catastrophe. An "ethics without humanity" in particular paved the way by justifying and shaping these events (Platen-Hallermund 1948, Wiesemann and Frewer 1996, and Frewer and Wiesemann 1999). The long history of conceptualization since the nineteenth century, it has been demonstrated, was the fount of eugenic, political, and ideological concepts (Proctor 1988, Sandmann 1990, Frewer 2000). What trends are discernible in the debate on medical ethics as it pertains to the sensitive subject of experimentation on humans? Here I closely examine this question with particular reference to the German journal *Ethik,* meaning "Ethics."[1]

Moral Discourse in Germany 1922–1938 in the Journal *Ethik*

The sponsor and publisher of the journal *Ethik* was originally the German Medical and National Association for Sexual Ethics, which evolved from the Moral Conviction Association founded in Halle and the Medical Association for Sexual Ethics. From about 1927 onward, reference was being made only to an "Ethics Association." The society was increasingly simplified structurally, and, from 1928 onward, this finally led to the journal *Ethik* being published by Emil Abderhalden alone.[2] The members of the Ethics Association were subscribers to the journal *Ethik*. Lübeck, for example, had one of the largest regional groups with more than sixty members and, even for the Weimar period, had representatives of many different religious denominations on its committee. The reports relating to the social class and profession of the members may be summarized as follows: 1926: approx. 500 members; 1929: 2,314 members; 1934: approx. 800 members; 1938: approx. 400 members, mainly members of the medical professions but also theologians and teachers, some members of the legal profession, and nurses.[3]

The first house journal devoted to the problems of ethics to be published by the Association under the guidance of Abderhalden bore the title *Ethik, Pädagogik und Hygiene des Geschlechtslebens* (Ethics, education, and hygiene in sexual life) and appeared in 1922 in three issues. This was the first international journal to have "ethics" in the title of a scientific publication run by physicians. At first glance, the chosen field of specialization may appear restricted, but this is mainly a reflection of our contemporary perspective. "Ethical Problems at the Inception and on the Transmission of Human Life" would perhaps be a more modern and wider definition of the subject matter of the journal. May 1, 1925, saw the appearance of Issue No. 1, in a "New Series," of *Sexualethik* (Sexual ethics). This was now called the "Organ of the German Medical *and National* Association for Sexual Ethics," indicating that the original institutional basis had been extended by the aforementioned broader social perspective. Based on the subsequently employed numbering system, the edition phase of *Sexualethik* is to be regarded as the very first volume: *Ethik. Sexual- und Gesellschafts-Ethik* (Ethics—Sexual and social ethics) of 1926 continued as "Volume II." Abderhalden introduced the "Organ of the Medical and National Association for Sexual and Social Ethics of the German-Speaking Countries" with the words: "The 1926 volume represents a broadening of the scope of the hitherto existing journal *Sexual Ethics*." With the introduction of social ethics, the Ethics Association was now also addressing the entire spectrum of social concerns, and the topics actually discussed ranged from general morality to problems of morals in housing policy, sports, or business ethics—but medical ethics still clearly remained the focus of attention. The title page of *Ethik*, although subsequently modified slightly in both general presentation and typeface, was published in essentially the same form until 1938. What were the positions adopted in the discussions and in the central subject matter of the journal *Ethik* as regards human experimentation?

Human Experimentation in the Forum of *Ethik*

An "Open Discussion Forum" initiated by Emil Abderhalden was devoted in 1928 to questions surrounding research ethics and the problems of human experimentation. Abderhalden's position is summed up in a prefatory statement:

> Any transmission of a disease to a healthy person for the purpose of studying its different phases or to establish whether a certain infectious pathogen or any substance derived therefrom is able to induce known disease symptoms is to be categorically rejected, unless the researcher concerned carries out the experiments on himself. Equally irreconcilable with medical ethics are experiments whose sole purpose is to confirm the results of an animal experiment in humans, without there being any prospect of a beneficial effect on any condition for the individual who is the subject of the experiment, there rather being the probability of a greater or lesser degree of harm. (Abderhalden 1928, 12)

Referring to the cases repeatedly held up to opprobrium in the journal *Biological Medicine*, Abderhalden makes his fundamental position clear:

> There remain, however, and this must be stated with complete frankness, enough cases which must unreservedly be condemned both from the medical and the general ethical standpoint. When reading such papers in which it is reported that certain experiments have been carried out that involve inflicting harm on healthy persons, even if these may be prostitutes,[4] the mentally ill etc.—a human being is and remains a human being!—one gains the impression that a certain development in medicine is being taken to extremes and should be curbed at all costs. (Abderhalden 1928, 12)

Writing in the journal *Ethik*, Abderhalden expanded on this statement and asked the question, to what extent may human experimentation be allowed? Three physicians put forward their views on this subject: Dr. Matthes, director of the Medical Clinic in Königsberg (Answer 1), Dr. W. His, dean of the medical faculty of the University of Berlin (Answer 2), and Dr. Erwin Liek, surgeon and popular writer, Danzig (Answer 3). Matthes distinguishes between experiments undertaken for the patient's direct benefit and those performed solely to clarify scientific questions. In the former case, trials with new medical remedies or surgical techniques, when conducted with the utmost circumspection, are ethically acceptable. To illustrate the latter case, the author presents an example in which he and a senior registrar of his clinic subjected themselves to experimentation. Although Matthes clearly states in his summary, "Experiments by which patients may be harmed, however, I consider to be completely inadmissible and have never tolerated them in my clinic" (Matthes 1928, 5[1]:19), no position is taken with regard to immoral experimentation that had actually been performed or to the medical problems that had prompted them. The "never . . . in my clinic" is the final sentence for Matthes. In the second contribution, the "do no harm principle" is the central consideration: "*Nihil nocere.*" According to His, therapeutic trials are necessary to "extend the therapeutic armamentarium," for which the physician has the right to carry out experiments on humans. The decisive factor, however, is the patient's consent. In a sense, for His the end also justifies the means: "[An experiment] is only ethically justified if there is major interest in its being performed and if the previous methods have been recognized to be ineffective or inadequate" (Matthes 1928, 5[1]:19). Interestingly, in a previous paragraph His had referred only indirectly to one of the biggest scandals of his time before Lübeck:

> In order to identify a curative effect, however, we need a comparison with untreated or differently treated cases. (...) The situation is very similar with nutritional therapy, which can be so eminently effective during childhood and has made such a great contribution to reducing childhood mortality. It is well recognized that especially the treatment of the pernicious condition of rickets by the provision of correct nutrition is making tremendous progress, but here too the value of the curative procedure can only be properly recognized on the basis of a comparison. (His 1928, 5[1]:19)

To pediatricians, these claims appear at first sight to be completely plausible, if one is unfamiliar with the relevant background. Interestingly, the contribution placed in third place by Abderhalden, as editor—without any reference to the previous article—debates exactly this example. Liek initially presented a broad sweep of argument both in terms of medical history and by reference to current debates in the "orthodox medicine versus 'quackery' controversy."[5] For him, the main problem was the loss of confidence due to structural problems inherent in an anonymous medicine that find their most acute expression in unjustified experimentation. Liek stated: "The real physician, the man who deserves this name, will have only one thing in mind with such experiments—the well-being of the patient, the restoration of health, the averting of risk to life" (Liek 1928, 5[1]:23). Like the other authors, Liek also draws on conventional Hippocratic notions: "I will establish rules of conduct only for the benefit and avail of the suffering, according to my abilities and my powers of judgment and shall refrain from all evil and unrighteous actions towards them" (5[1]:23). After describing major surgical interventions that had innovatively advanced the cause of medicine, he turns his attention to problem cases. He quotes from the *Deutsche Medizinische Wochenschrift* of 1927:

> We performed this [trial of Vigantol] on a material[6] of about 100 rats und 20 children. [...] If, on the other hand, florid rickets patients are kept in unfavourable locations in closed rooms, our experience has shown that the rachitic process can also remain florid for months even during the summer and there is not the slightest sign of recovery. We kept our experimental children under unfavourable conditions of diet and light, and if they exhibited signs of healing in a substantially shorter time than 3–4 weeks after the start of the Vigantol therapy, this is unquestioningly due to the effect of the medicine.

In this and in one other case, Liek responded in the only possible way: "As a physician, my judgement upon such doings can only be this: complete and unqualified rejection."[7] The quintessence for him—after a long description with numerous examples and touching on many other subsidiary topics—is found in the concluding passage: "No law and no supervision, no matter how strict, will prevent 'human experiments,' but only one thing, physicians remembering the nature of their vocation and the lived example" (Liek 1928, 5[1]: 23).

An analysis of these three examples reveals some interesting trends. Even though all three authors—and these are already the most committed—give reassurances by referring in a similar manner to the "[primum] *nihil nocere*" ("do no harm") of Hippocratic tradition, the arguments presented are, nevertheless, implicitly very complex in nature. If we look at these contributions critically, three types of argumentation of wider relevance can be discerned. A clinic director who places emphasis on the "not with me" and completely refrains from any further discussion of the problems, the physician who in the last analysis would also perform experiments on the basis of their priority and indirectly defends his colleagues, and the popular medical writer, who is actually the only one to really touch on the sore point and detects aspects of relevance to the problems inherent in practicing the doctor's profession: these positions in the debates conducted in *Ethik* represent variants of opinions quite frequently encountered in the history of medicine—but the extreme radicalization of Nazi medicine in regard to human experimentation cannot be anticipated here. Nevertheless, the slippery slope can be seen in the trend, that, for some authors, the ends legitimate the means and the slowly ongoing turn to the principle "*Salus publica suprema lex.*" An important step was the reductionistic perspective that regards human beings as research material. (See Roelcke 2003, Lederer 1995, and Roelcke and Maio 2004.)

"Preventing Going Too Far": Guidelines in the Debate of *Ethik*

In the fifth issue of volume 7, the May/June 1931 edition of *Ethik*, the subject "human experimentation" again took center stage. Dr. Heinrich Vorwahl, a medical historian and teacher from Hamburg, published the article "The Ethical Boundary of Experimentation," which is one of the very few pieces of evidence of how the official guidelines on human experimentation were received. In his introduction, Vorwahl referred directly to the consequences of the "Lübeck vaccination scandal"—the so-called *Lübeck danse macabre* (see Moses 1930)—in which more than seventy children were killed due to the use of an imperfect vaccine:

> The Lübeck affair has prompted the Reich Health Office to issue guidelines which have been welcomed as imposing restrictions on the "experimentation mania" of doctors. Indeed it cannot be denied that large sections of the population hold convictions that were given such mordant expression by B. Shaw long before this event. He calls the doctors fanatics and sorcerers who demand that the striving for scientific knowledge, even when employing the cruellest methods, must be *completely free from moral laws* and who claim that they could make man immune from all illness if only they were given unlimited power over our bodies. (Vorwahl 1931, 7[5]:458)

Vorwahl went on to quote a large number of examples that had instigated debates regarding the boundaries of science. The criticisms reported range from the rejection of sexual provocation of volunteers in studies on "psychoanalytic psychotechnique," through notions of inseminating female chimpanzees with human sperm in the natural manner, to hypothetical experiments on decapitated subjects in plans of the psychiatrist Hoche. In his autobiography, Alfred Hoche had expressed the wish "to conduct an experiment, in which severed heads are restored to consciousness by mechanical perfusion with a chemically adequate fluid." Vorwahl commented: "For this experiment, which he considers promising, he lacks *only* the apparatus. The only reservation he makes is"— and here there follows another quotation from Hoche—"that, since in the event of success the death sentence would be pronounced a second time on the beheaded subject, such experiments could only be performed on persons who had received several sentences of death." For Hoche, professor of psychiatry and well-respected author, this appears an adequate appraisal of the ethical consequences. Abderhalden had also invited Hoche, as a prominent personality, to participate in the "Open Discussion Forum" in the very next issue, "The Educational Tasks of the University Teacher," which clearly shows that he was certainly capable of accepting Hoche as an academic role model. And Vorwahl, despite the criticism that he expressed—indirectly through the style of presentation *rather* than explicitly—in the very next sentence even pays homage to Hoche as the coauthor of the book *Freigabe zur Vernichtung lebensunwerten Lebens* (Permission to destroy life devoid of value) (see Binding and Hoche 1920): "Despite all the appreciation we show for controversial moral issues such as euthanasia and the elimination of worthless life," however, as regards the limits on human experimentation, Vorwahl perceived a "violation of the boundaries not only of the sanctity of life, but also of death" (Vorwahl 7[5]:458) and came to the conclusion: "If general insights can also enrich scientific research and may thus indirectly be to the benefit of the living, physicians and educators must never forget that they are dealing with human beings. Kant's warning against treating man with his dignity as a mere means to an end should rule out all experimentation for its own sake, either on sick people or children, as part the educational process, unless born of desperate necessity" (Vorwahl 7[5]:459).

There is no additional evidence of further discussion or queries in the correspondence either in the journal *Ethik* or in papers in the estate of Abderhalden.[8] The extreme unrest in the wake of the Lübeck vaccination scandal has no further repercussions here. This may also have been due to the fact that in 1928, that is, relatively shortly before this, the more far-reaching "Open Discussion Forum" devoted to "Human Experimentation" already had been presented, and there was no editorial interest in raising this topic anew. Abderhalden certainly adopted a critical stance on the subject of "human experimentation," but, as a physiological researcher, he could have had no interest in mounting a campaign against research.

"Research Ethics without Conscience" in Progress

To what extent were the first beginnings of the "medical ethics without humanity" of the Nazi state already present in the final phase of the Weimar Republic? In 1932, Reichstag member Julius Moses wrote:[9]

> Medical ethics are beset by many complex problems. All of them are solved in the "Third Reich." Thick books have been written, for example, about euthanasia and sterilization. Again and again, physicians have experienced moral conflicts: Should dying be made easier for the mortally ill? In the "Third Reich" the conflict no longer exists: They are killed! Just as the medical ethics and morality of a civilized society are swept away by the barbaric savagery of the South Sea Islanders, the still much-vaunted idea of "fellowship among physicians" and "professional dignity" is simply thrown overboard. The socialist and Jewish physician is treated in the "Third Reich" like a pariah. [. . .] The national socialist radicalisation of the medical profession, therefore, is leading to an ethical decline in physicians' perception of their professional identity. (Moses 1932, 9[5]:1–4)

With tremendous acuity and prophetic vision, Moses anticipates here the arrival of the "ethics of the national community" of the Nazi state. The first steps starting from racial hygiene and performance medicine toward the eradication of the sick and needy are already being taken.

The change in the journal *Ethik* during the seizure of power and the early Nazi period is significant:

> It is apparent from numerous enquiries that many readers of *Ethik* had expected the journal to take some position regarding the rebirth of the German nation. If this has not been forthcoming, it is because I see in much of what has now been achieved and is now being aimed at for the future, the fulfillment of struggle lasting for years, under sometimes extremely difficult circumstances, which has been carried on within and outside the journal "Ethik." It thus follows quite naturally that the tremendous cleansing process which has taken place within the German people is to be most heartily welcomed. (Abderhalden, editorial, *Ethik* 1933, 9[6])

A letter addressed by Abderhalden to his close colleague and friend G. Bonne may serve as a useful barometer: "I am not an opponent of the present state, rather a comrade-in-arms." Abderhalden discerned common ground especially in the areas of prophylaxis, eugenics, and a "true socialism" (March 28, 1935, HAL EA 61). During the continued editorship of *Ethik* by Abderhalden in the period 1933–1938, the elements of National Socialist press policy emerge with growing clarity: In April 1936, Abderhalden received the official membership card of the Reich Chamber for Arts and Culture and thereby became a member of the Reich Chamber of Writers. Besides being subject to state regulation, Abderhalden was now in legal terms "by virtue of the affiliation of the Reich Chamber of Culture and Arts to the German Labour Front (DAF) indirectly a member of the DAF" (Frewer 2000, 99).[10]

"Gone Too Far": Experimentation Ethics in Nazi Germany

The journal *Ethik,* in its context, is an eminently valuable instrument of medical-historical analysis into questions concerning human experimentation in the period 1922–1938. The processes of debate highlight the development in these years of National Socialism and the increasing trend toward biologism. The subject is refracted into complexity especially by the personality of the editor Abderhalden, who held all the editorial powers to publish—or not publish—different contributions. For the period up to 1932, a differentiated discussion of the problems surrounding "human experimentation" can be seen to have taken place, as evidenced in the pages of *Ethik.* Later in the course of the 1930s, however, a pluralistic spectrum of opinion regarding the boundaries of human experimentation is seen to have increasingly receded in favor of biologistic moral concepts, and toward the end of the 1930s there is no longer any critical questioning of the problems of human experimentation in the form of an "Open Forum Discussion." A perceptible change in *Ethik* in the National Socialist state is undeniable; for example, his long-time colleague Albert Niedermeyer wrote to Abderhalden in November 1937: "I regard it as my duty to tell you, esteemed Privy Councillor, that I am by no means surprised by these consequences. Anyone who had known the journal *Ethik* in previous years could only observe with the profoundest regret how far it has departed in recent years from what you originally stood for" (Letter from A. Niedermeyer to E. Abderhalden, Nov. 6, 1937, HAL EA 245). Particularly during the 1930s, the standards of *Ethik*—like its size—declined slowly due to a number of factors (see Frewer 2001, 134, and Frewer 2000, 108–11). A substantial proportion of employees embraced the Nazi line; "open debates" with pro and contra argumentation were no longer possible. The tendentious tone creeping into the book reviews, which may appear to be of secondary importance but is, nevertheless, symptomatic, reveals the growing orientation toward the ethics of the national community and racial hygiene. Abderhalden's guidelines and statements on the subject of human experimentation in the 1928 issue of *Ethik* are certainly liberal and could still achieve a consensus today. But a development that is almost symptomatic of the debate on human experimentation in the 1930s is reflected directly by his personality. In volume 7 of the "Nova Acta Leopoldina/New Series," Abderhalden offered in 1939 a study on the theory of heredity employing the research instruments of physiological chemistry: "Race and Heredity Considered from the Perspective of Blood and Cellular Proteins." In 1938, the very year that the journal *Ethik* ceased publication, he approached the *Reichsforschungsrat* and the famous surgeon Ferdinand Sauerbruch to propose that research be conducted into racial characteristics with the aid of physiological chemistry and his "A.R." (Abderhalden Reaction) technique. From this developed the "Abderhalden-Sauerbruch-Verschuer Triangle," until finally it was Josef Mengele who was researching into the project "specific proteins" in Auschwitz.[11] The Abderhalden Reaction was taken up by race research, and we can trace lines of development from the medical ethicist Abderhalden leading to the human experiments in Auschwitz. Yet biological concepts can be identified both in the journal and in the writings of Abderhalden long before 1933—insofar as it is possible to speak of continuities *and* discontinuities, although Abderhalden certainly underestimated the radical nature and the ultimate extent of the implementation of Nazi ethics.

Julius Moses mentioned Emil Abderhalden in the same breath as Albert Moll, thereby characterizing him as one of the leading medical moral philosophers of the first half of the twentieth century. His theory, that "Abderhalden and others are probably fools to the National Socialists!" (see Wert 1989, 229), however, is thrown considerably into relief by the background just described. The subject of human experimentation is a special indicator of the continuities and discontinuities in moral theory and "practical ethos" from the Weimar Republic to the period of National Socialism. The development toward a biologically based ethics—from *salus aegroti* to *salus publica suprema lex*—can be traced both in the work of Abderhalden and in the journal *Ethik*. The collective morality of the national community was ultimately the cause and internal logic of an "ethics without humanity."

The "medical" experiments in the concentration camps Buchenwald (near Weimar), Dachau (near Munich), Sachsenhausen (near Berlin), Natzweiler (near Strasbourg) or Ravensbrück, and Auschwitz, saw the consequences of those theoretical concepts, a decline of German scientific culture and the total instrumentalization of human beings. (Cf. Dörner, Linne, and Ebbinghaus 1999; Frewer and Wiesemann 1999; Ley and Ruisinger 2001; Ebbinghaus and Dörner 2001; Sachse 2003; Frewer and Siedbürger 2004.)

Notes

See Frewer and Wiesemann 1999; Tröhler and Reiter-Theil 1997; Frewer and Winau 1997, Winau 1996, Wiesemann and Frewer 1996, Elkeles 1996; Hahn 1995, Tashiro 1991, Steinmann 1975, and Beecher and Dorr 1970. For this article in particular see Frewer 2003 and Frewer 2004.

1. For the background see Frewer 2000, 47–54, 77–91, and Frewer 2001.
2. Emil Abderhalden (1877–1950). Born in the Kanton St. Gallen, Abderhalden studied medicine in Basel from 1895 until 1901 (thesis at the Institute of Gustav von Bunge). After the state examination in 1902, he was the assistant of Emil Fischer at the University of Berlin. His research was in physiology and immunology, and he was a pioneer of biochemistry and protein research. From 1911 he was professor of physiology, Halle (Saale), 1932–1945, and president of the "Deutsche Akademie der Naturforscher" ("Leopoldina," founded 1652). He won several prizes and honors and was twice proposed for the Nobel Prize. See Frewer 1998; Frewer 2000; and, furthermore, IAV; HAL/EA; Gabathuler 1991; Kaasch and Kaasch 1997; Deichmann and Müller-Hill 1998; Frewer and Neumann 2001.

3. For development of the membership of the "Ethics Association," see Frewer 2000, 75, 47–76.

4. Abderhalden is presumably referring here to the controversy surrounding the experiments of Albert Neisser; see Frewer and Neumann 2001; Tashiro 1991; and Elkeles 1985.

5. Interestingly, a society dedicated to combating quackery was one of the financial supporters of the journal *Ethik*.

6. Interestingly, this reductionistic terminology can also be found in the American pediatric research context: Susan Lederer quotes in her important study on human experimentation in America an "illustration of an 'experimental material'" from an exposé on the experimental use of orphans from St. Vincent's Home, Philadelphia. From "Vivisection Animal and Human, Cosmopolitan, 1910"; see Lederer 1995, 81.

7. Liek 1928, Antwort 3, *Ethik* 5, no. 1: 23.

8. The subject of human experimentation is only once more addressed in a later issue.

9. Julius Moses (1868–1942), physician and politician; as Social Democrat, a member of the German parliament. Moses died in 1942 in the concentration camp Theresienstadt.

10. See Barch, Berlin-Zehlendorf, BDC RKK 2102, Box 001, File 03; membership card no. "A 9963" of the "Reichskulturkammer/Reichsschrifttumskammer," April 4, 1936, with a photo of Abderhalden.

11. Mengele did the research for the head of the "Kaiser-Wilhelm-Institut für Anthropologie, menschliche Erblehre und Eugenik," Otmar Freiherr von Verschuer; see Klee 2001; Kröner 1998.

References

Archives

BArch   Bundesarchiv, Standorte Koblenz bzw. Berlin-Zehlendorf
Akten Reichsschrifttumskammer/Reichskulturkammer
Personenbezogene Daten zu E. Abderhalen
Bestände des (ehem.) *Berlin Document Center* (BDC)
BGGM   Berliner Gesellschaft für Geschichte der Medizin (Archiv)
EA   Nachlass-Mappe von Emil Abderhalden in HAL
HAL   Hallisches Archiv der Leopoldina (Deutsche Akademie der Naturforscher, gegründet 1652), Halle (Saale)
IAV   International Abderhalden-Association, Wattwil (Schweiz)

Literature

Abderhalden, E. 1921. *Das Recht auf Gesundheit und die Pflicht sie zu erhalten.* Leipzig: S. Hirzel Verlag.

———. 1928. Versuche am Menschen, *Ethik* 5, no. 1: 13–16.

———. 1944. *Lehrbuch der Physiologie.* Munich: Urban und Schwarzenberg.

———. 1947. *Gedanken eines Biologen zur Schaffung einer Völkergemeinschaft und eines dauerhaften Friedens.* Zürich: Rascher Verlag.

Abderhalden, R. 1991. Emil Abderhalden—Sein Leben und Werk. *Schweizerische Ärztezeitung/Bulletin de médecins suisses* 72, no. 44: 1864 (1991).

Aly, G. 1987. Die Aktion T 4. *Die Euthanasiezentrale in der Tiergartenstrasse 4*. Berlin: Edition Hentrich.

Annas, G. J., and M. A. Grodin, eds. 1992. *The Nuremberg Code: Human Rights in Human Experimentation*. New York: Oxford University Press.

Baader, G., and U. Schultz, eds. 1980. *Medizin im Nationalsozialismus. Tabuisierte Vergangenheit—Ungebrochene Tradition?* Frankfurt: Mabuse-Verlag.

Bachmann, M. 1952. *Die Nachwirkungen des hippokratischen Eides*. Med. diss., Mainz.

Baker, R. B., ed. 1999. *The American Medical Ethics Revolution: How the AMA's Code of Ethics Has Transformed Physicians' Relationships to Patients, Professionals, and Society*. Baltimore: Johns Hopkins University Press.

Baur, E., E. Fischer, and F. Lenz. 1921. *Grundriss der menschlichen Erblehre und Rassenhygiene*. Munich: J. F. Lehmans.

Beck, C. 1995. *Sozialdarwinismus, Rassenhygiene und Vernichtung "lebensunwerten" Lebens. Bibliographie*. Bonn: Psychiatrie-Verlag.

Beecher, H. K., and H. I. Dorr. 1970. *Research and the Individual: Human Studies*. Boston: Little Brown.

Binding, K., and A. Hoche. 1920. *Die Freigabe der Vernichtung lebensunwerten Lebens, ihr Mass und ihre Form*. Leipzig: Felix Meiner Verlag.

Bleker, J., and N. Jachertz, eds. 1993. *Medizin im "Dritten Reich."* Köln: Deutscher Ärzte Verlag, 2, erweiterte Auflage.

Brand, U. 1977. *Ärztliche Ethik im 19. Jahrhundert*. Freiburger Forschungen zur Medizingeschichte, Neue Folge Band 5. Freiburg: Hans F. Schulz.

Brieger, G. H. 1982. Human Experimentation: History. In *Encyclopedia of Bioethics*, ed. W. T. Reich, 1:684–92. New York: Free Press.

Bromberger, B., H. Mausbach, K.-D. Thomann. 1990. *Medizin, Faschismus und Widerstand*. Frankfurt: Mabuse Verlag.

Deichgräber, K. 1983. *Der hippokratische Eid*. Stuttgart: Hippokrates.

Deichmann, U., and B. Müller-Hill. 1998. The Fraud of Abderhalden's Enzymes. *Nature* May 14, 1998; 393 (6681):109–11.

Deutsch, E., ed. 1979. *Das Recht der klinischen Forschung am Menschen*. Frankfurt a.M.: Peter Lang.

Dörner, K., K. Linne, and A. Ebbinghaus, eds. 1999. *Der Nürnberger Ärzteprozeß 1946/47. Wortprotokolle, Anklage- und Verteidigungsmaterial, Quellen zum Umfeld*. Im Auftrag der Hamburger Stiftung für Sozialgeschichte des 20. Jahrhunderts herausgegeben von Klaus Dörner (. . .) Bearbeitet von Karsten Linne. Einleitung von Angelika Ebbinghaus. Deutsche Ausgabe. Munich: Saur.

Ebbinghaus, A., and K. Dörner, eds. 2001. *Vernichten und Heilen. Der Nürnberger Ärzteprozess und seine Folgen*. Berlin: Aufbau Verlag.

Elkeles, B. 1985. Medizinische Menschenversuche gegen Ende des 19. Jahrhunderts und der Fall Neisser. Rechtfertigung und Kritik einer wissenschaftlichen Methode. *Medizinhistorisches Journal* 20: 135–48.

———. 1996. *Der moralische Diskurs über das medizinische Menschenexperiment im 19. Jahrhundert*. Jahrbuch des Arbeitskreises Medizinischer Ethik-Kommissionen in der Bundesrepublik Deutschland, Medizinethik 7. Stuttgart: Fischer.

Eser, A., M. v. Lutterotti, and P. Sporken, eds. 1989. *Lexikon Medizin, Ethik, Recht*. (Unter Mitw. von Franz Josef Illhardt u. Hans-Georg Koch). Freiburg [u.a.]: Herder.

Ethik. *Sexual- und Gesellschafts-Ethik*. 1926–1938. Herausgegeben von Geheimrat Prof.

Dr. E. Abderhalden, Halle a.d. Saale [Nachfolger von: "Ethik . . . " (1922) bzw. "Sexual-ethik" (1925)].

Evangelische Akademie Bad Boll, ed. 1982. *Medizin im Nationalsozialismus*, Protokoll-dienst 23/82, Bad Boll.

Fischer, G. 1979. *Medizinische Versuche am Menschen.* Göttinger Rechtswissenschaftliche Studien. Band 105, Göttingen: Verlag Otto Schwarz.

Frewer, A. 1998. *Ethik in der Medizin von der Weimarer Republik zum Nationalsozialismus. Emil Abderhalden und die Zeitschrift"Ethik."* Diss. med., Berlin.

———. 2000. *Medizin und Moral von der Weimarer Republik zum Nationalsozialismus. Die Zeitschrift "Ethik" unter Emil Abderhalden.* Frankfurt: Campus Verlag.

———. 2001. "Entwicklungsprozesse auf dem Weg zur Moral des NS-Staates: Diskus-sionen im Spiegel der Zeitschrift 'Ethik' 1922–1938." In Frewer and Neumann 2001, 141–64.

———. 2003. L'expérimentation sur l'homme à la lumière de la revue *Ethik* (1922–1938): Ruptures et continuités d'un débat en Allemagne. In *La médecine expérimentale au tribunal*, ed. C. Bonah, É. Lepicard, and V. Roelcke (Hrsg.), 133–55. Paris: Éditions des Archives Contemporaines.

———. 2004. Debates on Human Experimentation in Weimar and Early Nazi Germany as Reflected in the Journal *Ethik* (1922–1938) and Its Context. In *Twentieth Cen-tury Research Ethics: Historical Perspectives on Values, Practices and Regulations*, ed. V. Roelcke and G. Maio, 137–50. Stuttgart: Steiner Verlag.

Frewer, A., and F. Bruns. 2003. "Ewiges Arzttum" oder "neue Medizinethik" 1939–1945? Hippokrates und Historiker im Dienst des Krieges. *Medizinhistorisches Journal* 3/4: 313–36.

Frewer, A., and J. N. Neumann, eds. 2001. *Medizingeschichte und Medizinethik. Kontro-versen und Begründungsansätze 1900–1950.* Frankfurt: Campus Verlag.

Frewer A. and G. Siedbürger, eds. 2004. Zwangsarbeit und Medizin im Nationalsozialis-mus. Einsatz und Behandlung von "Ausländern" im Gesundheitswesen. Frankfurt: Campus Verlag.

Frewer, A., and C. Wiesemann, eds. 1999. *Medizinverbrechen vor Gericht: Das Urteil im Nürnberger Ärzteprozess gegen Karl Brandt und andere sowie aus dem Prozess gegen Generalfeldmarschall Erhard Milch.* Bearbeitet und kommentiert von U.-D. Oppitz. Erlanger Studien zur Ethik in der Medizin, Band 7. Erlangen und Jena: Verlag Palm und Enke.

Frewer, A., and R. Winau, eds. 1997. *Geschichte und Theorie der Ethik in der Medizin. Grundkurs Ethik in der Medizin*, Band 1. Erlangen und Jena: Palm und Enke.

Gabathuler, J. 1991. *Emil Abderhalden. Sein Leben und Werk.* Wattwil (St. Gallen): Inter-nationale Abderhalden-Vereinigung.

Hahn, S. 1995. "Der Lübecker Totentanz": Zur rechtlichen und ethischen Problematik der Katastrophe bei der Erprobung der Tuberkuloseimpfung 1930 in Deutschland. *Medizinhistorisches Journal* 30: 61–79.

Hanson, H. 1977. Emil Abderhalden als Lehrer, Forscher und Präsident der Leopoldina. Vorträge eines Gedenksymposiums aus Anlass seines 100. Geburtstages. *Wissen-schaftliche Beiträge der Martin-Luther-Universität Halle-Wittenberg* 26 (T 18): 7–23.

Helmchen, H., and R. Winau, eds. 1986. *Versuche mit Menschen.* Berlin: de Gruyter.

His, W. 1928. Versuche am Menschen. Antwort 2, *Ethik* 5, no. 1: 18–19.

Hubenstorf, M. 1989. "Deutsche Landärzte an die Front!" Ärztliche Standespolitik zwi-schen Liberalismus und Nationalsozialismus. In *Wert* (1989): 200–23.

Jones, J. H. 1981. *Bad Blood: The Tuskegee Syphilis Experiment.* New York: Free Press.

Kaasch, J., and M. Kaasch. 1995. Wissenschaftler und Leopoldina-Präsident im Dritten Reich: Emil Abderhalden und die Auseinandersetzung mit dem Nationalsozialismus. In *Die Elite der Nation im Dritten Reich: Das Verhältnis von Akademien und ihrem wissenschaftlichen Umfeld zum Nationalsozialismus*, ed. Seidler et al., 213–50. Acta historica Leopoldina Nr. 22, Halle (Saale).

———. 1996. Emil Abderhalden und seine Ethik-Mitstreiter. Ärzte, Wissenschaftler und Schriftsteller als Mitarbeiter von Abderhaldens Zeitschrift "Ethik." Teil I (1925–1933). *Jahrbuch 1995, Leopoldina (R. 3)* 41: 477–530.

———. 1997. Emil Abderhalden und seine Ethik-Mitstreiter. Ärzte, Wissenschaftler und Schriftsteller als Mitarbeiter von Abderhaldens Zeitschrift "Ethik." Teil II (1933–1938). *Jahrbuch 1996, Leopoldina (R. 3)* 42: 509–75.

Kaiser, W., W. Piechocki, and K. Werner. 1977. Die Gesundheitserziehung im wissenschaftlichen Werk von Emil Abderhalden. In In memoriam Emil Abderhalden. Vorträge eines Gedenksymposiums aus Anlaß seines 100. Geburtstages. *Wissenschaftliche Beiträge der Martin-Luther-Universität Halle-Wittenberg* 26 (T 18): 37–55.

Kater, M. H. 1986. *Ärzte und Politik in Deutschland 1818–1945.* Jahrbuch 1986 des Instituts für Geschichte der Medizin der Robert-Bosch-Stiftung, Band 6, Stuttgart, 1987, 34–43.

———. 1987. The Burden of the Past: Problems of a Modern Historiography of Physicians and Medicine in Nazi Germany. *German Studies Review* 10: 31–56.

———. 1989. *Doctors under Hitler.* Chapel Hill: University of North Carolina Press.

Katz, J. 1972. *Experimentation with Human Beings.* New York: Russell Sage Foundation.

Klasen, E.-M. 1984. Die Diskussion über eine "Krise" der Medizin in Deutschland zwischen 1925 und 1935. Diss. med., Mainz.

Klee, E. 1986. *Was sie taten—Was sie wurden, Ärzte, Juristen und andere Beteiligte am Kranken-oder Judenmord.* Frankfurt a.M.: Fischer.

———. 2001. *Auschwitz, die NS-Medizin und ihre Opfer* (Überarbeitete Neuausgabe). Frankfurt a.: Fischer-Taschenbuch-Verlag.

Koslowski, L., ed. 1992. *Maximen der Medizin.* Stuttgart: Schattauer.

Kröner, H.-P. 1998. *Von der Rassenhygiene zur Humangenetik. Das Kaiser-Wilhelm-Institut für Anthropologie, menschliche Erblehre und Eugenik nach dem Kriege.* Medizin in Geschichte und Kultur 20. Stuttgart [u.a.]: Verlag G. Fischer.

Kudlien, F. 1985. *Ärzte im Nationalsozialismus.* Köln: Kiepenheuer und Witsch.

Kümmel, W. F. 2001. Geschichte, Staat und Ethik. Deutsche Medizinhistoriker 1933–1945 im Dienste "nationalpolitischer Erziehung." In Frewer and Neumann 2001, 167–203.

Langstein, L. 1928. Zu den Angriffen gegen unsere therapeutischen Rachitisversuche. *Deutsche Medizinische Wochenschrift* 54: 491.

Lederer, S. E. 1995. *Subjected to Science: Human Experimentation in America before the Second World War.* Baltimore: Johns Hopkins University Press.

Ley, A, and M. M. Ruisinger, eds. 2001. *Gewissenlos Gewissenhaft: Menschenversuche im Konzentrationslager.* Erlangen: Specht Verlag.

Liek, E. 1924. Versuche am Menschen. Antwort 3, *Ethik* 5, no. 1: 19–26.

———. 1926. *Der Arzt und seine Sendung.* Gedanken eines Ketzers, Munich: Lehmann.

Lifton, R. J. 1985. *Ärzte im Dritten Reich.* Frankfurt: Materialien aus dem Sigmund-Freud-Institut, 9/1989.

Lilienthal, G. 1979. Rassenhygiene im Dritten Reich: Krise und Wende. *Medizinhistorisches Journal* 14: 114–34.

Luther, E. 1977. Ethische Aspekte im Leben und Werk Abderhaldens. In *In memoriam*

Emil Abderhalden. Vorträge eines Gedenksymposiums aus Anlaß seines 100. Geburt-stages. Wissenschaftliche Beiträge der Martin-Luther-Universität Halle-Wittenberg 26 (T 18): 7–23.

———. 1991. Emil Abderhaldens Lebensbilanz: Die Menschheit braucht dauerhaften Frieden. In *Äskulap oder Mars? Ärzte gegen den Krieg*, ed. T. M. Ruprecht and C. Jenssen. Bremen: Donat Verlag.

Mann, G. 1973. Rassenhygiene, Sozialdarwinismus. In *Biologismus im 19. Jahrhundert. Vorträge eines Symposiums vom 30.10.-31.10.70 in Frankfurt a.M.*, ed. G. Mann, 73–93. Stuttgart: Enke Verlag.

———. (1983): Sozialbiologie auf dem Wege zur unmenschlichen Medizin des Dritten Reiches. In: *Unmenschliche Medizin. Geschichtliche Erfahrungen—gegenwärtige Probleme und Ausblick auf die zukünftige Entwicklung.* Bad Nauheimer Gespräche der Landesärztekammer Hessen (22–43). Mainz: Verlag Kirchheim.

Matthes, M. 1928. Versuche am Menschen. Antwort 3, *Ethik* 5, no. 1: 16–17.

Meinel, C., and P. Voswinckel, eds. 1994. *Medizin, Naturwissenschaft und Technik im Nationalsozialismus. Kontinuitäten und Diskontinuitäten.* Jahrestagung der DGGMNT in Jena 1992. Stuttgart: GNT-Verlag.

Mitscherlich, A., and F. Mielke. 1947. *Das Diktat der Menschenverachtung.* Heidelberg: Lambertus.

———. 1949. *Wissenschaft ohne Menschlichkeit.* Heidelberg: Lambertus.

———. 1960. *Medizin ohne Menschlichkeit: Dokumente des Nürnberger Ärzteprozesses.* Frankfurt a.M.: Fischer.

Moll, A. 1899. Ärztliche Versuche am Menschen. *Die Woche* 3: 447–49.

———. 1902. *Ärztliche Ethik. Die Pflichten des Arztes in allen Beziehungen seiner Thätigkeit.* Stuttgart: Enke Verlag.

Moses, J. 1930. *Der Totentanz von Lübeck.* Radebeul bei Dresden: Madaus.

———. 1932. Der Kampf gegen das "Dritte Reich": Ein Kampf für die Volksgesundheit. *Der Kassenarzt* 9, no. 5: 1–4.

Numbers, R. L. 1979. William Beaumont and the Ethics of Experimentation. *Journal of the History of Biology* 12: 113–35.

Osnowski, R., ed. 1988. *Menschenversuche: Wahnsinn oder Wirklichkeit.* Köln: Kölner Voksblattverlag.

Pagel, J. L. 1905. *Zur Geschichte und Literatur des Versuchs am lebenden Menschen.* Verhandlungen der Gesellschaft deutscher Naturforscher und Ärzte. 76/2, p. 83.

Pappworth, M. H. 1967. *Human Guinea Pigs: Experimentation on Man.* London: Routledge and Kegan Paul.

———. 1968. *Menschen als Versuchskaninchen: Experiment und Gewissen.* Rüschlikon Zürich Stuttgart and Wien: Verlag Albert Müller.

Platen-Hallermund, A. v. 1948. *Die Tötung Geisteskranker in Deutschland* (Frankfurt a.M.: Verlag der Frankfurter Hefte).

Proctor, R. 1988. *Racial Hygiene: Medicine under the Nazis.* Cambridge, Mass.: Harvard University Press.

Reich, W. T., ed. 1995. *Encyclopedia of Bioethics.* 5 vols. New York: Free Press.

Roelcke, V. 2003. Zur Ethik der klinischen Forschung: Kontextualisierende und reduktionistische Problemdefinitionen und Formen ethischer Reflexion, sowie einige Implikationen. *Zeitschrift für ärztliche Fortbildung und Qualitätssicherung* 97, no. 10: 703–709.

Roelcke, V., and G. Maio, eds. 2004. *Twentieth Century Research Ethics: Historical Perspectives on Values, Practices and Regulations.* Stuttgart: Steiner Verlag.

Ruck, M. 2000. *Bibliographie zum Nationalsozialismus*. Darmstadt: Wissenschaftliche Buchgesellschaft.

Sachse, C., ed. 2003. *Die Verbindung nach Auschwitz. Biowissenschaften und Menschenversuche an Kaiser-Wilhelm-Instituten. Dokumentation eines Symposiums*. Göttingen: Wallstein.

Sandmann, J. 1990. Der Bruch mit der humanitären Tradition: Die Biologisierung der Ethik bei Ernst Haeckel und anderen Darwinisten seiner Zeit. *Forschungen zur Neueren Medizin- und Biologiegeschichte*. Band 2, herausgegeben von G. Mann und W. F. Kümmel, Akademie der Wissenschaften und der Literatur, Mainz. Stuttgart: Fischer.

Sass, H.-M. 1983. Reichsrundschreiben 1931: Pre-Nuremberg German Regulations concerning New Therapy and Human Experimentation. *Journal of Medicine and Philosophy* 8: 99–111.

Schoen, E. 1952. Das soziale Wirken Abderhaldens. In *Emil Abderhalden zum Gedächtnis*. Nova Acta Leopoldina N. F. Band 14, Nr. 103, 178–89.

Schwantje, M. 1919. *Friedensheldentum: Pazifistische Aufsätze aus der Zeitschrift "Ethische Rundschau" (1914/15)*. Berlin: Verlag Neues Vaterland.

Seidler, E., C. Scriba, and W. Berg, eds. 1995. *Die Elite der Nation im Dritten Reich. Das Verhältnis von Akademien und ihrem wissenschaftlichen Umfeld zum Nationalsozialismus*. Acta historica Leopoldina Nr. 22, Halle (Saale).

Sievert, L. E. 1996. *Naturheilkunde und Medizinethik im Nationalsozialismus*. Frankfurt: Mabuse Verlag.

Skramlik, E. v. 1952. Abderhalden als Forscher. In *Emil Abderhalden zum Gedächtnis*. Nova Acta Leopoldina N. F. Band 14, Nr. 103, 155–77.

Spicker, S. F., ed. 1988. *The Use of Human Beings in Research*. Philosophy and Medicine 28. Dordrecht: Kluwer Academic Press.

Stoll, S. 2003. Klinische Forchung und Ethik bei Paul Martini. *Zeitschrift für ärztliche Fortbildung und Qualitätssicherung* 97, no. 10: 675–79.

Tashiro, E. 1991. *Die Waage der Venus. Venerologische Versuche am Menschen am Menschen in der Zeit von 1885 und 1914*. Abhandlungen zur Geschichte der Medizin, Naturwissenschaften, Heft 64. Husum: Mathiesen Verlag.

Thom, A., and G. J. Caregorodcev, eds. 1989. *Medizin unterm Hakenkreuz*. Berlin (Ost): VEB Verlag Volk und Gesundheit.

Tröhler, U., and Reiter-Theil, S., eds. *Ethik und Medizin 1947–1997. Was leistet die Kodifizierung von Ethik?* Göttingen: Wallstein Verlag.

Vollmann, J./Winau, R. 1996.: Informed Consent in Human Experimentation before the Nuremberg Code. *British Medical Journal* 313: 1445–47.

Vollmer, H. 1927. Beitrag zur Ergosterinbehandlung der Rachitits. *Deutsche Medizinische Wochenschrift* 39: 1634–35.

Vorwahl, H. 1931. Die ethische Grenze des Experiments. Ethik 7, no. 5: 458–62.

Weindling, P. J. 1991. *Health, Race and German Politics between National Unification and Nazism, 1870–1945*. Cambridge: Cambridge University Press.

———. 1996. *Ärzte als Richter: Internationale Reaktionen auf die Medizinverbrechen des Nationalsozialismus während des Nürnberger Ärzteprozesses in den Jahren 1946–47*. In Wiesemann and Frewer 1996, 31–44.

[Der] Wert des Menschen. Medizin in Deutschland 1918–1945. 1989. Reihe Deutsche Vergangenheit, Band 34, herausgegeben von der Ärztekammer Berlin in Zusammenarbeit mit der Bundesärztekammer. Berlin: Edition Hentrich.

Wiesemann, C., and A. Frewer, eds. 1996. *Medizin und Ethik im Zeichen von Auschwitz—*

50 Jahre Nürnberger Ärzteprozeß. Erlanger Studien zur Ethik in der Medizin, Band 5. Erlangen und Jena: Verlag Palm und Enke.

Winau, R. 1996. Medizin und Menschenversuch. Zur Geschichte des "informed consent." In Wiesemann and Frewer 1996, 13–29.

Wistrich, R. 1982. *Who's Who in Nazi Germany.* London: Weidenfeld and Nicolson.

3 Experimentation on Humans and Informed Consent: How We Arrived Where We Are

Rolf Winau

The practice of experimenting on humans dates back to antiquity, but we know few details from that time. The notion of experimental research came to fruition only once medicine had detached itself from the dogmatism of the ancient and medieval eras—that is, once the physician's own eyes and what they observed, rather than the authority of the ancients, became the main point of reference for medical practice.

In the course of the eighteenth century we observe sporadic individual experiments, some tending to be rather bizarre. But we also see a number of experimenters who did much to advance the theory and methodology of experimentation. Here I will discuss the experiments performed by only two of these, James Lind and Anton Störck.

In 1747, Lind documented in a clinical test, aboard a sailboat, that citrus fruits were superior in combating scurvy. Lind, who can count as our representative of the establishment of the clinical experiment, otherwise still operates within the notions of the doctor-patient relation prevalent since antiquity. The doctor knows what is right for the patient and will not act to the patient's detriment.

Anton Störck's position ends up looking similar. Störck set new standards in experimental medicine through his research on hemlock. His methodology was new and exemplary, but neither he nor his critics worried about the patient's consent. This topic remained outside the categories of thought of the time (see Zumstein 1968).

Similarly, in theoretical literature there are only occasional references to informing and consenting. Johann Friedrich Gmelin, for example, remarks in his *Geschichte der Gifte* (History of the poisons) of 1776 that experiments were limited to being performed on "wrongdoers and our own person" (Gmelin 1776–77, 1:34).

Georg Friedrich Hildebrandt argued similarly in his *Versuch einer philosophischen Pharmakologie* (Essay in philosophical pharmacology). He called for a multi-tier system of experimentation: in vitro testing—animal testing—human testing. It is in this context that the theoretical writing of the Enlightenment epoch on the subject touches on, though only implicitly, the question of consent (Hildebrandt 1786, 78).

Hildebrandt similarly imposes detailed guidelines on the experimental healing of humans. In this context, however, the patient's right to information and the question of consent did not arise for him. In another set of detailed directions, published by Johann Christian Reil and, independently, by Adolph Friedrich Nolde in 1799, the question is left similarly unmentioned (Reil 1799, 26–44; Nolde 1799, 1 St., 47–97, 2 St. 75–116).

Summarizing this, we can say: the first phase of human testing leads to the development of a methodology of testing as well as to experimental healing, without leading to a notion of a patient's rights (see Winau 1971).

At first glance, informed consent appears to be a phenomenon of the most recent history of medicine, thematized at some point during the second half of the twentieth century. The date 1947 is often given as the *origin of informed consent*, when the notion arose in the context of the Nuremberg Codex. Another date often advanced is 1957, being the year of the first Supreme Court decision on the subject in the U.S.[1] The question, whether there were indeed discussions about informed consent before these dates, and, if so, how far back these discussions go in history, has been subject to much debate and controversy (Katz 1984; Pernick 1982). But in researching this issue, I found little such discussion in the sources.

Occasionally, formulations in eighteenth-century sources are open to rather easy misinterpretation. John Gregory is a good example; by and large, his arguments revolve around familiar notions of a paternalistic doctor-patient relationship. Single sentences picked out of context cannot really be adduced as documentation for a supposed call for patients' rights. Rather, scanning the eighteenth-century literature on the topic, we find the same line of argumentation repeated: informing patients is linked to the philosophical Enlightenment, often with direct reference to Kant's dictum of the "emergence of man from his self-caused immaturity." Johann Karl Osterhausen, for example, in his book *Über medicinische Aufklärung* (On medical enlightenment) of 1798, demands the "emergence of man from his self-caused immaturity in matters of his physical health." Scientific Enlightenment and popular Enlightenment are the two main pillars of his project. He mentions the Universal Rights of Man as "the most sacred thing on earth," but he doesn't take up the theme of patients' rights anywhere in his four-hundred-page work (Osterhausen 1798).

Quite clearly, then, neither the eighteenth nor the nineteenth century saw a great deal of discussion of a patient's rights or his autonomy, but rather the focus is on the duties of doctors. *Helping the patient and not hurting him* is the ethical maxim always in the background in these discussions.

This position dates back to the Hippocratic Oath. Even if the oath doesn't date back to Hippocrates, but was rather backdated to him at a later point, and even if we know little about its actual effectiveness as an ethical norm in antiquity and the Middle Ages, it still constitutes the essential foundation of medical activity for two millennia: the patient's health and the protection from harm are the doctor's mission. The patient's wishes and rights are not taken up; in one section they are explicitly pushed aside: "I will not give anyone a deadly substance, not even if they ask for it" (see Winau 1989; Winau 1994).

Given this background, it is not surprising that a discussion of informed consent was somewhat slow in developing.

In the rather voluminous literature on human testing before the second half of the nineteenth century, there is not one reference to the consent of test subjects. Testing done on convicted criminals is occasionally mentioned. This is where the transformation occurred: the forcible performance of experiments and the abuse of someone's vulnerable position is today roundly condemned as immoral (see Gerken 1976; Fischer 1977). A change in the question of informed consent came about only in the last decade of the nineteenth century, concurrently with a period of transformation in medicine itself. In 1890, Robert Koch introduced a medicine, of a type later known as "tuberculin," as a cure for tuberculosis, during the Tenth International Medical Conference. In the same year, Behring and Kitasato laid (and published) the foundations for serotherapy. The earliest documents of interest for our investigation refer to these events. As early as January 1891, the Prussian minister of the interior circulated a memorandum regulating the use of a tuberculin in the prison system. It marks the first time a public document makes reference to the will of the patient.

It reads as follows:

> The use of Professor Koch's substance on prisoners suffering from tuberculosis is recommended by the minister for spiritual, educational and medical matters only if and when the prison doctor is acquainted with the treatment, and only if the prison has a separate infirmary. Moreover, the doctor should be a resident in the institution, in order to be able to observe the diseased man as regularly as necessary. It is also necessary that Dr. Koch's substance be used only in recent and appropriate cases and never against the will of the sick person. (*Ministerialblatt für die gesamte innere Verwaltung in den Königlich Preussischen Staaten* 1891, 27)

This directive provided the occasion for the *Journal of the American Medical Association* (JAMA), referring to a report in the *British Medical Journal* in April 1891, to issue a memo under the title "Official Regulations as to Tuberculin in Germany and Italy," claiming that the Prussian minister had directed that "The remedy must in no case be used against the patient's will" (JAMA 1891, 492). What in the original memo had been a mere aside had in this article already been transformed into one of four core points of a Prussian regulation. More recent scholarship similarly mentions the Prussian memo, obviously referring only to the JAMA article, as the first general regulation: "No American legislation, however, went as far as the Prussian government, which in 1891 made a regulation that insured that tuberculin would 'in no case be used against the patient's will'" (Lederer 1995, 1).

The confusion over the memo's status notwithstanding, it is clear that the memo stresses explicitly the importance of the will of the patient, even if it is the will of a particular *type* of patient, one in prison. We do not yet know where this emphasis comes from. The second case is more dramatic. Testing on humans in venereology was a tradition reaching back to the eighteenth century. Consider, for example, John Hunter's experiments and those of Franz von Rinecker and Ernst Bumm, who tested the spreading of gonorrhea. All these experiments were publicized, but there is no record of consent on the part of the test subjects. In 1898, the Breslau dermatologist Albert Neisser published a series of experiments he already had run in 1892. In introducing these experiments, he speaks of the marvelous discovery of serotherapy, and claims to have had the idea before Behring and Kitasato. He then describes his own tests: he had injected eight young women, hospitalized for unrelated illnesses, with a cell-free serum procured from syphilitics in the hope of immunizing them. In four of the eight women, all described as *puella publica* (prostitutes), syphilis developed during a subsequent observation period of four years. Neisser, however, linked this to "natural" causes rather than due to his injections. On the contrary, Neisser took the development of the disease in them to mean that immunizing by serum injection was not in fact possible (see Tashiro 1991, 84–103).

The scientific community looked at Neisser's study rather positively, but when the *Münchener Freie Presse*, a liberal daily, reported on human testing under the title *Poor People in Hospitals* (published separately as a brochure, *Arme Leute in Krankenhäusern*, in 1900), a public outcry resulted.

Neisser's case had become public knowledge on January 26, 1899. As early as March the Prussian House of Representatives dealt with the case, which, according to the minister of culture, was by then already being examined by the scientific deputation for medical matters. Also in March, the chief prosecutor's office began investigating Neisser, though the statute of limitations made any charge against Neisser impossible. Eventually, disciplinary proceedings were opened, and these dealt primarily with whether Neisser had solicited the consent of his subjects. He himself explained that he had not done so, because the injections, in his opinion, did not require consent. "If I had gone through the formalities to cover myself, I certainly would have succeeded, for nothing is easier than to use friendly prodding to convince a person with no expertise to assent to just about anything. I would speak of true consent only if dealing with people who are capable, by their knowledge and observations, of assessing the full significance of the possible dangers" (Tashiro 1991, 93). Neisser was fined three hundred marks. The court's decision centered on the following sentence: "The defendant is charged with . . . inoculating . . . eight women without having obtained either their consent or the consent of their legal representatives" (Tashiro 1991, 95).

The conclusions that the Ministry of Culture drew from Neisser's case took the shape of an order to the supervisors of hospitals, policlinics, and other such medical establishments. The order, dated December 29, 1900, forbade medical procedures if

1. they were performed on minors,
2. the person in question had not signaled his or her consent to the procedure in an unambiguous way, or
3. this consent was not based on adequate preparatory disclosure concerning any adverse effects that might possibly result from the procedure.

Further, the order mandated the documentation of both disclosure and consent. (*Centralblatt für die gesamte Unterrichtsverwaltung in Preussen* 2: 188–89.)

This provoked fierce and polemical discussions, in which, underneath their differences, there was a shared recognition of informed consent as the basic prerequisite for human testing. It is uncertain, however, how far this discussion really effected a change in thinking within the medical profession. Albert Moll, in his *Doctor's Ethics* of 1902, denounced not only the continuing high number of experiments without consent, but also the cynical attitude taken in publications. Moll criticized testing on humans in a paper, *Zukunft* (The future), as early as 1899. He had lamented that doctors, "instead of taking a stand unequivocally," had been silent on the Neisser affair or glossed over it in a few words:

> The researcher, for example, is at the same time a doctor treating a patient. The case is of especial interest here, because these two functions can under certain circumstances come into conflict with one another. If the doctor is exclusively at the service of the patient who has entrusted himself to him, then the use of that particular case for the purposes of scientific research becomes impossible; if the doctor is however exclusively at the service of a scientific problem, he will easily tend to set aside the well-being of the individual entrusted to him. (Moll 1899, 215)

Even the patient's consent, Moll claimed, did nothing to take the responsibility off the experimenter. Moreover, children, the mentally ill, the unconscious, and the dying were for him exempt from any experimentation, since no effective consent could be solicited from them.

Further, Moll called for critical standards for the consent of hospital patients, since it was far too easy for a doctor to abuse his own authority and extort consent. Consent was valid only in so far as it was obtained from an independent person who was capable of assessing the potential ramifications of his or her decision. The arguments themselves have changed dramatically.

I will use two examples to illustrate that there was quite a difference of opinion in this discussion. Karl Ernst von Baer in the *Medicinischen Woche* (Medical weekly) of 1900 argued instead against any attempt to curb the doctor's authority. "If these gentlemen [i.e., all those critical of Neisser] had their way, then medicine would suffer a setback to the days of Hippocrates, and natural healers, homeopaths, and charlatans would take the place of actual doctors" (Baer 1900, 91).

To link the discussion of informed consent with the practice of charlatans was a canny rhetorical shift recentering the discussion as one concerning natural healing and quack doctors. On one side were equated the doctor, medical progress, the right to perform human testing without outside control. On the other were quack doctors, regression, and any criticism of the doctor. This almost certainly impressed doctors of the time, who wanted to enlist on the side of progress.

Even Julius Pagel, a doctor working with the poor in Berlin, and a level-headed man, wrote that same year that

> for doctors, the basic question whether Neisser had the ethical right to do his tests, is not actually relevant. For them, the only necessities that arise from the Neisser case are those of gathering in solidarity around the researchers amongst them, of holding high the banner of Science, and protecting such research from erroneous attacks coming from both within and from outside their profession. Only by so doing can we prevent the dissolution of the noble endeavor of our profession, which has been our glory at all times, namely, the prevention of illness and being of use to the suffering. That is the only ethical imperative arising from the Neisser case. (Pagel 1900, 269–70)

Four years later, however, at the convention of natural scientists in Breslau, Pagel gave a talk surveying the topic "On Experimentation on Live Humans." In it he admitted that the experimenters had "in their excitement for the advancement of science" lost track of the "magnitude of their experiments and had inflicted unavoidable damage on the test subjects." Again, he mentions the Neisser case: "Whoever has actually read Neisser's paper, will think it incomprehensible that anyone dared criticize it. Much to the contrary, every man inspired by the progress of science should be grateful for Neisser's painstaking, deliberate work . . . and should recognize that Neisser slipped in his care on only one point, namely when he assumed the tacit consent of his subjects rather than expressly soliciting it" (Pagel 1905, 227). Here we find again the two central concepts, which rise like a barrier before any discussion of ethics: namely, the progress of science and the greater good of humanity. The doctor stands forth as representative of both of these; his role is not that of making a critical interrogation of his own activity. Nonetheless, Pagel has to admit by the end of his talk that in general the permission of test subjects has to be obtained and that experimentation on people who cannot give such permission—the unconscious and the dying—is not licit.

This intense discussion quickly diminished. Whether the directives given by the Prussian ministry disappeared as quickly from the files and from the consciousness of doctors, we cannot say. They certainly appear to have done so.

In this period, nonetheless, discussions about the patient's consent had made progress in the different clinical fields. Sensational experimental surgical procedures, such as one by Victor Cornil in Paris in 1891 concerning the transferability of cancers, and also similar ones in Berlin performed by Ernst von Bergmann and Eugen Hahn, although arising in different contexts, had raised the profession's consciousness of the problem.

As early as 1895, Ernst König, who later became a professor at the University of Berlin, wrote in an essay entitled *Der Arzt und der Kranke* (Doctor and patient): "It is self-evident that in any procedure that is . . . painful or somehow dangerous, the consent of the sick person or the sick person's relatives must be procured" (König 1895, 5). Any course of therapy that involves pain or surgery is possible only with the explicit permission of the patient. "We deem it therefore . . . legally impermissible to perform any operation connected with bloodletting, with pain, or with danger without special agreement on the part of the patient" (6). In 1907, William Osler at the Congress of American Physicians and Surgeons expressed the opinion that by then the limits of justifiable testing on humans had been rather clearly established. Such tests, he claimed, were necessary but had to be preceded by preparatory animal testing and were contingent upon the "full consent" of the patient. Moreover, every patient involved in the experiment should be able at least potentially to profit from the experimental treatment. For tests on subjects in perfect health, Osler made a similar stipulation: full disclosure about the experiment and complete voluntariness (Osler 1907, 7–11).

But neither the debate about the Neisser case, nor the discussions among surgeons, nor Osler's statement led to a comprehensive overhaul of medical praxis. This becomes evident when we look at Germany at the end of the 1920s. Papers and magazines from the camp of persons in favor of natural healing and biological medicine picked up stories of cases published in medical journals that appeared to document highly irregular behavior toward test subjects, children in particular (see Steinmann 1975). Arno Nohlen of Dusseldorf, for example, is cited as having injected soot into dying children in order to induce an artificial anthracosis. H. Vollmer at the Kaiserin-Auguste-Viktoria-Haus in Berlin experimented with Vigantol, which had been recently discovered, "on a sample of 100 rats and 20 children," both kept in unfavorable dietary and light conditions (Vollmer 1927, 1634–35). Julius Moses, a deputy for the Social Democrat Party, chose *Vorwärts* as the basis for his campaign against "the rage in experimentation" (*Gegen die Experimentierwut*—the title of one of his numerous articles), before bringing the subject to the attention of the Reichstag (Moses 1928a).

Once again, the parliamentary debate was echoed by a general discussion within the medical profession. Once again, it split that profession into two camps. The experimenters who had been attacked by Moses resisted, and their superiors, Arthur Schlossmann and Leo Langstein, supported them. Langstein claimed that their success justified the experiments. Failure to gain consent was of only minor importance (Langstein 1928, 491). The discussion quickly turned political: "Dr. Moses who, along with a few doctors, stands fully outside of the medical profession as a whole, seems to think he has found a good opportunity to pin something on the profession, to rouse the rabble against doctors, and thus to move us closer to the final goal of social democracy, the socialization of all medicine" (Steinmann 1975, 36).

The discussion within the ranks of the Berlin Medical Association was somewhat more serious. The association decided after intense deliberation to establish a fact-finding committee and passed a resolution on July 16, 1928. I quote the final two paragraphs in full:

> There must not be any legal limit set on scientific research, lest it come to a halt; we simply cannot test new therapeutic procedures or make new medical discoveries useful to the sick without testing on humans. Nonetheless, in so doing, a doctor must be constantly aware of his responsibility for the life and health of his patient. Any trial on humans must be limited to what is absolutely necessary, must be well grounded theoretically and scientifically, and must be well defined biologically. Every doctor who performs such tests must have and keep "nil nocere" as his highest law, for the well-being of the patient is more important than science. Moreover, medical ethics commands that the patient or a legal representative be informed of the spirit and purpose of the particular therapeutic test.
>
> Furthermore, the Berlin Medical Association, with respect to recent experiences, expresses its expectation that in the future tactfulness will continue to be shown in scientific publications, and that valid feelings of the public will be respected. (*Berliner Ärzt–Correspondenz* 1928, 278–80)

Of course, what this paper calls for is not consenting but, at least, informing.

Inspired by the discussion, Emil Abderhalden, who was a doctor and the publisher of the magazine *Ethik,* started polling his colleagues for their opinions on human testing. The results display the split we have already encountered, namely unconditional supporters and critics of experimentation on humans. The survey tells us nothing about the question of informed consent.

For the discussion about informed consent, another event became critical, namely the BCG disaster in Lübeck. In February 1930, more than seventy people died after being inoculated for tuberculosis with BCG (Bacillus Calmette-Guérin). I will not touch here on the legal aftermath and the discussion of the classification of inoculation as a form of testing on humans. One thing, however, is important for this discussion: the classification of inoculation as a form of testing on humans depended for the court on the informed consent of the parents, and the court investigated whether informed consent had indeed been given.[2]

In March of 1930, the Reich's Health Council convened for a special session devoted to the question of testing on humans. After hearing expert witnesses and after extensive discussion, the council adopted "Guidelines for New Forms of Therapy and Tests Performed on Humans." These were published with slight alterations on February 28, 1931. The guidelines not only distinguish between new forms of therapy and scientific experimentation, both of which are clearly defined, but also demand that new therapies and tests "conform with the principles of medical ethics and the rules of medical art and science." They state categorically: "Medical ethics forbids any exploitation of persons in socioeconomic distress." They also demand informed consent, even for simple treatment. And it has the following to say about human testing:

Undertaking such a test without informed consent is impermissible under any circumstances. Any test on humans that could have been replaced with a test on animals is to be rejected. Tests on humans may only be performed once all documentation necessary for its clarification has been obtained and safeguards have been taken, be this by laboratory tests or tests on animals. Given these preconditions, any baseless and haphazard testing is naturally illegal. Experiments performed on children or adolescents under the age of 18 are not allowed if they will endanger the welfare of the child or adolescent in the slightest. Experiments on the dying are incompatible with the principles of medical ethics and thus not permitted.

In one of its last paragraphs, the paper indicates that "academic instruction [should] take every opportunity" to point out this problem. In the cover letter to the guidelines from the secretary of the interior, we read among other things that "doctors active in institutions for inpatient treatment or in outpatient service should be bound to these rules and so indicate with their signatures upon entry into the profession" (Schreiben des Reichsministers des Inneren vom 28.2.1931 an die deutschen Landesregierungen).

However, much as in the case of the order from 1900, these guidelines remained without effect in Germany, unable as they were to prevent the medical crimes committed in the context of the Third Reich.

The discussion of informed consent did not come about through the Nuremberg Doctors' Trial, or through the Nuremberg Codex of 1947. Only very much later did German doctors once again face up to the questions of medical ethics.

Notes

1. For more on the history of informed consent, See P. S. Appelbaum, C. W. Lidz, and A. Meisel 1987; Elkeles 1989; and R. R. Faden and T. L. Beauchamp 1986.

2. The final draft of the guidelines for new therapeutic treatment and human testing was handed down to local governments along with a cover letter by the secretary of the interior on 02/28/1931. See Steinmann 1975, 126.

References

Appelbaum, P. S., C. W. Lidz, and A. Meisel. 1987. *Informed Consent: Legal Theory and Clinical Practice.* New York: Oxford University Press.

Arme Leute in Krankenhäusern. 1900. München.

Baer, K. E. von. 1900. Der Fall "Neisser." *Deutsche Medicinische Woche* 1: 89–91.

Berliner Ärzte–Correspondenz. 1928. Sitzungsbericht der Sitzung der Ärztekammer. Berlin am 16.6.1928. 33: 278–80.

Centralblatt für die gesamte Unterrichtsverwaltung in Preussen. 1901. 2: 188–89.

Elkeles, B. 1989. Die schweigsame Welt von Arzt und Patient. Einwilligung und Aufklärung in der Arzt-Patient-Beziehung des 19. und frühen 20. Jahrhunderts. *Med. G G* 8: 63–91.

Faden, R. R., and T. L. Beauchamp. 1986. *A History and Theory of Informed Consent.* New York: Oxford University Press.

Fischer, Chr. 1977. Zur Theorie des Arzneimittelversuchs am Menschen in der ersten Hälfte des 19. Jahrhunderts, Diss. med., Mainz.

Gerken, G. 1976. Zur Entwicklung des klinische Arzneimittelversuchs am Menschen, Diss. med., Mainz.

Gmelin, F. 1776–77. *Geschichte der Gifte.* Leipzig, Nuremberg.

Hildebrandt, G. F. 1786. *Versuch einer philosophischen Pharmakologie.* Braunschweig.

JAMA (Journal of the American Medical Association). 1891. Official Regulations as to Tuberculin in Germany and Italy. 16: 492.

Katz, J. 1984. *The Silent World of Doctor and Patient.* New York: Free Press.

König, E. 1895. Der Arzt und der Kranke. *Zeitschr. f. sociale Medizin* 1: 1–11.

Langstein, L. 1928. Zu den Angriffen gegen unsere therapeutischen Rachitisversuche. *Dtsch.med.Wschr.* 54: 491.

Lederer, S. E. 1995. *Subjected to Science: Human Experimentation in America before the Second World War.* Baltimore: Johns Hopkins University Press.

Ministerialblatt für die gesamte innere Verwaltung in den Königlich Preussischen Staaten. 1891. 52: 27.

Moll, A. 1899. Versuche am lebenden Menschen. *Die Zukunft* 29: 213–18.

Moses, J. 1928a. 100 Ratten und 20 Kinder: Arbeiterkinder als Experimentierkarnickel. *Vorwärts* v. 03/08/1928.

———. 1928b. Kinder als Versuchsobjekte. Gegen die Experimentierwut. *Vorwärts* v. 03/22/1928.

Nolde, A. F. 1799. Erinnerung an einige zur kritischen Würdigung der Arzneymittel sehr notwendige Bedingungen. *Hufelands Journal* 8: 1. St. S. 47–97, 2. St. S. 75–116.

Osler, W. 1907. The Evolution of the Idea of Experiments in Medicine. *Transactions of the Congress of American Physicians and Surgeons* 7: 7–11.

Osterhausen, Johann Karl. 1798. *Über medicinische Aufklärung.* Zürich.

Pagel, J. 1900. Zum Fall Neisser. *Deutsche Medizinalzeitung* 21: 269–70.

———. 1905. Über den Versuch am lebenden Menschen. *Deutsche Aerzte-Zeitung,* 193–98, 217–28, 227.

Pernick, M. S. 1982. "The Patient's Role in Medical Decision-Making: A Social History of Informed Consent in Medical Therapy," in *Making Health Care Decisions,* vol. 3, ed. President's Commission for Study of Ethical Problems in Medicine and Biomedical and Bioethical Research. Washington, D.C.: U.S. Government Printing Office.

Reil, J. C. 1799. Beitrag zu den Principien für jede künftige Pharmekologie. *Röschlauns Magazin* 3: 26–44.

Schreiben des Reichsministers des Inneren vom 28.2.1931 an die deutschen Landesregierungen.

Steinmann, R. 1975. Die Debatte über medizinische Versuche am Menschen in der Weimarer Zeit. Diss. med., Tübingen.

Tashiro, E. 1991. *Die Waage der Venus, Venerologische Versuche am Menschen zwischen Fortschritt und Moral.* Husum.

Vollmer, H. 1927. Beitrag zur Ergosterinbehandlung der Rachitis. *Dtsch.med.Wschr.* 53: 1634–35.

Winau, R. 1971. Experimentelle Pharmakologie und Toxikologie im 18. Jahrhundert. *Med. Habil.schr.* Mainz.

——. 1989. Der Hippokratische Eid und die ärztliche Ethik. In *Praxis der Nierentransplantation III,* ed. F. W. Albert, 99–107. Stuttgart, New York.

——. 1994. The Hippocratic Oath and Ethics in Medicine. *Forensic Science International* 69: 285–89.

Zumstein, B. 1968. *Anton Störck und seine therapeutischen Versuche.* Zürich: Juris-Verlag.

4 The Silence of the Scholars

Benno Müller-Hill

Science lives in the present. Its past does not interest scientists. One does not cite papers that are more than three years old, and the textbooks contain little history. Everything that was shown to be incorrect is forgotten—all the more so if it was not incorrect, but amoral and inhuman. Those who were close to such crimes claim not to have known anything. The student defends his teacher, and the colleague his colleague. History of Science, where the past may be quietly remembered, is a field far away from the active scientist.

I am not an historian of science. I am a chemist by training and a molecular biologist by choice. Yet in the late seventies I became interested in the history of human genetics. I discovered that almost nothing was written about human genetics in Nazi Germany. Neither German nor international historians of science had written books or articles about the subject. This seemed most astonishing, if one recalled that German human geneticists had produced the fundaments of racial ideology and thus supported the ideology of the Nazis. I spent a full year visiting archives, reading the scientific journals of that time, and interviewing the geneticists who had been active during those twelve years.

Then in June 1984 I published my book on the topic: *Tödliche Wissenschaft. Die Aussonderung von Juden, Zigeunern und Geisteskranken 1933–1945* (Murderous science: Elimination by scientific selection of Jews, Gypsies, and others in Germany 1933–1945). The book was not reviewed—there was almost total silence. The first review appeared February 1985 in *Nature*. Then a review appeared in the *Frankfurter Allgemeine,* and that was it for Germany. I went back into molecular biology and tried at the same time to keep track of the history of genetics.

Examples of Science and Oblivion

Max Delbrück on German Geneticists

In 1947 H. J. Muller asked Max Delbrück to find out which German geneticists had been Nazis. Delbrück went to Berlin and gave a talk in the Harnack House of the Kaiser Wilhelm-Gesellschaft (KWG). The building next to it was the home of the Kaiser Wilhelm-Institut für Anthropologie, menschliche Erblehre und Eugenik, of which Eugen Fischer and Ottmar von Verschuer had been directors. Josef Mengele, a postdoctoral student of von Verschuer, had regularly entered through its door, which was ornamented with the head of Athene, before he went to Auschwitz and several times while he was active at Auschwitz. And what did Delbrück communicate to Muller? He said that those who were good in genetics were not Nazis (Fischer 1985, 213). Was this generalization true for Fischer and von Verschuer? I doubt it. This was an easy way out.

Sterilizing the Unwanted

On July 14, 1933, the law demanding the sterilization of the unwanted, *Gesetz zur Verhütung erbkranken Nachwuchses* (Law to prevent reproduction by persons with hereditary diseases) was announced in Germany (Gütt, Rüdin, and Ruttke 1934). It said that certain other persons should also be sterilized against their will. These were in particular people of low intelligence (*Schwachsinnige*), schizophrenics, manic-depressives, alcoholics, and some others. The exact numbers of those sterilized are known for the years 1934, 1935, and 1936: altogether, close to 200,000. If we assume that the annual numbers did not change, altogether 350,000 persons were sterilized before the war began and the law ended. To this number have to be added those who were sterilized illegally: about 600 "colored" children, the children of French "colored" soldiers, an unknown number of Gypsies, and others. Finally, the 2 percent who died during the operation should be remembered (Müller-Hill 1984). Ernst Rüdin defended the law until his death in 1952.

Similar laws had been active in the U.S. and were announced somewhat later in the Scandinavian states. The German law was praised internationally as being progressive (Kühl 1997). It was suspended in Germany after 1945, but for many years its victims were not regarded as victims. Hans Nachtsheim, a subdirector (*Abteilungleiter*) of the Kaiser Wilhelm-Institut für Anthropologie in Berlin, defended the law in the late 1950s and early 1960s. One should not forget that these same human geneticists also asked for a law that would allow the sterilization of persons defined as antisocial (*asozial, gemeinschaftsfremd*). According to the planned law, two M.D.s and one police officer were sufficient to decide whether such a person should be sterilized and put into a concentration camp. The law never became reality—the Department of Justice was adamantly against it (Müller-Hill 1984).

Collecting the Brains of the Murdered

On October 28, 1940, Julius Hallervorden, a professor of brain anatomy, went to the extermination center in the Brandenburg jail (Peiffer 1997). He was present when fifty children were murdered by carbon monoxide. He dissected their brains immediately after and kept thirty-seven of these. Later he received several hundred such interesting brains in his institute. After the war he became subdirector (*Abteilungsleiter*) of the Max-Planck-Institut für Hirnforschung (Brain Research) in Frankfurt. There he published many papers on the brains. He had some problems with foreign colleagues but not in Germany. Certainly it was not Hallervorden's idea to kill the children. He did not open the carbon monoxide valve. But to profit from the murder in such a way? Hallervorden's science seems to be excellent. This makes the situation even worse in my eyes.

Planning the Genocide of the Gypsies

Dr. Robert Ritter, a psychiatrist, held a position in the Reichsgesundheitsamt (National Institute of Health) (Müller-Hill 1987). Together with a group of collaborators he planned the genocide of the Gypsies. According to his view, fewer then 10 percent of the Gypsies were true Gypsies; more than 90 percent of them were the descendants of the lowest criminal European subproletariat. His institute wanted to define every Gypsy according to the group to which he or she belonged: Were they pure Gypsies who were to be allowed to survive, or were they mixed Gypsies who were to be sterilized and put into work camps? This work was financed by the Deutsche Forschungsgemeinschaft (DFG) (the German research granting agency). Ritter died in 1951, shortly after court proceedings against him began. He had a collaborator, Sophie Ehrhardt, who in 1959 became a professor at Tübingen University. She kept material from the Gypsy studies of Ritter's institute; in 1966 she asked the DFG for grant money to work on it (*Populationsgenetische Untersuchungen an Zigeunern*). The referees were in favor of supporting her proposal, but soon thereafter some Gypsies found out about the project and protested. The grant finally was not awarded, but Ehrhardt remained a professor. She died in 1990, five years after a legal prosecution found her not guilty.

In 1983, when I discovered the records of the DFG in the *Bundesarchiv* in Koblenz, I wrote to the president of the DFG, Eugen Seibold, and asked him to consider whether the DFG should not pay for the library of the House of the Sinti and Roma (the Gypsy people) that was being planned in Heidelberg, to recompense for the planning of the genocide. To the best of my knowledge the DFG never even commented on the fact that its own precursor had financed the planning of the genocide of the Gypsies.

Dr. Mengele, "My Collaborator in Auschwitz"

The same day that I discovered the DFG reports of Ritter in the Bundesarchiv, I also discovered the reports von Verschuer wrote to the DFG in 1943 and 1944. Most devastating were a few sentences (Müller-Hill 1988 [1984]): von Verschuer called Mengele "my collaborator . . . in Auschwitz." In another sentence he stated that "the research will be done together with Dr. Hillmann, a collaborator of the Institute of Biochemistry," where Adolf Butenandt was director. This implied the likely possibility that Butenandt, who later became president of the Max-Planck-Gesellschaft (MPG), knew something about the experiments Mengele was doing for von Verschuer. This was too much. The MPG tried to keep silent about these sentences and what they implied. They refused categorically to take a closer look. This changed only after Hubert Markl, president of the MPG, appointed a committee in 1999 to investigate the questionable past of the KWG. The high point of this development was a meeting in June 2001, one to which the MPG had invited some of the surviving twins of Mengele's experiments in Auschwitz. Markl apologized that it had taken so many years to invite them and to acknowledge the bad past (Markl 2001).

Discussion of the Cases Presented

Most of the medical scientists I mentioned here were not directly involved in murder. Those who formulated the sterilization law or were involved in it never felt responsible for the unhappiness and possible death they created for so many people. They excused themselves by saying that it was their responsibility to support such a law. If it was misused, this was not their affair. And what about the six hundred "colored" children they inspected before they were sterilized? There was no prosecution.

And Max Delbrück, who received a Nobel Prize for Medicine in 1969? Should he in 1947 have gone to the building next to the Harnack House and talked with Hans Nachtsheim? Perhaps he did so, and it was the wisdom of Nachtsheim he was propagating. The law was based on bad science and so it became unimportant. Of course there is something to it. Today we know that schizophrenia is not simply recessively inherited. In the thirties monozygotic twins were shown to be about 90 percent concordant for schizophrenia. Now this value is down to 50 or even 30 percent. It is not clear to me what the explanation is: different definition of schizophrenia or incompetence of the psychiatrists? Ernst Rüdin, who discovered the nonexistent recessiveness in schizophrenia and who was one of the persons responsible for the law, never expressed any guilt.

The same is true for Hallervorden. But what if he had once touched the carbon monoxide valve? If he had visited Auschwitz to collect the brains of some murdered Jews, brains considered "interesting"? Is Hallervorden excused because his science was so good? Or is he simply excused because so many other German and Austrian brain anatomists also received such brains? I was told confidentially by some Swedish colleagues at a conference that a Swedish brain anatomist received large amounts of a certain brain part from the euthanasia organizers.

In the meanwhile it was proposed that the name of Hallervorden-Spatz syndrome should be changed. I spoke out against such a change. It seemed to me that the name of Hallervorden and his director Spatz should be remembered just for what they did while the euthanasia action was going on.

Today informed consent is important, but it does not suffice. A law that forbids asking for the genotype of a person seeking health insurance or a job is still missing in the U.S. and in Germany. At the moment only a very few people are hurt by the absence of such a law, but this may change. Such a law is essential—in its absence we may move into a society where the ruling class is a genetically determined race.

General Discussion

Other cases I mention here indicate how easy it is to be seduced into using "human material" or data that should not be used. This seduction is today as extensive as it was then. In 1989 I participated at a conference on "Bioethics and the Holocaust" at the University of Minnesota. There a speaker suggested that Sigmund Rascher's data might be used if those data can save lives. I recall that Rascher forged his thesis and murdered many people at low pressure or in ice-cold water. At the conference the majority of speakers agreed that the data might be used. Jay Katz, Robert L. Berger, and I were the only participants against this proposition. Yet in the printed version (Caplan 1992), those who had earlier been for the use of Rascher's data had changed their minds. Now the majority was against the use of such data. I find this most important. Material and data that have been obtained by murder or violence should not be touched. Hallervorden, Verschuer, and Ehrhardt would not have had their reputations tarnished if they had not used this type of material and data. This should be the message: Do not touch such material, and speak out against its use.

It is profoundly disquieting that no scientist involved in the practice of "race hygiene" in Nazi Germany ever wrote or published an article or a book about these misdeeds. Not a single scientist I talked to saw anything wrong in what was done. I can understand that nobody wanted to accuse himself and later be prosecuted. I can understand that nobody wanted to indicate that a colleague had done anything wrong. But they seriously believed that everything had been in order. As stated before, the two institutions the precursors of which were involved in these crimes, the Deutsche Forschungsgemeinschaft and the Max-Planck-Gesellschaft, until recently claimed that the evil past was not their affair. For more than half a century they were silent. Apparently it is necessary for everyone involved to be dead before one can talk freely about the past.

What was true for human genetics was true for all other fields. The Federal Republic was built on silence. This silence was massively attacked for the first time by the students of 1968. Of course the students soon thereafter forgot what they had wanted. Today, finally, this silence does not exist any more.

There is another important lesson to consider: Science prospers when it is not being kept secret. Secrecy slowly destroys science. It is extremely unlikely that von Verschuer did not know what Mengele did in Auschwitz. And Butenandt talked to von Verschuer (Müller-Hill 2003). To claim that one does not know what is going on is harmful for science. Secrecy is the plague of science.

References

Caplan, Arthur L., ed. 1992. *When Medicine Went Mad: Bioethics and the Holocaust.* Totowa, N.J.: Humana Press.

Fischer, P. 1985. *Licht und Leben. Ein Bericht über Max Delbrück, den Wegbereiter der Molekularbiologie.* Konstanz: Universitätsverlag.

Gütt, A., E. Rüdin, and F. Ruttke. 1934. *Gesetz zur Verhütung erbkranken Nachwuchses vom 14. Juli 1933.* Munich: Lehmanns Verlag.

Kühl, S. 1997. *Die Internationale der Rassisten.* Frankfurt: Campus Verlag.

Markl, H. 2001. Ansprache des Präsidenten der Max-Planck-Gesellschaft zur Förderung der Wissenschaften, Hubert Markl, Berlin 7. Juni 2001. Referat für Presse und Öffentlichkeitsarbeit der MPG.

Müller-Hill, B. 1984. *Tödliche Wissenschaft, die Aussonderung von Juden, Zigeunern und Geisteskranken 1933–1945.* Reinbek: Rowohlt.

———. 1987. Genetics after Auschwitz. *Holocaust and Genocide Studies* 2: 3–20.

———. 1988 [1984]. *Murderous Science: Elimination by Scientific Selection of Jews, Gypsies and Others in Germany 1933–1945.* Translation of Müller-Hill 1984. Oxford: Oxford University Press. Reissued by Cold Spring Harbor Laboratory Press in 1998.

———. 2003. Selective Perception: The Letters of Adolf Butenandt, Nobel Prize Winner and President of the Max Planck Society. In *Comprehensive Biochemistry* 42: 548–79.

Nachtsheim, Hans. 2003. In *Das Personenlexikon zum Dritten Reich*, ed. E. Klee. Frankfurt: Fischer.

Peiffer, J. 1997. Hirnforschung im Zwielicht: Beispiele verführbarer Wissenschaft aus der Zeit des Nationalsozialismus. In *Abhandlungen zur Geschichte der Medizin und der Naturwissenschaften*, ed. R. Winau and H. Müller Dietz. Husum: Matthiesen Verlag.

5 The Ethics of Evil: The Challenge and the Lessons of Nazi Medical Experiments

Arthur L. Caplan

Taking the Nazis' Ethical Arguments Seriously

Most histories of medical ethics locate the origins of bioethics in the ashes of the German concentration camps. The Nuremberg Code is frequently held up in courses and textbooks on medical ethics as the "constitution" of human subjects research. But very little is said about the actual experiments that generated this document. And even less is said about the moral rationales those involved in the horrific research gave in their defense. Why?

One reason is that the events of the Holocaust are so horrid that they speak for themselves. What more is there to say about mass murder and barbaric experimentation except that it was unethical?

Another is that many scholars have dismissed the research done in the camps as worthless. Those involved in conducting it have been dismissed as lunatics and crackpots. What point is there is discussing the ethics of research that is nothing more than torture disguised as science (Berger 1990)?

Yet another reason for the failure to grapple with Nazi moral rationales is that there has been a tradition of trying to offer psychological explanations for the behavior of those involved in the killing, so that moral explanations seem unnecessary. Those who went to work at the gas chambers and dissection rooms did so through adaptations of personality and character that make their conduct understandable but make it difficult to hold them morally accountable for their conduct (Lifton 1986; Browning 1993).

And there is always the fear that to talk of the ethics of the research done in the camps is to lend barbarism a convenient disguise. It is simply wrong to look at the ethical justifications for what was done because it confers a false acceptability on what was manifestly wrong.

Perhaps the most important reason for the absence of commentary on the ethics of the research done in the camps is that such questions open a door that few bioethicists wish to enter. If moral justifications can be given for why someone deemed mass murder appropriate in the name of public health or thought that it was right to freeze hapless men and women to death or decompress them or infect them with lethal doses of typhus—then to put the question plainly—what good is ethics?

Debunking the Myths of Incompetence, Madness, and Coercion

It is comforting to believe that health care professionals from the nation that was, at the time, the world's leader in medicine, who had pledged an oath to "do no harm," could not conduct brutal, often lethal, experiments upon innocent persons in concentration camps. It is comforting to think that it is not possible to defend in moral terms wound research on the living. It is comforting to think that anyone who espouses racist, eugenic ideas cannot be a competent, introspective physician or scientist. Nazi medical crimes show that each of these beliefs is false (Caplan 2004).

It is often believed that only madmen, charlatans, and incompetents among doctors, scientists, public health officials, and nurses could possibly have associated with those who ran the Nazi party. Among those who did their "research" in Auschwitz, Dachau, and other camps, some had obvious psychological problems, were lesser scientific lights, or both (Lifton 1986). But there were also well-trained, reputable, and competent physicians and scientists who were also ardent Nazis. Some conducted experiments in the camps. Human experimentation in the camps was not conducted only by those who were mentally unstable or on the periphery of science. Not all who engaged in experimentation or murder were inept (Kater 1990; Proctor 1992; Caplan 1992, 2004).

Placing all of the physicians, health professionals, and scientists who took part in the crimes of the Holocaust on the periphery of medicine and science allows another myth to flourish—that medicine and science went "mad" when Hitler took control of Germany. Competent and internationally renowned physicians and scientists could not willingly have had anything to do with Nazism. However, the actions as well as the beliefs of German physicians and scientists under Nazism stand in glaring contrast to this myth (Proctor 1988; Kater 1989).

Once identified, the myths of incompetence and madness make absolutely no sense. How could flakes, crackpots, and incompetents have been the only ones supporting Nazism? Could the Nazis have had any chance of carrying out genocide on a staggering, monumental scale against victims scattered over half the globe without the zealous help of competent biomedical and scientific authorities? The technical and logistical problems of collecting, transporting, exploiting, murdering, scavenging, and disposing of the bodies of millions from dozens of nations required competence and skill, not ineptitude and madness.

The Holocaust differs from other instances of genocide in that it involved the active participation of medicine and science. The Nazis turned to biomedicine specifically for help in carrying out genocide after their early experience using specially trained troops to murder in Poland and the Soviet Union proved impractical (Browning 1993).

Another myth that has flourished in the absence of a serious analysis of the moral rationales proffered by those in German biomedicine who participated in the Holocaust is that those who participated were coerced. Many doctors, nurses, and scientists in Germany and other nations have consoled themselves about the complicity of German medicine and science in genocide with the fable that once the Nazi regime seized power, the cooperation of the biomedical and scientific establishments was secured only by force (Lifton 1986; Proctor 1988; Kater 1989). Even then, this myth has it, doctors', scientists', and public health officials' cooperation with Nazism was grudging.

The myths of incompetence, madness, and coercion have obscured the truth about the behavior of biomedicine under Nazism. Most of those who participated did so because they believed it was the right thing to do. This helps to explain the relative silence in the field of bioethics about both the conduct and the justifications of those in biomedicine who were so intimately involved with the Nazi state.

Why Does Bioethics Have So Little to Say about the Holocaust?

If one dates the field of bioethics from the creation of the first bioethics institutes and university programs in the United States in the mid-1960s, then the field is roughly twenty-five years old. Incredibly, no book-length bioethical study exists that examines the actions, policies, abuses, crimes, or rationales of German doctors and biomedical scientists.

There has been almost no discussion of the roles played by medicine and science during the Nazi era in the bioethics literature. Rather than see Nazi biomedicine as morally bad, the field of bioethics has generally accepted the myth that Nazi biomedicine was either inept, mad, or coerced.

By subscribing to these myths, bioethics has been able to avoid a painful confrontation with the fact that many of who committed the crimes of the Holocaust were competent physicians and scientists who acted from strong moral convictions. Not one of the doctors or public health officials on trial at Nuremberg pleaded for mercy on the grounds of insanity. A few claimed they were merely following legitimate orders, but almost no one alleged coercion (Nuremberg Trial Transcripts 1946).

When called to account at Nuremburg and other trials for their actions, Nazi doctors, scientists, and public health officials were surprisingly forthright about their reasons for their conduct. The same cannot be said for the ethical evaluations offered in Germany and in the Western world for their crimes.

The puzzle of how it came to be that physicians and scientists who committed so many crimes and caused so much suffering and death did so in the belief that they were morally right cries out for analysis, discussion, and debate. But it is tremendously painful for those in bioethics to have to undertake such an analysis.

Those who teach bioethics often presume, if only tacitly, that those who know what is ethical will not behave in immoral ways. What is the point of doing bioethics, of teaching courses on ethics to medical, nursing, and public health students, if the vilest and most horrendous of deeds and policies can be justified by moral reasons? Bioethics has been speechless in the face of the crimes of Nazi doctors and biomedical scientists precisely because so many of these doctors and scientists believed they were doing what was morally right to do.

Experimentation in the Camps

There were at least twenty-six different types of experiments conducted for the explicit purpose of research in concentration camps or using concentration camp inmates in Germany, Poland, and France during the Nazi era (Caplan 1992). Among the studies in which human beings were used in research were studies and analyses of high-altitude decompression on the human body; attempts to make seawater drinkable; the efficacy of sulfanilamide for treating gunshot wounds; the feasibility of bone, muscle, and joint transplants; treatment of burns caused by incendiary bombs; the efficacy of polygal for treating trauma-related bleeding; the efficacy of high-dose radiation in causing sterility; the efficacy of phenol (gasoline) injections as a euthanasia agent; the efficacy of electroshock therapy; the symptoms and course of noma (starvation-caused skin gangrene); the postmortem examination of skeletons and brains to assess the effects of starvation; the efficacy of surgical techniques for sterilizing women; and the impact of stress and starvation on ovulation, menstruation, and cancerous growths in the reproductive organs of women. A variety of other studies were carried out on twins, dwarves, and those with congenital defects. Some camp inmates were used as subjects to train medical students in surgery. Jewish physicians in one camp surreptitiously recorded observations about the impact of starvation on the body.

The question of whether any of these activities carried out in the name of medical or scientific research upon unconsenting, coerced human beings deserves the label of "research" or "experimentation" is controversial (Berger 1990). When the description of research is broadened further to include the intentional killing of human beings in order to establish what methods are most efficient, references to "research" and "experimentation" begin to seem completely strained. Injecting a half-starved young girl with phenol to see how quickly she will die or trying out various forms of phosgene gas on camp inmates in the hope of finding cheap, clean, and efficient modes of killing so the state can effectively prosecute genocide is not the sort of activity associated with the term "research."

But murder and genocide are not the same as intentionally causing someone to suffer and die to fulfill a scientific goal. Killing for scientific purposes, while certainly as evil as murder in the service of racial hygiene, is, nonetheless, morally different. The torture and killing that were at the core of Nazi medical experiments involves not only torture and murder but also the exploitation of human beings to serve the goals of science. To describe what happened in language other than that of human experimentation blurs the nature of the wrongdoing. The evil inherent in Nazi medical experimentation was not simply that people suffered and died but that they were exploited for science and medicine as they died.

A summary report prepared for the American military about the hypothermia experiments has been cited in the peer-reviewed literature of medicine more than two dozen times since the end of World War II. Not only was the data examined and referenced—it was applied. British air-sea rescue experts used the Nazi data to modify rescue techniques for those exposed to cold water (Caplan 1992). The force of the question, "should the data be used?" is diminished not only because there are reasons to doubt the reliability and exclusivity of the data, but also because the question has already been answered—Nazi data has been used by many scientists from many nations.

There is another moral issue that does not hinge on the answer to the question of whether the research was well designed or the findings were of enduring scientific value. How did physicians and scientists convince themselves that murderous experimentation was morally justified?

No one understood the need for justification more clearly than the doctors and scientists put on trial after the conclusion of the war for their crimes. The defendants admitted that dangerous and even lethal experiments had been conducted on unconsenting persons in prisons and other institutions. Some protested attempts by the prosecution, in its effort to highlight the barbarity of what they had done, to demean or disparage the caliber of their research. No one apologized for their role in various experiments conducted in the camps. Instead, those put on trial attempted to explain and justify what they had done, often couching their defense in explicitly moral terms.

The Ethics of Evil

Probably the most succinct precis of the moral arguments brought forward by physicians, public health officials, and scientists in defense of their participation both in experimentation in the concentration camps and in the "final solution" can be found in the transcripts of the Nuremberg trials. The first group of individuals to be put on trial by the Allies were physicians and public health officials. The role they had played in conducting or tolerating cruel and often lethal experiments in the camps dominated the trials (Caplan 1992). As it happens, the same arguments that were brought forward in defense of the camp experiments were also used to justify participation in mass murder and attempts at the forced sterilization of camp inmates. A review of the major moral arguments presented by defendants at the Nuremberg trials sheds light not only on the moral rationales that were given for the hypothermia and phosgene gas experiments, but also for the involvement of biomedicine in the broad sweep of what the prosecution termed "crimes against humanity."

One of the most common moral rationales given at the trials was that no wrong had been done because those who were subjects had volunteered. Prisoners might be freed, some defendants argued, if they survived the experiments. The prospects of release and pardon were mentioned very frequently during the trial since they were the basis for the claim that people participated voluntarily in the experiments (Nuremberg Trial Transcripts 1948). Following this line of thinking, experimentation was justified because it might actually benefit the subjects.

The major flaw with this moral rationale is simply that it was false. A British newspaper, the London *Sunday Observer*, in 1989 found a man who had survived the hypothermia experiments that involved prolonged submersion in tanks of freezing water. He had been sent to Dachau because of his political beliefs.

He said that the researchers told him that if he survived the hypothermia experiments and then the decompression experiments, he might be freed. He was not. He said no prisoners were. However, he was given a medal by the Reich on the recommendation of the experimenters. The medal was given in recognition of the contributions he had made to medical science!

Another of the key rationales on the part of those put on trial was that only people who were doomed to die were used for biomedical purposes (Nuremberg Trial Transcripts 1948). Time and again the doctors who froze screaming subjects to death or watched their brains explode as result of rapid decompression stated that only prisoners condemned to death were used. It seemed morally defensible to physicians and scientists to learn from what they saw as the inevitable deaths of camp inmates.

A third ethical rationale for performing brutal experiments upon innocent subjects was that participation in lethal research offered expiation to the subjects. By being injected, frozen, or transplanted, subjects could cleanse themselves of their crimes. Suffering prior to death as a way to atone for sin seemed to be a morally acceptable rationale for causing suffering to those who were guilty of crimes.

The problem with this ethical defense is that those who were experimented on or made to suffer by German physicians and scientists were never guilty of any crime other than that of belonging to a despised ethnic or racial minority or of holding unacceptable political views. Even if those who were experimented upon or killed had been guilty of some serious crime, would it have been moral to use medical experimentation or the risk of death as a form of punishment or expiation? It is hard to see how these goals square with the goals of medicine or health care. It is impossible to see how such a position is persuasive with respect to incompetent persons and minor children.

A fourth moral rationale, one that is especially astounding even by the standards of self-delusion in evidence throughout the trial proceedings, was that scientists and physicians had to act in a value-neutral manner. They maintained that scientists and doctors are not responsible for, and have no expertise about, values and thus could not be held accountable for their actions: "if the experiment is ordered by the state, this moral responsibility of experimenter toward the experimental subject relates to the way in which the experiment is performed, not the experiment itself" (Nuremberg Trial Transcripts 1946).

Some researchers felt themselves responsible only for the proper design and conduct of their research. They felt no moral responsibility for what had occurred in the camps because they did not have any expertise concerning moral matters. They claimed to have left decisions about these matters to others. In other words, they argued that scientists, in order to be scientists, could not take normative positions about their science.

The fifth moral justification many of the defendants presented for what had happened was that they had done what they did for the defense and security of their country. All actions were done to preserve the Reich during "total" war (Nuremberg Trial Transcripts 1948). "Germany was engaged in war at that time. Millions of soldiers had to give up their lives because they were called upon to fight by the state. The state employed the civilian population for work according to state requirements. The state ordered employment in chemical factories which was detrimental to health. . . . In the same way the state ordered the medical men to make experiments with new weapons against dangerous diseases" (Nuremberg Trial Transcripts 1946).

Total war, war in which the survival of the nation hangs in the balance, justifies exceptions to ordinary morality, the defendants maintained. Allied prosecutors had much to ponder in thinking about this defense in light of the firebombing of Dresden and Tokyo and the dropping of nuclear bombs on Hiroshima and Nagasaki.

The last rationale is the one that appears to carry the most weight among all the moral defenses offered. Many who conducted lethal experiments argued that it was reasonable to sacrifice the interests of the few in order to benefit the majority.

The most distinguished of the scientists who was put on trial, Gerhard Rose, the head of the Koch Institute of Tropical Medicine in Berlin, said that he initially opposed performing potentially lethal experiments on camp inmates to create a vaccine for typhus. But he came to believe that it made no sense not to risk the lives of a hundred or two hundred men in pursuit of a vaccine when a thousand men a day were dying of typhus on the Eastern front. What, he asked, were the deaths of a hundred men compared to the possible benefit of getting a prophylactic vaccine capable of saving tens of thousands? Rose, because he admitted that he had anguished about his own moral duty when asked by the Wehrmacht to perform the typhus experiments in a concentration camp, raises the most difficult and most plausible moral argument in defense of lethal experimentation.

The prosecution encountered some difficulty with Rose's argument. The defense team for Rose noted that the Allies themselves justified the compulsory drafting of men for military service throughout the war, knowing many would certainly die, on the grounds that the sacrifice of the few to save the many was morally just. Moreover, they also pointed out, throughout history medical researchers in Western countries used versions of utilitarianism to justify danger-ous experiments upon prisoners and institutionalized persons.

Justifying the sacrifice of the few to benefit the majority is a position that must be taken seriously as a moral argument. In the context of the Nazi regime it is fair to point out that sacrifice was not borne equally by all as is true of a compulsory draft that allows no exceptions. It is also true that many would ar-gue that no degree of benefit should permit intrusions into certain fundamental rights.

Crude utilitarianism is a position that sometimes rears its head in contem-porary bioethical debate. For example, some argue that we ought not spend scarce social resources on certain groups within our society, such as the elderly, so that other groups, such as children, may have greater benefits. Those who want to invoke the Nazi analogy may be able to show that this form of crude utilitarian thinking does motivate some of the policies or actions taken by con-temporary biomedical scientists and health care professionals, but they need to do so with great caution.

In closely reviewing the statements that accompany the six major moral ra-tionales for murder, torture, and mutilation conducted in the camps—freedom was a possible benefit, only the condemned were used, expiation was a possible benefit, a lack of moral expertise, the need to preserve the state in conditions of total war, and, the morality of sacrificing a few to benefit many—it becomes clear that the conduct of those who worked in the concentration camps was sometimes guided by moral rationales. It is also clear that all of these moral arguments were nested within a biomedical interpretation of the danger facing Germany.

Physicians could justify their actions, whether direct involvement with eu-thanasia and lethal experiments or merely support for Hitler and the Reich, on the grounds that the Jew, the homosexual, the congenitally handicapped, and the Slav posed a threat—a biological threat, a genetic threat—to the existence and future of the Reich. The appropriate response to such a threat was to elimi-nate it, just as a physician must eliminate a burst appendix by means of surgery or dangerous bacteria by use of penicillin (Caplan 2004).

Viewing specific ethnic groups and populations as threatening the health of the German state permitted—and, in the view of those on trial, demanded—the involvement of medicine in mass genocide, sterilization, and lethal experimen-tation. The biomedical paradigm provided the theoretical basis for allowing those sworn to the Hippocratic principle of nonmalfeasance to kill in the name of the state.

The Neglect of the Holocaust and Nazism in Bioethics

Why has the field of bioethics not attended more closely to the Holo-caust and the role played by German medicine and science in the Holocaust? Why have the moral arguments bluntly presented by the Nazis received so little attention? These are questions that do not admit of simple answers.

The crimes of doctors and biomedical scientists revealed at the Nuremberg trials were overwhelming in their cruelty. Physicians and scientists supervised, and in some cases actively participated in, the genocide of millions, directly engaged in the torture of thousands, and provided the scientific underpinning for genocide. Hundreds of thousands of psychiatric patients and senile elderly persons were killed under the direct supervision of physicians and nurses. Numerous scientists and physicians, some of whom headed internationally renowned research centers and hospitals, engaged in cruel and sometimes lethal experiments on unconsenting inmates of concentration camps.

Ironically, the scale of immorality is one of the reasons why the moral reasoning of health care professionals and biomedical scientists during the Nazi era has received little attention from contemporary bioethics scholars. It is clear that what Nazi doctors, biologists, and public health officials did was immoral. The indisputable occurrence of wrongdoing suggests that there is little for the ethicist to say except to join with others in condemnation of what happened.

But condemnation is not sufficient. After all, many of those who committed crimes did so firm in their belief in the moral rectitude of their actions. While bioethics cannot be held accountable for every horrible act that a physician chooses to explain by using moral terms, those who teach bioethics in the hope that it can affect conduct or character must come to terms with the fact that biomedicine's role in the Holocaust was frequently defended on moral grounds.

Guilt by association has also played a role in making some bioethicists shy away from closely examining what medicine and science did during the Nazi era. Many doctors and scientists who were contemporaries of those put on trial at Nuremberg denied any connection between their own work or professional identities and those in the dock. Contemporary doctors and scientists are, understandably, even quicker to deny any connection between what Nazi doctors or scientists did and their own activities or conduct. Many scholars and health care professionals, in condemning the crimes committed in the name of medicine and the biomedical sciences during the Holocaust, insist that all those who perpetrated those crimes were aberrant, deviant, atypical representatives of the health and scientific professions. Placing these acts and those who did them on the fringe of biomedicine keeps a needed distance between then and now.

To suggest that the men and women currently engaged in research on the human genome or in transplanting fetal tissue obtained from elective abortions are immoral monsters on a par with a Josef Mengele or a Karl Brandt is to miss the crucial point that the Nazis carried out genocide for moral reasons and from a biological worldview that has little connection with the values that motivate contemporary biomedical physicians and scientists. Abortion may or may not be a morally defensible act, but it is a different act from injecting a Jewish baby with gasoline in order to preserve the racial purity of the Reich. Scholars in bioethics may have avoided any analysis of Nazi medicine simply because they feared the wrath of those who felt belittled, insulted, or falsely accused by any connection being drawn between their behavior and that of Nazi doctors, nurses, and scientists.

Yet, by saying little and thereby allowing all Nazi scientists and doctors to be transformed into madmen or monsters, bioethicists ignore the fact that the Germany of the first half of this century was one of the most "civilized," technologically advanced, and scientifically sophisticated societies on the face of the globe. In medicine and biology pre–World War II Germany could easily hold its own with any other scientifically literate society of that time. Indeed, the crimes carried out by doctors and scientists during the tenure of the Third Reich are all the more staggering in their impact and are all the more difficult to interpret precisely because Germany was such a technologically and scientifically advanced society.

The Holocaust is the exemplar of evil in our century. The medical crimes of that time stand as the clearest examples available of moral wrongdoing in biomedical science. Bioethics may have been silent precisely because there seems to be nothing to say about an unparalleled biomedical immorality, but silence leads to omission. By saying little about the most horrific crimes ever carried out in the name of biomedicine and the moral views that permitted these crimes to be done, bioethics contributes to the most dangerous myth of all—that those engaged in evil cannot do so motivated by ethical beliefs. The challenge to bioethics and indeed all of ethics is to subject the beliefs that led to such horror to close critical scrutiny.

References

Berger, R. L. 1990. Nazi Science: The Dachau Hypothermia Experiments. *New England Journal of Medicine* 322: 1435–40.

Browning, Christopher. 1993. *Ordinary Men: Reserve Police Battalion 101 and the Final Solution in Poland.* New York: Harper Collins.

Caplan, A. L. 1992. *When Medicine Went Mad: Bioethics and the Holocaust.* Totowa, N.J.: Humana Press.

——— 2004. Medicine's Shameful Past. *Lancet* 363: 1741–42.

Harvard Law School Library Nuremberg Trials Project. Nuremberg Trial Transcripts. Trial One. The Doctors' Trial. 1946. http://nuremberg.law.harvard.edu/php/docs_swi.php?DI=1&text=transcript.

Kater, Michael H. 1990. *Doctors under Hitler.* Chapel Hill: University of North Carolina Press.

Lifton, Robert Jay. 1986. *The Nazi Doctors: Medical Killing and the Psychology of Genocide.* New York: Basic Books.

Michalczyk, J. J. 1994. *Medicine, Ethics, and the Third Reich: Historical and Contemporary Issues.* Kansas City, Mo.: Sheed and Ward.

Proctor, Robert N. 1992. *Racial Hygiene.* Cambridge, Mass.: Harvard University Press.

Steinfels, P. 1986. Biomedical Ethics and the Shadow of Nazism: A Conference on the Proper Use of Nazi Analogy in Ethical Debate. *Hastings Center Report* 6: 1–19.

6 Unit 731 and the Human Skulls Discovered in 1989: Physicians Carrying Out Organized Crimes

Kei-ichi Tsuneishi

A Brief History of Unit 731

The Tōgō Unit

Unit 731 was officially inaugurated in the town of Ping Fan (near Harbin) in China in August of 1936 (Kōseishō [Ministry of Health and Welfare] 1982).[1] Preparatory activities were already underway in the fall of 1932, however, in a shoyu (soy sauce) factory in a small village about one hundred kilometers southeast of Harbin (Endō 1981). In that year, Shirō Ishii, the man who would later become the head of Unit 731, launched and became the director of the Army Medical College's Epidemic Prevention Research Laboratory (EPRL) in Tokyo (Rikugun gun'i gakkō 1936). During the next year, in addition to his official activities in EPRL, Ishii headed the construction of the unit's headquarters in China. Experiments on human beings began in the fall of 1933 as an activity within the Kantō Army (Endō 1981). The researchers who participated in these operations were all military physicians, and each used an alias. This unit was called by the code name Tōgō, after the alias Ishii used at that time. The use of aliases indicated how much importance the researchers attached to maintaining the secrecy of their activities.

EPRL was the control center, and the Tōgō Unit (as well as successors such as Unit 731 and related units) carried out its commands—including experiments on humans. Another key function of the laboratory was to serve as a link between civilian research facilities and military ones such as Unit 731.

Two factors contributed to the necessity of maintaining secrecy about operations during the three years beginning in 1933. One was that the experimenters wanted to hide the purpose of the unit's organization: that they were performing experiments on humans. The second imperative was to protect the emperor; that is, this facility was doing research on human beings as part of a feasibility study, and responsibility must not extend to the emperor if its staff either failed or was found out. Failure on the part of the emperor's military would tarnish the image of his infallibility, and for members of Japan's army at that time such a thing was impermissible.

The aim of the feasibility study for conducting experiments on humans had two aspects:

1. To find out whether it was possible to procure a continuous supply of test subjects and to determine whether continuous experimentation on humans was feasible.
2. To make sure that Ishii's project—experiments on humans for the development of biological weapons—could be pursued successfully.

Experiments to inoculate people against the illness associated with anthrax germs were already being carried out in the operations prior to 1936. Of greater note were the methodical experiments on humans using cyanide. Approximately ten people were subjected to these experiments each time they were performed (Kai 1948).[2]

Six times from 1934 to 1936, the project directors had the test subjects drink cyanide and observed the circumstances leading to their deaths. The following procedures were characteristic of these cyanide experiments on humans:

1. Photographs were taken.
2. Autopsies were performed.
3. Verification of a lethal dose was noted.
4. The cyanide was mixed with beer, wine, or coffee.
5. The subjects were Russian spies (derogatorily known as Russkies), as well as spies that the Special Service Agency had used and deemed no longer necessary.

Procedures 1–3 show that the experiments were performed not in order to murder the victims, but to pursue "medical" purposes. The motivation for procedure 4 was to make the subjects drink the difficult-to-swallow cyanide without any resistance and without causing them any apprehension about being made to drink a toxic substance. The use of spies as victims at this time—procedure 5—indicates that the procurement of test subjects, thought to have begun after Unit 731 was established, actually began during the period of the Tōgō Unit.

The medical objectives of the cyanide experiments were, except for procedure 3, to determine the effect murder by cyanide had on the human body. We can surmise this from the testimony of Kōzō Okamoto, a scholar of pathology from Kyoto University, at an investigative council held in July 1948:

> The unit physicians inoculated about 15 prisoners at one time. In order to study the conditions of the patients' illness they murdered them on the 3rd day, 4th day, and so on after its onset and before death, and then performed autopsies on the corpses. The bodies had most likely been poisoned with potassium cyanide since the cause of death was suffocation, but because Okamoto was only directly to perform research on the subjects after they were dead, he had no idea who these poisoned criminals were. (Kai 1948)

Cyanide was not the only substance used; other researchers used chloroform. Yoshio Onodera, who had performed experiments on humans in Unit 1644 in Nanjing, provided the following testimony on July 24th: "We performed studies on approximately 100–150 people. Shunji Satō analyzed the logs [term used to refer to human subjects—K. T.] and Onodera performed research on the developmental conditions of tuberculosis. In the end we injected them with chloroform and *put them to sleep*. They died from the injection. During his tenure there, they did not use potassium cyanide" (italics in the original text—Editor) (Kai 1948).

In 1947, Shirō Kasahara, who performed experiments on humans who had epidemic hemorrhagic fever (EHF, now called hemorrhagic fever with renal syndrome) in Unit 731, responded to an American inquiry about this by saying that "he put them to sleep with chloroform" (Hill and Victor 1947, Table T).[3]

Some physicians murdered their victims with potassium cyanide, and then dissected them, while others used chloroform. It may be assumed that these different approaches were due to the experiments' objectives. We can surmise that the reason they performed potassium cyanide experiments to such an extent when the Unit was first created was that before beginning their real research, they were looking for a method by which to murder their test subjects that would not contradict the medical data. Scrupulous precautions are a requirement of all research, but how should we judge the scrupulosity shown in these instances—cases where the goal is the opposite of usual research? It is obvious how extremely narrow the perspective of these "specialized fools" had become. But this circumstance is also emblematic of how frightening it is when researchers go deeper and deeper into the particulars of their work while becoming more and more distant from what is common sense in ordinary society.

Official Start of Unit 731

In August 1936, Unit 731 was created as a formal unit of the Japanese army, and the Tōgō Unit ceased to exist. The center of operations was moved to facilities built about thirty kilometers south of Harbin. These facilities not only had medical research and experimentation rooms but were also furnished with places for interning test subjects, that is, a jail (wards 7 and 8). The research and experimentation rooms were built surrounding the jail, and the researchers performed their daily research while watching over the test subjects.[4]

There was no change in the level of "scrupulous precaution" after Unit 731 came into existence. The procurement of test subjects for Unit 731 was entrusted to the military police and the Special Service Agency. According to the unit's demands, a health examination determined when people would be sent by either to the unit (Kai 1948, vol. 5, April 28).

The group in charge of test subjects was headed by a physiologist, Hisato Yoshimura, who joined the unit from Kyoto University in 1938. He was called the "scientific devil" within the unit. The group Yoshimura headed was composed of two sections, each with two subgroups. One section carried out medical exams, and the other was in charge of supervising prisoners, dispatching prisoners to experimentation rooms, and processing their admission to the unit. The heads of the two subgroups in charge of the medical exams were both physicians. One of these, Tadashi Miyagawa, joined Unit 731 in April 1944. He was in charge of X-rays of the test subjects. After the war he became a professor in Tokyo University's Medical Department and lived to the age of 88. His obituary stated, "Miyagawa led a life that pioneered the medical use of radiation. He contributed to the development of the medical use of the cyclotron to treat brain tumors and other diseases" (*Mainichi shinbun*, Jan. 4, 2002). The second subgroup was in charge of blood and immunity exams as well as the health maintenance of test subjects. Not everyone sent to Unit 731 was subjected to experiments. These were carried out only on healthy people, and after they were accepted into the program the maintenance of their health was a priority.

Why did Yoshimura become the head of this group? He was a physiologist. Physiology is a counterpart of pathology, the study of the etiology of illness. There were four pathologists in Unit 731, and their task was to determine whether a prisoner's cause of death during an experiment in which he had been infected with a pathogen was actually due to the pathogen. The field of physiology, on the other hand, pertains to understanding why a living being lives. Yoshimura wrote, "The purpose of a physiologist's scholarship is to scientifically explain from a variety of aspects what *the phenomenon of a normal life* is" (italics in the original) (Yoshimura 1984, 143). Physiology is the academic discipline that studies the characteristics of human health. Yoshimura was suitable, therefore to take responsibility for the departments that controlled wards 7 and 8.

In these wards medical exams were carried out with scientific rigor to determine how a test subject should finally be killed. But a rigorously "scientific" mentality that does not take into account the dignity of its victims as human beings—that ignores such values—is perverse science. In the case of Unit 731, it is not difficult to make this judgment; it is not difficult because the perversion of science in Unit 731 was obvious. But recently it seems that a more subtly perverse science is being put before us. Taking shape in ways more difficult for us to recognize, it too disregards the value of human beings and reverses what science should be. An example is human cloning that masquerades as "therapy for infertile persons."

The military personnel of Unit 731, who were not themselves physicians, referred to Yoshimura as a "scientific devil." A person who photographed the progress of experiments on humans testified: "In the spring of 1944 there were prisoners on the second floor of ward 7. About seventy of them, taking keys off a guard and singing revolutionary songs, created quite a disturbance. All of them were killed with gas. Yoshimura, who was in Kobe at the war, was a scientific devil, a cold-blooded animal" (Kai 1948, vol. 6, May 22; and my interviews with Dr. Masahiko Meguro from 1981 to 1988).

According to testimony, many of these prisoners were undergoing various experiments; they were killed by a gas attack so that the experimental data they embodied could be retained. Yoshimura was called a "devil" not only because of the strictness with which he conducted experiments: his cruelty was exhibited in an incident in which he soaked the fingers of a three-day-old child in water containing ice and salt.

There were several hundred prisoners in the jails of Unit 731 in the summer of 1945 after Japan was defeated. Every one of them was murdered. The following testimony describes those circumstances:

> On August 11 and 12, after the end of the war, approximately 300 prisoners were disposed of. The prisoners were coerced into suicide by being given a piece of rope. One quarter of them hung themselves, and the remaining three quarters who would not consent to suicide were made to drink potassium cyanide and killed by injection. In the end all were taken care of. The prisoners were made to drink potassium cyanide by mixing it with water and putting it into bowls. The injections were probably chloroform. (Kai 1948, vol. 6, May 27)

The murdered people were cremated and buried at the facilities of Unit 731.

The Human Skulls Discovered in 1989

In July 1989 a great quantity of human bones was discovered in Tokyo at the construction site for the Ministry of Health and Welfare's Research Center for Preventive Hygiene. This area had been the home of the Army Medical College from 1929 until 1945. The police first announced that the bones were from thirty-five bodies, but in 1992 Hajime Sakura, an expert involved with the case, announced that they were from more than one hundred bodies (Sakura 1992). He said the bones were those of people of Asian descent, but not of just one ethnic group. Several ethnic groups were intermingled. Moreover, the bones were not over one hundred years old; they had been there for more than fifteen years.

Sakura's data indicated that the bones found in 1989 were those of foreigners of Asian descent who had been buried during the period in which the Army Medical College was located there. The fact that they were buried did not mean that they had been interred there formally, but that they were hidden to suppress evidence. This was the same method of disposal used by Unit 731 on murdered test subjects.

The police treated the discovery of the bones as they would any dead body or bodies by investigating the cause of death and events leading up to it. But a week after the bones were discovered, the police announced that they uncovered no evidence about the events surrounding their deaths. They concluded that even if these people had been victims of a crime, they had been in the ground for over fifteen years, and the statute of limitations had passed. They concluded that the remains were those of people who had been found dead on the street and disposed of in this manner.

The reality was different. Sakura's investigation made two points clear (Sakura 1992):

1. There were marks on most of the skulls that led him to believe that they had been severed with a scalpel or a saw during practice brain surgeries at an experimental stage. The bones had been in the earth for over fifty years, but in Japan in the 1940s, brain surgeries that severed a part of the skull had not yet been performed.
2. There were gashes from a sword on several of the skulls, and others had been pierced by bullets from a pistol.

Sakura's first point indicated that the skulls had either been used for experimentation or practice where brain surgeries were performed. The second suggested that they were victims of crimes, at least medical crimes.

There is no direct connection between these experiments or crimes and Unit 731. What these bones do indicate is that the barbarism of Unit 731 did not stand out as anything exceptional among military doctors in Japan. We can presume that these bones mean that physicians in the Japanese army practiced upon or performed experiments on the brains of people on the battlefield, or that physicians who had some relationship with the Army Medical College did, and that the evidence was destroyed and buried there.

The testimony of Ken Yuasa, an army physician who confessed to killing Chinese captives while training others in surgery, supports this conjecture. According to Yuasa's testimony, in order to quickly prepare physicians trained primarily as internists for the work needed as surgeons on the battlefield, they were gathered together every few months to perform atrocities called "surgery drills" on the battlefields of China. They would capture citizens, shoot them in the thigh with a bullet, and undertake drills to see how long the extraction of a bullet would take. If someone were frostbitten, they would perform an operation to sever the frostbitten part (Yuasa 1981).

These surgery drills were not just limited to one region of the country, but practiced widely. In most cases the victims were locals arrested by the military and delivered to the Army's medical division. This indicates that the surgery drills were not performed according to individual whim but that the army military division and military police undertook these activities methodically within the entire army. It is likely that the skulls obtained from surgery drills were collected and sent to the Army Medical College under the control of the army physicians. If this is the case, the skulls were definitely those of victims of war crimes.

Open Secret

In my own research published in 1981, after analyzing research reports from 1943 and 1944 concerning hemorrhagic fever with renal syndrome published by Masaji Kitano, Ishii's successor as unit director from August 1942 to May 1945, and other researchers, I concluded that their results were based on experiments done on human beings. I substantiated that Yoshimura performed experiments on humans in his laboratory work on frostbite (Tsuneishi 1981). It was not difficult to prove their experiments on human beings through analysis of the papers they themselves published. It needed only some medical knowledge to reveal this. Any qualified physician could have reached the same conclusions as mine from these reports.

Kitano contributed to an article about hemorrhagic fever with renal syndrome in publications for the Defense Agency in 1969. He wrote, "Smordentiv was not able to infect standard experiment animals such as mice, marmots, rabbits, and monkeys with either the blood or urine of patients. He *too* performed experiments on humans to do research on the etiology of diseases" (my emphasis) (Kitano 1969, 194). Smordentiv was a Soviet researcher who worked on EHF in the 1940s and identified the virus for experiments on humans. In Kitano's 1969 recollections, he *also* confessed to having performed experiments on humans, as had the other researcher. The results of these reports were announced in Defense Agency publications in which Kitano did not try to hide that experiments had been performed on human beings.

In 1968, the year before Kitano's publication, Naeo Ikeda, a physician with Unit 731, published his own research in a paper entitled "Experimental Studies on Epidemic Hemorrhagic Fever: *Pediculus vestimenti* and *Xenopsylla cheopis* as Suspected Vectors of the Disease" (Ikeda 1968). According to this report, experiments having to do with infections were carried out in the army hospital in Kokka on the border between China and the Soviet Union in January 1942. These experiments on humans confirmed that EHF was carried by lice and fleas to the local people. Five percent of the people who were infected with the disease died. This unequivocal report, which admitted that human experiments had been performed with pathogenic inoculations that can cause death, passed the inspection of referees and was published in a scholarly journal. That experiments on humans had taken place in Unit 731 was self-evident to Ikeda and to the Association for Infectious Diseases that accepted his research. It was the acquisition of data difficult to obtain without human experiments that was important rather than any ethical issues. But because the research was never confirmed by recreating the experiments, it was meaningless.

Yoshimura, the "scientific devil" of Unit 731, wrote: "My research during the war was published in English journals of physiology after the war and influenced European and American scholars. Present-day research that evolved from my own is performed not only in Japan but also in universities and research centers worldwide and has produced results" (Yoshimura 1984, 305). Yoshimura conducted research during the war at Unit 731 in China on low-temperature physiology, including the elucidation of mechanisms concerned with frostbite. After the war ended, he organized the Japanese Society of Biometeorology; his China research was the beginning of his work on how physiology relates to environmental stress.

Articles Yoshimura published in English in the *Journal of Japanese Physiology* reported how humans reacted to zero-degree water (Yoshimura and Iida 1950–52). The experiments had consisted of soaking the middle finger of the right hand in zero-degree water and then observing the changes in skin temperature for thirty minutes. Approximately a hundred Chinese men and women between the ages of fifteen and seventy-four were the subjects of these experiments. "Approximately" is Yoshimura's own word, which raises doubt about the rigor of the experiments.

Yoshimura's English article was criticized in newspapers and elsewhere because of the statement, "We performed experiments by soaking 3-day-old infants in zero-degree water." Yoshimura and his fellow researchers responded, "Though detailed studies could not be attained on children below 6 years of age, some observations were carried out on babies. . . . [T]he reactions were detected on the 3rd day after birth, and . . . increased rapidly with the lapse of days until at last it was nearly fixed after a month or so" (Yoshimura and Iida 1952, pt. 2, 177–78). Data was recorded about a child's physiological reactions when the child's middle finger was soaked in ice water for thirty minutes on the third day, at the first month, and at sixth months.

When a reporter from the Osaka office of the *Mainichi shinbun* contacted Yoshimura by telephone for a report on the infant experiments, he responded:

> Everyone misunderstands. I'm being criticized for having done experiments on an infant, but this was the child of a staff member of Yakudai [Pharmaceutical College] who had been sent to the Unit. They were experiments to investigate what kind of physiological reactions take place in the blood vessels when the skin is touched by cold water and from what point there is resistance to this and what we can do in this situation. I used the child of my staff member with his own encouragement. The child was not the child of a prisoner. (Tsuneishi and Asano 1982, 227–28)

He then related how excited all the staff was about this research and that it was their eagerness that allowed one of them to offer the child to the experimental body. That Yoshimura said the child he used for the experiments was not the child of prisoner but the child of his staff member indicates that he was aware that these experiments were not usual practice.

Should we forgive the parents their excessive enthusiasm in giving their three-day-old infant up to experiments? What does it mean that these people participated in experiments and did research as scientists? I do not accept Yoshimura's explanation to the reporter: everything can be forgiven as a misunderstanding because there was "enthusiasm" for his scientific research. Yoshimura showed his lack of understanding in the way he replied to the reporter. All the staff members in Yoshimura's account have died, and we can no longer ascertain the truthfulness of his explanations.

If we accept Yoshimura's claim that the child was not the child of a prisoner, a different problem arises: Why did he not use his own children? According to Yoshimura's memoirs, *Kiji kaiko* (Seventy-seven years in retrospect), he had four children. Of those four, two were born before he went to Unit 731, and two were born while he was at the unit. If we follow Yoshimura's own logic, the reason he did not offer his children to their experiments was because he was not enthusiastic about his own research.

But the fact of the matter is that Yoshimura did not use his assistant's child: he used the children of people who had been captured by the unit.

The three researchers about whom I have just reported did not try to hide their experiments on humans. When I first began researching Unit 731, I anticipated enormous work exposing these experiments. However, as we see in investigating Kitano's *Ryūkōsei shukketsu netsu ni tsuite: Dai tōa sensō rikugun eiseishi* (On epidemic hemorrhagic fever: The history of army hygiene during the Greater East Asia War), much can be accomplished with a little bit of effort; we can say it was easier than expected. We can also say that most of the researchers in Unit 731 were not involved in a special cover-up about the experiments in which they took part. While they have never revealed their crimes to society with the object of criticizing themselves, they have discussed and revealed various facts within their own medical fields. Consequently, it has not been difficult to ascertain—especially in terms of research pertaining to EHF and frostbite—who did what kind of human experiments.

Because almost everyone in the Japanese medical world knew about the experiments on humans in Unit 731 (Naito 1947), the researchers in the unit were able to report later on their own work in medical papers; even after the war, reports were published that were unmistakably about the results of experiments on humans, and reminiscences about the unit were written up in medical journals. From this we can be certain that everyone in the Japanese medical community knew about the experiments of Unit 731.

Organized Crimes

Even in the twenty-first century, the Japanese medical community continues to ignore the barbarism doctors committed between 1930 and 1945. After 1945 the community showed indifference toward articles published in medical journals based on data obtained through such brutal practices.

It would be a mistake for us to attribute this solely to the insensitivity of the Japanese medical community. The problem was not just the independent actions of Yoshimura, Okamoto, and others—the scandal had institution-wide implications. For example, professors from Kyoto University and Tokyo University were the subjects of the American army's inquiry into Unit 731's experiments (Hill and Victor 1947). These professors were not members of Unit 731, but they were senior consultants to Ishii's Tokyo research site, EPRL. At Ishii's request, they sent students Yoshimura and Okamoto to the unit, knowing that they would perform experiments on humans.

The experiments on frostbite that Yoshimura performed were central to his research at Kyoto University. Tachiomaru Ishikawa, who was dispatched to the unit at the same time as Yoshimura, wrote: "When an epidemic was raging in Manchuria's Nōan area, we performed autopsies on fifty-seven corpses which had been stricken with the disease. This was a world record in terms of the number of corpses" (Ishikawa 1944). Kenji Kiyono, one of Ishikawa's teachers, sent his students with the hope that they would research diseases of which Japan had seen few cases.

The truth is that teachers such as Kiyono intended for their students to perform experiments on humans. The students carried out this barbarism—which couldn't be done in Japan proper—in China, Japan's colony. The wishes of the teacher were communicated to the students in China through EPRL, and the results of those experiments were sent back to their teacher through the same channel.

What are we to make of the fact that none of this was a secret in the Japanese medical world but it was unknown for so long in the nonmedical world? It is possible that people in the medical world did not feel there was a reason to "expose" or "reveal" something that was not a secret. Even if this is true, we must strongly denounce the insensitivity of ignoring the highly unusual nature of performing experiments on humans—experiments hidden from the nonmedical world. Or, to look at it another way, if the experiments continued to be hidden because of their unusual nature, this means there has been no change in the sense of privilege and authority physicians demonstrate even after they had been informed of the experiments performed on humans by their fellow physicians.

But once we look back on their activities, we find that the probability is great that physicians have not felt an obligation to hide anything in particular about their experiments on humans during and after the war. That may be why it is quite easy to prove the existence of human experimentation in the unit through openly published research papers. We are forced to conclude that, although people outside the medical world would consider it an act of atrocity if humans are victimized, subjected to tests, or murdered in this way, people within the medical community who do this as everyday work might not consider these acts to be unusual in any way.

These murderous experiments were performed within a network formed by the Army's Unit 731 and the national medical colleges, with EPRL as the mediator. The murderers were the physicians in the army research facilities, but it was not just the physicians who received the "benefits" of these acts; it was also the public researchers who were their teachers. Excuses for their behavior took the following forms: (1) researchers who actually dirtied their own hands with these experiments did it for the nation and the army, and (2) their actions contributed to the progress of science and medicine.

Without consulting anyone, the medical world took upon itself the right to decide all these things and forced the "results" of their research on society. But is this not the situation today as well? I emphasize that it is not a question of research "results" being good or bad, but rather a societal deficiency in which the medical community determines how those "results" are achieved. I am troubled that we continue to ignore the barbarism of the twentieth century even now, in the twenty-first century. And I am concerned that this is an indication that the Japanese medical community is neglecting its social responsibilities. This is not just an issue of whether overt barbarism like that which existed at Unit 731 could possibly occur again, but the fact that we still lack the means to discover and prevent barbarism in a more subtle form from occurring.

Notes

1. This report was submitted to the Diet on April 6, 1982.

2. Bunsuke Kai, chief of 1st Section of Investigation of the Metropolitan Police Department, recorded every day reports by each of the investigators of the Teigin (Imperial Bank) case, a bank robbery in Tokyo in January 1948. The Teigin case was an incident in which twelve persons were killed with cyanide, and money was taken. Researchers on toxic substances in the former Japanese Army and members of Unit 731 were suspected. But in August a painter was arrested and sentenced to death. He denied his guilt in the Teigin case until his death at age ninety-five in the prison hospital in 1992.

3. Hill was Chief, Basic Sciences, Camp Detrick, Maryland.

4. Interview with Dr. Sueo Akimoto by Tsuneishi. Akimoto was a member of the Unit since 1944, performing research on serology without human experimentation. He gave up his career as a researcher—he could have returned to his work at Tokyo University, after returning to Japan—because of his regret that he had not been able to oppose others' experimentation on human beings.

References

Endō, Saburō. 1981. *Nitchū jūgo-nen sensō to wataskushi* (I and the fifteen-year war with China). Tokyo: Nitchū shorin.

Hill, Edwin V., and Joseph Victor. 1947. Memorandum to Gen. Alden C. Waitt, Chief, Chemical Corps from Dr. Edwin V. Hill, Chief, Basic Sciences, Camp Detrick, Subject: Summary Report on B. W. Investigations, Dec. 12, 1947. Fort Detrick archives. (The other investigator was Joseph Victor, and this report is called the "Hill & Victor Report." I received the copy at Fort Detrick in Sept. 1986.)

Ikeda, Naeo. 1968. Ryūkō-sei shukketsu-netsu ni tsuite no jikken-teki kenkyū: Byōgen baikai dōbutsu toshite no *Pediculus vestimenti* to *Xenopsylla cheopis* (Experimental studies on epidemic hemorrhagic fever: *Pediculus vestimenti* and *Xenopsylla cheopis* as suspected vectors of the disease). *Nihon densenbyō gakkaishi* (Japanese Journal of Infectious Diseases) 42, no. 5: 125–30.

Ishikawa, Tachiomaru. 1944. Pesuto ni tsuite (Concerning plague). *Nihon byōri gakkaishi* (Japanese Journal of Pathology) 34, nos.1 and 2: 17–20.

Kai, Bunsuke. 1948. Teigin sōsa shuki (Report on the Teigin case).

Kitano, Masaji. 1969. *Ryūkōsei shukketsu-netsu ni tsuite: Dai tōa sensō rikugun eiseishi* (On epidemic hemorrhagic fever: The history of army hygiene during the Greater East Asia War). Jieitai eisei gakkō, vol. 7.

Kōseishō (Ministry of Health and Welfare). 1982. *Kantōgun bōeki kyūsui-bu ryaku-reki* (Brief history of the Kwantung Army's epidemic prevention and water supply section).

Naitō, Ryoichi. 1947. Case No. 330, Yamaguchi, Motoji, November 1946–April 1947, Supreme Commander for the Allied Powers. Legal Section. Law Division. (1945–1952). Record Group 331: Records of Allied Operational and Occupation Headquarters, World War II, 1907–1966, ARC Identifier: 339605. April 4, 1947.

Rikugun gun'i gakkō. 1936. *Gun'i gakko gojū-nen-shi* (Fifty-year history of the Army Medical College).

Sakura, Hajime. 1992. *Toyama jinkotsu no kantei hōkokusho* (Shinjuku) (Report on the Investigation of Human Skulls Discovered at Toyama [Shinjuku Ward]). Online at http://www.geocities.co.jp/Technopolis/9073/.

Tsuneishi, Kei-ichi. 1981. *Kieta saikin-sen butai* (The biological warfare unit that disappeared). Tokyo: Kaimei-sha.

Tsuneishi, Kei-ichi, and Tomizō Asano. 1982. *Kieta saikin-sen butai to jiketsu shita futari no igakusha* (The biological warfare unit and two physicians who committed suicide). Tokyo: Shinchō-sha.

Yoshimura Sensei Kijukaiko Kinen Gyōjikai, ed. 1984. *Yoshimura Sensei kijukaiko kinen* (A retrospective of Yoshimura [Hisato's] seventy-seven years).

Yoshimura, Hisato, and Toshiyuki Iida. 1950–52. Studies on the Reactivity of Skin Vessels to Extreme Cold. *Japanese Journal of Physiology* 1 and 2. (Part 1, 1950. Part 2, 1952. Part 3, 1952.)

Yuasa, Ken. 1981. *Kesenai kioku* (Indestructible memories). Tokyo: Nitchū shuppan.

7   Biohazard: Unit 731 in Postwar Japanese Politics of National "Forgetfulness"

Frederick R. Dickinson

Japan and its citizens have an international reputation for historical amnesia. The battle by the Ministry of Education, Science, and Technology to tame references to wartime atrocities in Japanese textbooks has made the headlines in Western, as well as Asian, capitals over the last quarter century. These controversies have been accentuated in recent years by Prime Minister Junichirō Koizumi's highly public annual pilgrimages to the main Japanese war memorial, Yasukuni Shrine, where the spirits of Japanese war criminals remain enshrined. Western fascination with Japanese historical "amnesia" is manifest in a spate of English-language studies highlighting a peculiar Japanese brand of "forgetfulness." [1]

Among the most dramatic examples of Japanese amnesia is the failure to come to terms with Japan's history of wartime medical experiments. Between 1932 and 1945, special Japanese units in China subjected thousands of Chinese, Korean, Mongolian, Russian, and American prisoners of war to a range of experimentation aimed at developing new techniques in medical treatment and biological warfare. Word of these experiments was slow to emerge after 1945 and, together with Japan's record of wartime forced labor and "comfort" women, and with specific events such as the Nanjing Massacre and the Bataan Death March, became the object of Japanese government censorship of textbooks. A dearth of English-language analyses of Japanese wartime experiments relative to investigations of the Holocaust and of the activities of Dr. Mengele reinforces the impression that the Japanese record remains under tight wraps. According to one recent English-language title from the popular press, "until the 1990s, almost nothing at all was written or discussed publicly about the Japanese bio-war crimes" (Barenblatt 2004, xx).

What is the actual record of postwar Japanese discussions of wartime biological warfare (BW) experiments? How does that record shed light upon the larger pattern of Japanese debate over the wartime past? Although most analyses of this debate highlight the peculiar magnitude of Japanese "forgetfulness," Japanese discussions of the past might most profitably be viewed less in terms of a singular Japanese "amnesia" than as a reflection of the particular atlas of politics in post-1945 Japan. In fact, the political polarization in post-1945 Japan may be said to have facilitated, rather than hindered, exposure of highly sensitive information.

Exposing the Unthinkable in Japan

Contrary to the impression imparted by much of the discussion over Japanese textbooks, evidence of Japanese wartime atrocities did not emerge in just the last two decades. Rather, the fifty-three-count indictment of the International Military Tribunal for the Far East specifically highlighted such crimes as the "Rape of Nanking," the "Bataan Death March," and the massacre of Chinese civilians at Canton in 1938.[2] Like questions about the role of the Japanese emperor in the prosecution of the war, information about Japanese wartime bacteriological experiments was purposely suppressed by occupation authorities during the tribunal (Williams and Wallace 1989a, 176–79). But the issue was by no means unknown to the Japanese public.

There were hints of wartime medical experimentation on the continent even before the start of the Tokyo trials in May 1946. In January 1946, Tokyo papers quoted Japanese communist leaders' allegations that a "Japanese Medical Corps" had inoculated American and Chinese prisoners-of-war with bubonic plague virus (Williams and Wallace 1989a, 141). Less than four years later, formal word from Moscow that twelve Japanese soldiers had been tried and convicted in a six-day war crimes tribunal in Khabarovsk in December 1949 generated greater discussion. All twelve men had been members of Unit 731, the most notorious Japanese BW unit, which had been established in Manchuria in 1939, and were charged with "preparing and applying bacteriological weapons" (Williams and Wallace 1989a, 220–23). Both national dailies, the *Asahi shinbun* and the *Mainichi shinbun,* reported on the surprising Soviet announcement in late December. And a variety of local and specialty papers picked up the story.[3] The trials became the subject of the first two Japanese publications on Unit 731, Kyō Shimamura's *Sanzennin no seitai jikken* (3,000 Human Experiments; Shimamura 1967) and Seizaburō Yamada's *Saikinsen gunji saiban* (Military Tribunal on Biological Warfare; Yamada 1974).

One year after the appearance of Yamada's study of the Khabarovsk trials, a television documentary produced the first revelations of Unit 731 from Japanese sources. On the eve of the thirtieth anniversary of V-J Day, the largest Japanese commercial network, Tokyo Broadcasting System (TBS), aired a primetime half hour segment on Unit 731 based upon three years of research and interviews of twenty former Unit 731 employees by documentary filmmaker Haruko Yoshinaga. Although the first installment of "Akuma no 731 butai" (The Devil's Unit 731) offered mostly tantalizing images of respected doctors clamming up or running from the camera, two one-hour prime-time follow-ups in August and November of 1976 sparked an international sensation. These segments not only recorded the testimony of four former Unit 731 employees but included their allegations that they had escaped indictment by the International Military Tribunal in return for divulging their research to American authorities.[4] The November 1976 piece was highlighted both in the *Washington Post* and on *Sixty Minutes*.[5]

The TBS documentary opened the floodgates in Japan for research on Japanese wartime BW experimentation. Five years later, a wave of scholarly books on BW experimentation appeared, marking the 1980s as the heyday of Japanese research on the subject. Mystery writer Seiichi Morimura began the surge with a serialized story about Unit 731, titled *Shi no utsuwa* (Death receptacle; Morimura 1981b). Just several months later, Morimura published an analytic work on the subject, replete with photographs and charts obtained from former unit members and prewar medical journals. *Akuma no hōshoku* (The Devil's insatiability) was produced by a respected mainstream publishing house (Kōbunsha) and became a best-seller (Morimura 1981a). It inspired a fourth TBS documentary on Unit 731 in 1982 and was the source of a 90-minute movie about Japanese wartime BW produced in Hong Kong and later reintroduced into Japan.[6] Morimura's impact was accentuated by a second analytical work that appeared in the same year—Kei-ichi Tsuneishi's *Kieta saikinsen butai* (The biological warfare unit that disappeared), which was based upon wartime research reports of the second in command at Unit 731, Masaji Kitano (Tsuneishi 1981).

Together, Morimura and Tsuneishi seized the leadership of the scholarly treatment of Japanese BW experimentation. In 1982, both men published sequels to their original treatises. Morimura added new material from American archives to produce *Zoku akuma no hōshoku* (The Devil's insatiability—Supplement; Morimura 1982). And Tsuneishi produced further evidence of postwar medical research based upon wartime human experiments in *Saikinsen butai to jiketsu shita futari no igakusha* (The biological warfare unit and two physicians who committed suicide; Tsuneishi 1982). In 1983, Morimura published the third installment of his study, this time including materials from China (Morimura 1983).

The 1980s also witnessed a flood of testimonials by former Unit 731 employees. In 1982, a former female member of the Unit 731 staff offered memories and photographs in *"Shōgen" 731 Ishii butai* (Eyewitness: Unit 731; Gunji 1982). On the thirty-eighth anniversary of V-J Day in 1983, a former driver for Unit 731, Sadao Koshi, produced *Hi no maru wa akai namida ni* (Red tears of the red sun; Koshi 1983; Saikin butai moto taiin ga jitsuroku, 9). In 1989, a freelance journalist published a collection of testimonials by four former employees, which he had discovered in the Chinese memorial hall to Unit 731 outside of Harbin (Takitani 1989; Saikinsen 731 butai no katsudō, 3). In the same year, on the fiftieth anniversary of the Nomonhan Incident, the *Asahi shinbun* carried testimonials of three former members identifying the incident as the first Japanese battlefield use of biological agents (Nomonhan jiken ni "saikinsen" no shōgen, 3).

If the 1980s marked the appearance of the first substantive Japanese research on Japanese BW experimentation, the 1990s ushered in a new era of public consciousness of the issue. In 1992, the story emerged from the realm of private programming to the Japanese national network, NHK. In April of that year, NHK aired a two-part documentary on Japanese BW mastermind Shirō Ishii. Based upon newly discovered records of the Khabarovsk Trial from KGB files and materials from the Dugway, Utah, Proving Grounds, the main American testing ground for biological warfare, "731 saikinsen butai" (731 biological warfare unit) revealed how Japanese experiments were actually conducted and highlighted the Soviet–American rivalry over records (Harris 1994, 224).[7] In July 1995, a team of researchers released more evidence of the effect of Japanese experimentation in a collection of translated Chinese documents (Mori and Kasukawa 1995). Several months later, the *Asahi shinbun* reported the first joint Sino-Japanese symposium on wartime Japanese experimentation. Convening over five days in the city of Harbin, Manchuria, the symposium drew together approximately one hundred participants from both countries, including former members of Unit 731 (731 butai kyūmei e Nitchū kyōdō shinpo, 9).

Three important new discoveries in the Japanese record fueled the growing public consciousness of the 1990s. In 1989, the bones of suspected victims of Japanese wartime experimentation were unearthed from the grounds of the former Army Medical College in Tokyo.[8] Four years later, in January 1993, Kei-ichi Tsuneishi uncovered from military records in the Japanese National Archives the first documentary evidence of Japanese preparations for use of biological weapons on the battlefield.[9] In August of the same year, a team of Japanese researchers affiliated with Nihon no sensō sekinin shiryō sentā (the Center for Japanese War Responsibility) discovered in the administrative journal of the Army General Staff in the National Defense Agency Library documentary evidence of the use of biological weapons throughout China. The finding made front-page news on the forty-eighth anniversary of V-J Day (731 butai no saikinsen: Nihongawa shiryō de urazuke, 1; "Pesuto mōi" to hōkoku, 27).

Both the discovery of bones and Tsuneishi's disclosure of documentary evidence of Japanese preparations for biological warfare inspired the organization of an unprecedented national exposition of Japanese wartime experimentation between July 1993 and December 1994. The "731 butai ten" (Unit 731 Exhibit) displayed eighty-some implements and described wartime experiments with models constructed from the testimonies of former Unit 731 employees. Although originally scheduled for one year, the exhibit ultimately ran for eighteen months, toured sixty-four Japanese cities, and attracted 240,000 visitors (Kasahara et al. 1997, 16; Jibun ni muen no horā ja nai, 15; Seitai jikken o mokei de saigen, 24).

Meanwhile, the administrative journal of the Army General Staff that had been unearthed in the library of the National Defense Agency spurred fact-finding missions to China and a new publication. In 1994, following evidence from the journal, a private citizens' group visited Manchuria and obtained corroborating testimony from Chinese citizens of Japanese use of cholera and plague-carrying fleas (Mochi o tabe, zenshin ga aokuroku nari, shinda, 30). In 1995, two prominent members of the group that had discovered the General

Staff evidence published their findings in a booklet produced by one of Japan's most powerful publishing houses, Iwanami (Yoshimi and Ikō 1995; 731 butai no saikinsen kenshō, 14).

Hiding the Unthinkable in the United States

Non-Japanese audiences are less likely to be familiar with this history of revelations of Japanese BW than with the record of struggle over inclusion of such material in Japanese primary and secondary textbooks. Japanese textbook screening became a focus of intense international interest particularly after highly public political debates in the Japanese Diet in the early 1980s (Nozaki and Inokuchi 2000, 113).[10] The series of long and protracted lawsuits brought against the Japanese government by celebrated textbook author Saburō Ienaga between 1965 and 1997 ensured the Western press's almost permanent association of the Japanese state with censorship.[11] The very visible recent initiative by Tokyo University professor Nobukatsu Fujioka to fashion a "New Education," which purges Japanese textbooks of references to the "dark" past (covered in more detail below), has persuaded many Western observers of the intractable nature of intellectual debate generally in Japan.[12]

Central review of textbook content certainly distinguishes Japan from most Western industrialized states. But in the context of the above record of postwar revelations of wartime BW experimentation, the notion of Japanese historical "amnesia" seems overblown. In light of America's postwar record of revelation concerning wartime BW experimentation, it appears irrelevant.

The scale of Japanese wartime BW experimentation was certainly striking. At the peak of his power, Shirō Ishii directed over five thousand soldiers and scientists. Ping Fan (Unit 731) alone comprised over 150 buildings, including a one-thousand-seat auditorium, an athletic field, and other amenities for the three thousand employees stationed there (Harris 1994, 47, 52). But American wartime facilities were, at their height, just as impressive. The principal American BW facility, Camp Detrick, an old army base in rural Maryland, expanded between April and December 1943 from a rural outpost to a metropolis of 250 buildings and living quarters for five thousand people (Miller, Engelberg, and Broad 2001, 39).[13]

The known record of American experimentation on human subjects pales, of course, by comparison with the estimates of those killed in north China through willful Japanese extermination between 1932 and 1945.[14] Yet the virtual absence of academic discussion on American wartime efforts is remarkable. Investigative reporter Seymour Hersh weighed in with the first important glimpse of the American program in a 1968 volume titled *Chemical and Biological Warfare: America's Hidden Arsenal* (Hersh 1969). But unlike the Japanese case, this initial revelation did not mark the beginning of a wave of scholarship on American wartime experimentation.[15] Rather, we know more today from Japanese and American scholars about postwar American efforts to extract information about Japanese wartime experimentation than we do about American wartime programs themselves. Increasing interest has been generated in recent years in the tale of possible American use of biological agents in the Korean War (see, e.g., Endicott and Hagerman 1998). But the American appetite for such investigations is so low that the publishers of a celebrated British study of Unit 731 saw fit to excise the Korean War chapter highlighting U.S. collaboration with Japanese BW experts in Korea in the American edition of their work (for more on possible American use of biological weapons in the Korean War, see the essay by G. Cameron Hurst in this volume).[16]

Politics of Exposure in Japan

Observers are correct to pinpoint a clear record of official Japanese textbook censorship after 1945. But the notion that "the late 1950s and 1960s saw the textbook production and adoption system becoming more and more like the state-authored textbook system that was in place during World War II" (Nozaki and Inokuchi 2000, 105) is absurd. In post-1945 Japan, final selection of school texts remains in the hands of local school boards, not the state. Thus, even the most notorious recent "revisionist" text by Atarashii rekishi kyōkasho o tsukuru kai (the Society for History Textbook Reform), which won government approval in 2001, was blocked from local adoption in that year by a coalition of grassroots organizations (McNeill and Selden 2005).

Far from evidence of a collective national "amnesia" regarding Japanese wartime atrocities, the record of struggles over school texts seems more indicative of what may be considered the most salient context of the post-1945 debate over wartime BW experimentation: turbulent Japanese politics. Postwar battles over historical memory have been part and parcel of the tumultuous political conflicts spurred by the wrenching debate over national identity after 1945.

Although celebrated as the first Asian power to industrialize and shed the trappings of Western imperialism, modern Japan has confronted the monumental challenge of fashioning an entirely new national trajectory four times in the span of one hundred years. The founders of modern Japan shaped from the remains of a feudal realm a modern nation-state upon a German model. Following the destruction of Imperial Germany in 1918, party politicians led Japan upon a new trajectory of democracy and internationalism. Enemies of 1920s liberalism steered the nation toward a "Greater East Asian" world order in the 1930s. And when the "Asian" order collapsed in 1945, Japanese citizens confronted once more the question of what it meant to be Japanese.

Unlike the first three attempts, the post-1945 effort to redefine the nation proceeded under the artificial auspices of military occupation. As students of postwar Japan have observed, the overwhelming military, political, and economic presence of the United States in Japan after 1945 guaranteed an unprecedented polarization of Japanese politics (Dower 1993). On one side stood the conservative Liberal Democratic Party (LDP) and its political and bureaucratic allies. With the direct political and financial backing of the United States, these forces seized a monopoly of power and pursued rapid economic development at home and pledged allegiance to an international coalition of states led by the United States abroad. On the other side stood a diverse assortment of forces on the left (the Socialist and Communist Parties, militant unions, and student, teacher, and intellectual associations), who rejected both the LDP monopoly of power and unbridled pursuit of economic growth at home and Japan's military alliance with the United States.

Revelations about Japanese wartime BW experimentation, like many intellectual debates in postwar Japan, were a direct consequence of early political battles between Left and Right. Japanese socialists, communists, union organizers, students, and liberal intellectuals had originally viewed the United States as a liberating force for destroying Japanese militarism and releasing Japanese political prisoners. But as American policy took a conservative turn after 1947–48 (the so-called reverse course), the Japanese Left staked a position that would define the intellectual mainstream for over two decades. In a series of statements on the "Peace Problem," over fifty of Japan's most respected academics in 1950 challenged the conservative Japanese administration, rejected the prospect of a "separate peace" with the United States, and championed, instead, a policy of equal distribution of wealth at home and "neutrality" abroad. Printed in the left-leaning monthly journal *Sekai*, the policy statements were widely popular among the public.[17]

If the Japanese Left after 1947 became concerned with the conservative turn of Japanese politics and the overwhelming American political, economic, and military power behind it, that concern increasingly defined their intellectual pursuits. As already noted, initial word of wartime Japanese experimentation on Chinese and American POWs was circulated by members of the Japanese Communist Party in January 1946. That was the month that Japanese communist leader Sanzō Nozaka returned to Japan after having spent nine years in the Soviet Union and five years in the Chinese communist stronghold, Yenan, in northern China. At the Seventh Congress of the Communist Party of China in the spring of 1945, Nozaka had declared that it was he and the "progressive forces" of the Japanese Communist Party (JCP) in Japan, not the "pro-Anglo-American faction" dominated by financial magnates, members of the imperial household, bureaucrats, generals, and leaders of the Seiyūkai and Minseitō parties, that constituted the most reliable basis for democracy in Japan (Swearingen and Langer 1968, 81–82). Revelations of Japanese wartime BW experimentation in January 1946 were, in other words, one step in the larger attempt by the Japanese Communist Party to reconstruct its base of support in postwar Japan.

Having recognized the political potential of the BW issue in 1946, the JCP would become the most energetic early champion of "historical truth" about Japanese wartime experimentation. The Khabarovsk trials of late 1949 caused a minor sensation in Japan, but nowhere more so than in the principal organ of the Japanese Communist Party, *Akahata*. Among the mainstream national dailies, the Khabarovsk affair ran on the front page of the *Mainichi shinbun* morning edition next to a United Press dispatch on MacArthur's request for an investigation of Japanese internees under Soviet control, but did not run at all in the *Yomiuri shinbun* (Williams and Wallace 1989a, 226–27). The story gained increasing momentum in the left-leaning *Asahi shinbun*, which ran it the entire week, first on the third page, then with four consecutive days of front-page billing (see *Asahi shinbun*, Dec. 25, 27–30, 1949). But *Akahata* provided the most detailed coverage of all, spending a week, first to print the indictment of the twelve prisoners in full, then to feature interviews with men with purported connections to Unit 731.[18]

Among those interviewed by *Akahata* was Hideo Takeyama, who had been a staff writer for the *Nippon shinbun*. The Soviet Army had founded this newspaper thirteen days after the Japanese surrender in Khabarovsk to distribute to Japanese prisoners of war. Among its editorial staff was Haruki Aikawa who, upon returning to Japan, joined the editorial board of *Akahata* (Swearingen and Langer 1968, 233). Given that Soviet exposure of Japanese BW experimentation ran directly counter to American policy to maintain silence upon the matter, contemporaries and historians have stressed the political nature of the trials.[19] Likewise, the high-profile *Akahata* coverage of the tribunal may be interpreted in the largest sense as a JCP challenge to the American-dominated occupation and the conservative turn of politics in Japan. Indeed, American authorities aggressively countered the news emerging from Khabarovsk as Soviet propaganda.[20] General MacArthur himself publicly denied any evidence of Japanese experimentation on human beings in December 1950 (*New York Times*, Dec. 27, 1949, cited in Williams and Wallace 1989a, 231).

The late 1960s and early 1970s were characterized by increasing volatility in Japanese national discourse, principally spurred by growing U.S. involvement in Vietnam. Journalists such as Katsuichi Honda became national heroes through trenchant criticism of American "imperialism" and its devastating effects upon Vietnam.[21] But even more problematic from the perspective of the Japanese Left became the complicity of the Japanese government in American atrocities. According to one participant in the student movement of the era, in contrast to the Korean War era, Japan seemed to possess "independent political and economic power and seemed to take the initiative to commit itself to the Vietnam War." Increasingly, the anti–Vietnam War movement considered the greatest problem facing Japan to be "the structure of Japanese society itself" (Field 1997, 15).

It was no coincidence that Katsuichi Honda turned his attention in the early 1970s from the tale of Vietnamese suffering to the story of Japanese wartime atrocities. Disturbed by American actions in Vietnam, but also increasingly by official Japanese support, he envisioned the as-yet-hidden record of Japanese wartime behavior as another critical front in the intensifying battle for political balance in post-1945 Japan. In 1971, Honda traveled to China to begin a series of articles in Japan's most widely read national daily, *Asahi shinbun*, on the Nanjing Massacre. The series was based upon interviews with survivors and other data collected in the mainland and was ultimately reissued in volume form in *Chūgoku no tabi* (Journey to China; Honda 1972) and *Tennō no guntai* (The emperor's military; Honda 1975).

At the same time that Honda began reporting on American atrocities in Vietnam in Japan's largest-circulation daily, historian Saburō Ienaga published a highly critical account of Japanese involvement in the Second World War with Japan's most influential popular publishing house, Iwanami shoten. *Taiheiyō sensō* (The Pacific War), like Ienaga's high school history textbook, *Shin Nihonshi* (A new Japanese history), focused upon the "dark side" of Japan's wartime experience, and even included references to Japanese wartime BW experimentation. Given Ienaga's battles with the Japanese Ministry of Education since 1952 over approval for his history textbook, *The Pacific War* may be viewed, like Honda's exposé of the Nanjing Massacre, as a direct challenge to the conservative politics of post-1945 Japan. Indeed, Ienaga filed his first lawsuit over his history text against the national government in 1965, just three years before the appearance of *The Pacific War*. And the text of *The Pacific War* left no doubt about Ienaga's political aims: "The Japan–U.S. military alliance revives prewar roles, albeit with different stars. America has assumed the Japanese mantle of anti-Communist crusader in Asia and helpmate Japan functions as a strategic base. This arrangement again projects internal security laws outward across Asia and employs lethal force against radical ideas" (Ienaga 1978, 244).

The conservative establishment clearly viewed the wide dissemination of sordid tales of Japan's wartime past and direct criticism of postwar U.S.–Japan relations in such popular venues as the *Asahi shinbun* and in books by Iwanami shoten with alarm. Katsuichi Honda's revelations were roundly criticized in the conservative monthly *Bungei shunjū* (Lie 1993, 22). And the national government would continue to resist Ienaga's challenges until 1997, when the Japanese Supreme Court passed final judgment on Ienaga's third lawsuit.[22]

The heyday of Japanese research on wartime BW experimentation corresponded with the growing volatility of the national discourse in the aftermath of the Vietnam War. Private broadcasting network TBS aired the first three Unit 731 documentaries at the height of public discussion over Honda's exposé of the Nanjing Massacre. And the wave of published research on Japanese BW experimentation that marked the early 1980s came in the wake of a new LDP initiative to crack down on "progressive" historians following impressive victories at the polls. The 1980 general election had given the LDP a large majority in both houses of the Diet and spurred a vigorous new challenge of textbook writers considered to have ties with the Japan Trade Union, the Communist Party, or various democratic education movements. (For a discussion of this initiative, see Nozaki and Inokuchi 2000, 113.) The pivotal work by Sei-ichi Morimura and Kei-ichi Tsuneishi emerged within the context of this heightened conflict between Left and Right in Japan.

The JCP continued to play a critical role in the intensifying battle between liberal intellectuals and conservative politicians in the early 1980s. Both of Morimura's first two books, the fictional treatment of Unit 731, *Death Receptacle,* and the analytical work *The Devil's Insatiability,* were originally serialized in the Communist Party journal *Akahata.* "Death Receptacle" ran through the May 1981 Sunday issues of the magazine, and "The Devil's Insatiability" trickled out in seventy-four installments between July and October 1981 (Morimura 1982a, 54, 188). Through Morimura's introduction, one of the more dramatic American investigations of the Japanese BW issue, a seminal article by former editor of the *China Monthly Review* John W. Powell, in the *Bulletin of Atomic Scientists,* was also published in *Akahata* in October 1981 (Powell 1981; for a discussion of the publication in Japanese of the article, see Morimura 1982a, 188–97). In the wave of discussion that followed the initial publication of *The Devil's Insatiability,* Morimura noted that much of the cooperation that he had received from former staff members of Unit 731 had come from those who, following Japan's defeat, had become members of the Japanese Communist Party (Morimura 1982a, 95).

By the 1980s, however, the JCP no longer played the central role in disseminating information about wartime Japanese BW experimentation. The work of both Morimura and Tsuneishi was ultimately distributed in the Japanese popular press.[23] Morimura's *The Devil's Insatiability* eventually sold more than 1.5 million copies (Brackman 1987, 198). And new revelations appeared in a variety of sources. After first running in Japanese in *Akahata,* the seminal Powell article of 1981 reemerged in the June 1982 issue of *Bunka hyōron* (Morimura 1982a, 235). In the same month, TBS aired a fourth documentary on Unit 731. A flood of testimonials by former Unit 731 employees appeared in new publications and the national print media. And by 1992, the story of Ishii and Unit 731 came to the national network, NHK.

The 1990s witnessed a new level of participation by ordinary citizens in the effort to expose the history of Japanese wartime BW experimentation. In 1993, a private group in Shizuoka City released a ninety-minute film based upon the testimonials of victims of Japanese experimentation. Organized in 1980 and dedicated to exposing the history of Japanese aggression in film, the one-thousand-member Eiga "shinryaku" jōei zenkoku renrakukai (National Liaison Association for Showing "Aggression" in Film) sent fifty of its members on nine fact-finding tours of China and Korea over a five-year span to produce "Saikin-sen butai, 731" (Biological Warfare Unit 731).[24]

As described in the contribution by Kei-ichi Tsuneishi in this volume, the 1989 unearthing of bones on the grounds of the Army Medical College spurred the formation of Gun'i gakkō de hakken sareta jinkotsu mondai o kyūmei suru kai (the Association to Investigate the Problem of Human Remains Discovered at the Army Medical College). In August 1991, this group, too, sent a delegation of high school teachers and citizens to China on an investigative tour. Inspired by a suggestion from their Chinese hosts, the same group began planning for the Unit 731 exhibit that toured Japan's major cities between July 1993 and December 1994. Organizing committees were established in each prospective exhibit spot, largely in the hands of enterprising twenty-somethings. Parallel exhibits were planned by nonaffiliated youth. Students from Tokyo Women's College, Sophia University, and Toritsu High School created their own exhibits at their schools' culture festivals (*bunka matsuri*) in the spring of 1994. And by setting up a Unit 731 emergency number (110-ban), the organizers of the national exhibit solicited the participation of an unprecedented number of former Unit 731 members.

The national exhibit spawned a series of smaller expositions throughout the nation. Tokyo's Nakano Ward sponsored a "Rikugun Nakano gakkō to 731 butai ten" (Nakano Army Academy and Unit 731 Exhibit) at Nakano train station in September 1994. Among the attractions was a picture-story show of Japanese wartime experimentation created and performed by second-year students from Ishikawa Middle School in Hachiōji (731 butai no jittai, kami shibai ni, 29). In 1995, students of Shōwa High School in Saitama Prefecture attended the first joint Sino-Japanese symposium on wartime Japanese experimentation at Harbin. There they delivered the preliminary conclusions of their independent research on the mouse-breeding industry of their native Saitama. The mice, it was discovered, were sent to Manchuria during the war as agents in spreading the plague. After two years of interviews of over one thousand Saitama households, the students displayed their final results in a three-day exhibit at Kasukabu City Culture Hall.[25] Their research was also published as *Kōkōsei ga ou nezumi mura to 731 butai* (High schoolers in search of the mouse village and Unit 731; Endō 1996).

In June of the same year, an assembly of 220 professors, lawyers, doctors, and private citizens gathered in Tokyo to found the Association to Expose the Historical Facts about the Japanese Military's Biological Warfare (Nihongun ni yoru saikinsen no rekishi jijitsu o akiraka ni suru kai) (Kyū Nihongun no saikinsen, asu jittai kyūmei suru kai, 26). Among the members was thirty-year old Naoko Mizutani, whose great-uncle had, on his deathbed three years earlier, presented three hundred pages of material documenting his involvement with the Japanese biological warfare unit in Nanjing, China—Unit 1644 (Tekishutsu shita zōki, suketchi shita, 14). In July 1996, Mizutani accompanied other members of the group to Manchuria in a preliminary step toward aiding Chinese victims of Japanese biological warfare to bring suit against the Japanese government (Saikinsen butai o tsuikyū suru Mizutani Naoko san, 3).

Shifting Framework of Japanese Academic Debate

The erosion of the LDP monopoly of power and reconstitution of the Japanese Socialist Party after the fall of the Berlin Wall in 1989 has shifted the reference of academic debate in Japan in recent years. But it has not, by any means, mitigated the polarization of that debate. If the battle lines following the end of the Cold War are no longer drawn as starkly between intellectual Left and political Right, they have intensified within the intellectual establishment itself. If postwar history reveals the steady diffusion of Japanese wartime BW experimentation into mainstream discourse, it also discloses a growing conservative backlash within academe to the "mainstreaming" of Japanese wartime atrocities. Although novelist Fusao Hayashi had, as early as 1961, attracted notable attention by describing the "Greater East Asia War" as a war of "liberation" in the pages of the popular monthly *Chūō kōron*,[26] it has only been more recently that respected members of Japanese academe have been able to marshal forces for a concerted challenge of the intellectual Left.

Japanese military historian Ikuhiko Hata jumped into the high-profile debate between Saburō Ienaga and the Japanese government in 1987 and 1991, when he testified in the Tokyo High Court on behalf of the Japanese Ministry of Education. Hata, in fact, appeared expressly to refute Ienaga's references to Japanese wartime BW experimentation (Kasahara et al. 1997, 17–19). Hata would ultimately join Tokyo University professor Nobukatsu Fujioka and Electro-Communications University professor Kanji Nishio in the new national organization, the Society for History Textbook Reform, formed in 1996 to counter the "masochistic" (*jigyakuteki*) view of history purportedly promoted by the intellectual Left. The organization represents an impressive coalition of literary, media, academic, and business figures that has already achieved a level of mass exposure and support. The revisionist cartoons validating the "Greater East Asia War" produced by one of the most celebrated figures of the coalition, Yoshinori Kobayashi, were runaway bestsellers between 1998 and 2003 (Kobayashi 1998, Kobayashi 2001, Kobayashi 2003). And, although they were blocked for adoption by local school boards in 2001, the revisionist history and civics texts produced by the Society for History Textbook Reform have, since that time, slowly made inroads into the classroom. Added to regular over-the-counter figures, they have sold nearly one million copies (McNeill and Selden 2005).

Conclusion

To the Japanese scholars who have labored to unearth the facts of Japanese wartime BW experimentation and to American observers of contemporary Japanese society, the "New Education" movement represented by Fujioka and Kobayashi is understandably cause for concern. But, contrary to the impression imparted by many Western analyses of this initiative, it is less a reflection of a unilateral "Japanese movement to 'correct' history" (this is the title of Gavan McCormack's article on the venture; McCormack 2000) than a glimpse of one side of a turbulent debate over Japan's wartime past that has raged since the imperial declaration of surrender in August 1945. That debate is a direct product of the deep political polarization that has characterized Japan since military defeat and foreign occupation. Although the polarization has, on the one hand, spurred efforts to obscure the "darkest" aspects of the Japanese wartime record, it has served just as readily as a powerful catalyst for greater disclosure. The Japanese Left, particularly the Communist Party, looked to revelations of Japanese wartime BW experimentation, in part, to help reinvigorate its political base after 1945. And the great wave of Japanese scholarship on Japanese wartime experimentation in the 1980s sprang from the increasingly volatile intellectual debates surrounding the Vietnam War. By contrast, revelations of American BW experimentation have been slow in coming, in part due to the absence of an equally polarized debate over national identity in the United States.

The increasing prominence of conservative intellectuals in the Japanese national discourse is an unmistakable reflection of the post–Cold War decline of the Left in Japan. But it is also, in part, a product of the continuing vitality of the "critical" vision that marked mainstream Japanese scholarship on modern Japanese history through the 1970s. Professor Fujioka was inspired to mobilize in 1996 not from a position of strength. He was appalled to learn that all seven history textbooks approved by the Ministry of Education at that point for use in junior high schools contained references to wartime "comfort women." Fujioka and his cohorts were, in other words, reacting against the clear advance of the plight of Japan's "comfort women" in Japanese national consciousness.

Although national debates continue to rage around both the stories of Japanese wartime BW experimentation and of Japan's "comfort women," contrary to the experience of the United States, one can plot a clear record of progress in postwar Japanese revelation and consciousness of wartime BW experimentation, on a par with the advance symbolized by the tale of comfort women. Western laments about Japanese "historical amnesia" invariably focus upon official Japanese government policies and the actions and pronouncements of conservative politicians and intellectuals. The cluster of history textbooks approved by the Ministry of Education, Science and Technology in the spring of 2005 was clearly more conservative than those given the green light in the previous round of evaluations in 2001. And the continuing official refusal to countenance appeals for legal restitution for wartime acts, whether it be to Chinese victims of biological warfare, to former "comfort women," or to ex-POWs impressed into slave labor, are obvious setbacks for history, as well as for the plaintiffs.

But a spotlight on official policy reveals only part of the story of public memory. As the American expert on Unit 731, John W. Powell, has observed, the Japanese government is not alone in its attempt to conceal dark aspects of the wartime past. To do so is the hallmark of almost any government (Morimura 1982a, 128). And when it comes to legal restitution, the question of official recognition of wartime sins is vastly complicated by formal treaties and international law. Pressures on national governments to maintain a lid on a Pandora's box of legal demands against the state are, understandably, substantial.

Despite official Japanese resistance to restitution, the widespread Japanese public exposure to an increasingly tangible record of wartime BW experimentation in the 1990s marks a genie that cannot be returned to its bottle. The latest laments over Japanese "historical amnesia" ironically confirm the advances in Japanese public awareness. Japanese courts continue to resist compensation to Chinese victims. But lawsuits raised against the Japanese government since 1993 have been possible only because of new documentation unearthed in Japan and the assistance of Japanese private citizens. Problems in the evaluation of history textbooks in 2005, moreover, were of a fundamentally different character than those in the 1980s. Whereas twenty years ago the Ministry of Education actively excised references to Japanese "aggression," biological warfare, and "comfort women," by 2005, critics lamented not government action, but inaction—namely, failure to vigorously insert references to wartime atrocities into texts.

This change of emphasis symbolizes the most substantial advance in official policy vis-à-vis wartime atrocities over the last twenty years. In the contentious debate over textbook content, Tokyo now officially recognizes the historical reality of most Japanese war crimes: the Nanjing Massacre, comfort women, mass suicide in the Battle of Okinawa, and so on (Hicks 1997, 106). On the issue of biological warfare, the Ministry of Health and Welfare confirmed the existence of Unit 731 in the cabinet committee of the National Diet in April 1982 (731 butai kyokumitsu bunsho, 10). And the Japanese Supreme Court recognized the legality of references to Unit 731 in textbooks in the final ruling of Saburō Ienaga's third lawsuit in 1997 (Dai-sanji Ienaga soshō: 4 kasho no ihō kakutei, 1).

A study of the postwar politics of revelation of Japanese wartime medical experiments does not engage the issues of the causes of those initiatives and cannot predict the degree to which we might see questionable medical practices surfacing again in Japan's future. But by shifting the focus from the purported "culture" to the politics of Japanese "forgetfulness" after 1945, it does suggest that an important indicator of future developments may be found less in certain Japanese cultural practices (as is often stressed in the literature on Japanese bioethics—see, most recently, Engelhardt and Rasmussen 2002), than in the political lay of the land. The politics of exposure of wartime Japanese BW experimentation remains as vital as ever and continues to enrich Japanese public consciousness regarding this dark chapter of national history. Likewise, critical issues of bioethics (brain death, stem cell research, etc.) have become the focus of heated political debate.

One might even argue that the substantial exposure of Japanese citizens by the 1990s to the history of wartime BW experimentation has facilitated Japanese sensitivity to contemporary issues of bioethics. It is clearly difficult in today's Japan to ponder weighty issues of medical ethics without being reminded of the disturbing history of wartime experimentation. Thus, the Aug. 3, 1991, *Asahi shinbun* carried, side-by-side, an article questioning the all-too-convenient new standard of "brain death" for purposes of organ donation (for an echo of this argument, see Tetsuo Yamaori's essay in this volume) with one describing efforts by the national legislature and private citizens to obtain information about the Army War College bones belonging to suspected victims of Japanese wartime experimentation (Gun'i gakkō ato no jinkotsu Chūgoku mo chūshi, 19; Jinken mushi no nōshi ishoku, 19). An eighteen-year-old preparatory student who attended the national Unit 731 exhibit observed in 1994: "That war is bad goes without saying. But as someone intending to go to medical school, [this exhibit] made me think hard about what we consider today medical ethics" (Jibun ni muen no horā ja nai, 15).

In 1998, Japanese moviegoers flocked to a charming and delightfully humorous film about a rural family doctor that also pointedly asked, in the context of the history of wartime BW experimentation, how far physicians should go to preserve public health. Beautifully crafted by the award-winning veteran director Shōhei Imamura, *Kanzō sensei* (Dr. Akagi) follows the frenetic efforts of Dr. Akagi (known to neighbors as "Dr. Liver") to contain the spread of hepatitis in wartime Kyūshū, Japan. Obsessed with finding a cure, Dr. Akagi at one point contemplates extracting the liver of a live Dutch POW for experimentation. But he suspects that his son, a medical doctor in Manchuria, has access to the most advanced knowledge on liver disease because of tests on live subjects. Unable to countenance the horrors of an ambitious research agenda, the trusted doctor ultimately abandons his search for a general cure to return to the simple, if frenzied, life of catching each new flare-up of hepatitis through house calls.

The candid reference in a major Japanese feature film to wartime BW experimentation and a serious ethical dilemma that continues to plague medical practitioners is enough to belie the notion of a "forgetful" Japan. It is, moreover, a tantalizing hint of the rich philosophical terrain from which the active Japanese debates on medical ethics emerged in the 1990s. As William LaFleur notes in his introduction, the origins of this very volume lie in this widespread discussion of Unit 731 and contemporary medical ethics in 1990s Japan. We would all do well to heed Gernot Böhme's compelling point (in this volume) that we do not yet have the proper philosophical safeguards in place to avoid a repetition of history. But one might argue that the horrible reality of Japanese wartime experimentation in "dark medicine" and the clear postwar record of exposure of those crimes, at the very least, make Japanese professionals currently debating the weighty issues of bioethics all the wiser.

Notes

1. Ian Buruma (1994), George L. Hicks (1997), Laura Hein and Mark Selden (2000). Norma Field asks, "Why did these impulses for a self-critical renewal fail to flourish?" (Field 1997, 13). This view is not confined to Western commentators (see Wakamiya 1999).

2. For a quick overview of the fifty-three counts, see Higurashi 2002, 286–87.

3. For example, the *Gifu Times*, the *Chūgoku shinbun*, and the Japanese Communist Party daily, *Akahata* (see Williams and Wallace 1989a, 226–27).

4. Shishashitsu: Akuma no 731 butai, 20; Shishashitsu: zoku akuma no 731 butai, 20; Akuma no 731 butai: Futatabi rupo hōei, 9. Yoshinaga had already made a name for herself and TBS with other documentaries on such controversial issues as the story of right-wing sponsorship of the leftist student group Zengakuren (titled "Yuganda seishun" [Twisted youth]) (Kawatani 1996, 12).

5. Saar 1976. Reference to *Sixty Minutes* in Akuma no 731 butai: Futatabi rupo hōei, 9.

6. The new TBS documentary was titled "Soko ga shiritai: Akuma no 731 butai" (This Is What I'd Like to Know: The Devil's Unit 731) and introduced an American survivor of the camp (Akuma no 731 butai: Futatabi rupo hōei, 9; Shishashitsu: Soko ga shiritai, akuma no 731 butai, 24). The Hong Kong film, titled *Kuroi taiyō 731 butai* (Black

sun, Unit 731), was translated into Japanese and given four public showings a day at Nitchū Gakuin in Tokyo on October 7 and 8, 1992 (Kantōgun saikinsen butai no jittai egaita eiga kōkai, 26).

7. The two-part series was produced by Takashi Inoue and aired on two consecutive nights, April 13 and 14, at 10 p.m. (NHK dokyumento "731 saikinsen butai," 19). Similar to the BBC in Britain, NHK is a publicly owned radio and television broadcasting agency, which means that it is both independent and linked to the government in a way commercial broadcasters are not.

8. The discovery was even highlighted in the *New York Times* (Sanger 1990; Gun'i gakkō ato no jinkotsu Chūgoku mo chūshi, 19). Although it was originally reported that the bones came from 35 bodies, that number was eventually revised to over 100 (see chapter by Kei-ichi Tsuneishi in this volume).

9. Significantly, Japanese historian Ikuhiko Hata, who had earlier aided the Japanese Ministry of Education's legal case against Saburō Ienaga's inclusion of references to Japanese BW experimentation in high school history textbooks, confirmed the authenticity of these documents in 1994 (see 731 butai kyokumitsu bunsho: Zenkoku 40 kasho de junkaiten, 10).

10. Nozaki and Inokuchi note that, from July through September 1980, more than two thousand reports on Japanese textbook screening appeared in the press in nineteen Asian countries.

11. For sustained analysis of the Ienaga textbook controversy, see Hicks 1997, chap. 7.

12. Gavan McCormack sees Fujioka as epitomizing a "troubling" current situation in Japan in which "liberalism and rationalism are used to conceal a mode of reasoning that is both antiliberal and antirational" (McCormack 2000, 70–71).

13. It should be noted that the official history of Fort Detrick places the wartime high of employees at the facility at only 2,300 (Clendenin 1968, 26).

14. For a summary of those estimates, see Harris 1994, 66–67. The two most celebrated cases of American experimentation on human subjects during the war are the Tuskegee Syphilis Study (1932–72) and the Chicago Malaria Study. Neither of these projects, however, was related to the principal U.S. experimentation in BW agents conducted by the United States Army Chemical Warfare Service.

15. The one notable follow-up to Hersh was the 1988 piece by Stanford University historian Barton J. Bernstein (Bernstein, 1988).

16. Namely, chap. 17 of the British edition of Williams and Wallace, *Unit 731*, titled, "Korean War," pp. 235–85, is missing in the American edition published by the Free Press (Williams and Wallace 1989a; Williams and Wallace 1989b; Harris 1994, 283n36).

17. Following soon after the outbreak of the Korean War, the December 1950 issue of *Sekai*, in which the third Peace Problems Symposium statement was printed, doubled its circulation (Dower 1993, 9).

18. By contrast, the full eighteen volumes of raw data used by Soviet prosecutors to make their case have yet to be made available to researchers (Harris 1994, 229).

19. According to the most authoritative account, the USSR conducted the tribunal in an effort to justify the large numbers of Japanese POWs yet to be repatriated to Japan from Siberia (Harris 1994, 226–28).

20. The December 27, 1949, United Press quoted the American representative to the Allied Council for Japan and acting U.S. political advisor to Douglas MacArthur, William Sebald, describing the Khabarovsk trials as a likely "fiction" designed as a "smoke screen" to deflect attention from the thousands of Japanese POWs in Soviet custody still unaccounted for (see Kasahara et al. 1997, 23n14; Powell 1980, 15n1).

21. Honda wrote a series of articles on Vietnam, "Sensō to hito" (War and people), that ran for five months in the *Asahi shinbun* in the mid-1960s. Published in one volume in 1968, *Senba no mura* (The villages of war) became a best seller in Japan, and over 50,000 English-language copies were shipped overseas (see Lie 1993, 16).

22. Although the final ruling rejected Ienaga's most fundamental contention that government textbook screening was unconstitutional, it did accept the legality of his references to Unit 731 (Nozaki and Inokuchi 2000, 119; Dai-sanji Ienaga soshō: 4 kasho no ihō kakutei, 1).

23. Morimura published with Kōbunsha and Kadokawa. Tsuneishi's research appeared with Shinchōsha.

24. The film became the fifth in a series, titled *Katararenakatta sensō—Shinryaku* (The war that could not be told—Aggression; Kyū Nihongun saikinsen butai, eiga ni, 3).

25. The display was titled "731 butai ten in Kasukabu" (Unit 731 Exhibit in Kasukabu; Yonezawa 1996, 31).

26. Later published as *Daitōa sensō kōtei ron* (In affirmation of the Greater East Asia War) (Hayashi 1964).

References

Akuma no 731 butai: Futatabi rupo hōei (The Devil's Unit 731: Another report televised). *Asahi shinbun,* June 21, 1982, evening edition, p. 9.

Barenblatt, Daniel. 2004. *A Plague upon Humanity: The Hidden History of Japan's Biological Warfare Program.* New York: HarperCollins.

Bernstein, Barton J. 1988. America's Biological Warfare Program in the Second World War. *Journal of Strategic Studies* 2, no. 3: 292–317.

Brackman, Arnold. 1987. *The Other Nuremberg: The Untold Story of the Tokyo War Crimes Trials.* New York: Quill.

Buruma, Ian. 1994. *The Wages of Guilt: Memories of War in Germany and Japan.* New York: Farrar, Straus, and Giroux.

Clendenin, Richard M. 1968. *Science and Technology at Fort Detrick, 1943–1968.* Fort Detrick, Md.: Fort Detrick, Historian, Technical Information Division.

Dai-sanji Ienaga soshō: 4 kasho no ihō kakutei (Ienaga's third lawsuit: Legal abridgements recognized in four places). *Asahi shinbun,* Aug. 30, 1997, p. 1.

Dower, John W. 1993. Peace and Democracy in Two Systems: External Policy and Internal Conflict. In *Postwar Japan as History,* ed. Andrew Gordon, 3–33. Berkeley: University of California Press.

Endicott, Stephen, and Edward Hagerman. 1998. *The United States and Biological Warfare: Secrets from the Early Cold War and Korea.* Bloomington: Indiana University Press.

Engelhardt, H. Tristram, and Lisa M. Rasmussen, eds. 2002. *Bioethics and Moral Content: National Traditions of Health Care Morality: Papers Dedicated in Tribute to Kazumasa Hoshino.* Boston: Kluwer.

Endō, Mitsushi. 1996. *Kōkōsei ga ou nezumi mura to 731 butai* (High schoolers in search of the mouse village and Unit 731). Tokyo: Kyōiku shiryō shuppankai.

Field, Norma. 1997. War and Apology: Japan, Asia, the Fiftieth, and After. *Positions: East Asia Cultures Critique* 5, no. 1: 2–49.

Gun'i gakkō ato no jinkotsu Chūgoku mo chūshi (China also keeps a close watch on human remains from the site of the Medical College). *Asahi shinbun,* Aug. 3, 1991, evening edition, p. 19.

Gunji, Yōko. 1982. *"Shōgen" 731 Ishii butai* (Eyewitness: Unit 731). Tokyo: Tokuma shoten.

Harris, Sheldon H. 1994. *Factories of Death: Japanese Biological Warfare 1932–45 and the American Cover-up.* New York: Routledge.

Hayashi, Fusao. 1964–65. *Daitōa sensō kōtei ron* (In affirmation of the Greater East Asia War). 2 vols. Tokyo: Banchō shobō.

Hein, Laura, and Mark Selden. 2000. *Censoring History: Citizenship and Memory in Japan, Germany, and the United States.* New York: M. E. Sharpe.

Hersh, Seymour. 1969. *Chemical and Biological Warfare: America's Hidden Arsenal.* New York: Doubleday.

Hicks, George L. 1997. *Japan's War Memories: Amnesia or Concealment?* U.K.: Ashgate.

Higurashi, Yoshinobu. 2002. *Tōkyō saiban no kokusai kankei* (International relations of the Tokyo Trials). Tokyo: Bokutakusha.

Honda, Katsuichi. 1968. *Senba no mura* (The villages of war). Tokyo: Asahi shinbunsha. First appeared as a series of articles on Vietnam, "Sensō to hito" (War and People), that ran for five months in the *Asahi shinbun* in the mid-1960s.

———. 1972. *Chūgoku no tabi* (Journey to China). Tokyo: Asahi shinbunsha.

———. 1975. *Tennō no guntai* (The emperor's military). Tokyo: Asahi shinbunsha.

Ienaga, Saburō. 1978. *The Pacific War, 1931–1945: A Critical Perspective on Japan's Role in World War II.* New York: Random House. English-language version of *Taiheiyō sensō* (Tokyo: Iwanami shoten).

Jibun ni muen no horā ja nai (Not a horror entirely unrelated to us). *Asahi shinbun,* June 13, 1994, p. 15.

Jinken mushi no nōshi ishoku (Brain-dead transplantation that ignores human rights). *Asahi shinbun,* Aug. 3, 1991, evening edition, p. 19.

Kantōgun saikinsen butai no jittai egaita eiga kōkai (Public showing of a film depicting a biological warfare unit of the Guandong Army). *Asahi shinbun,* Oct. 7, 1992, p. 26.

Kasahara, Tokushi, et al., eds. 1997. *Rekishi no jijitsu o dō kakutei shi dō oshieru ka* (How to establish and teach historical fact). Tokyo: Kyōiku shiryō shuppankai.

Kawatani, Tadao. 1996. Review of Yoshinaga Haruko, *Nazo no dokuyaku* (The mysterious poison). *Asahi shinbun,* Apr. 28, 1996, p. 12.

Kobayashi, Yoshinori. 1998, 2001, 2003. *Senso ron I, II, III* (On war, I, II, III). Tokyo: Gentōsha.

Koshi, Sadao. 1983. *Hi no maru wa akai namida ni* (Red tears of the red sun). Tokyo: Kyōiku shiryō shuppankai.

Kyū Nihongun no saikinsen, asu jittai kyūmei suru kai (Meeting tomorrow to investigate the reality of biological warfare perpetrated by the imperial army). *Asahi shinbun,* June 28, 1996, p. 26.

Kyū Nihongun saikinsen butai, eiga ni (Biological warfare unit of the Imperial Japanese Army: On film). *Asahi shinbun,* Nov. 30, 1993, evening edition, p. 3.

Lie, John, ed. 1993. *The Impoverished Spirit in Contemporary Japan: Selected Essays of Honda Katsuichi.* New York: Monthly Review Press.

McCormack, Gavan. 2000. The Japanese Movement to "Correct" History. In Hein and Selden, 53–73.

McNeill, David, and Mark Selden. 2005. Asia Battles over War History: The Legacy of the Pacific War Looms over Tokyo's Plans for the Future. *Japan Focus,* Apr. 13, 2005. http://japanfocus.org/257.html (accessed Apr. 15, 2005).

Miller, Judith, Stephen Engelberg, and William Broad. 2001. *Germs: Biological Weapons and America's Secret War.* New York: Simon and Schuster.

Mochi o tabe, zenshin ga aokuroku nari, shinda (After Eating the Rice Cakes, They Turned Black and Blue All Over and Died). *Asahi shinbun,* Sept. 6, 1994, p. 30.

Mori, Masataka, and Yoshiya Kasukawa, 1995. *Chūgoku shinryaku to 731 butai no saikinsen* (Invasion of China and the biological warfare of Unit 731). Tokyo: Akashi shobō.

Morimura, Seiichi. 1981a. *Akuma no hōshoku* (The Devil's insatiability). Tokyo: Kōbunsha.

———. 1981b. *Shi no utsuwa* (Death receptacle). Tokyo: Kadokawa.

———. 1982a. *"Akuma no hōshoku" nōto* (Notes on "The Devil's insatiability"). Tokyo: Banseisha.

———. 1982b. *Zoku akuma no hōshoku* (The Devil's insatiability—Supplement). Tokyo: Kōbunsha.

———. 1983. *Akuma no hōshoku, dai-sanbu* (The Devil's insatiability—Part III). Tokyo: Kakugawa.

731 butai kyokumitsu bunsho: Zenkoku 40 kasho de junkaiten (Top secret documents of Unit 731: Traveling exhibit in 40 locations across the nation). *Asahi shinbun,* July 2, 1993, evening edition, p. 10.

731 butai kyūmei e Nitchū kyōdō shinpo (Sino-Japanese symposium to investigate Unit 731). *Asahi shinbun,* Sept. 16, 1995, evening edition, p. 9.

731 butai no saikinsen: Nihongawa shiryō de urazuke (Unit 731 biological warfare: Confirmation in Japanese sources). *Asahi shinbun,* Aug. 14, 1993, p. 1.

731 butai no jittai, kami shibai ni (Reality of Unit 731: In a paper-picture story). *Asahi shinbun,* Sept. 16, 1994, p. 29.

731 butai no saikinsen kenshō (Verification of Unit 731 biological warfare). *Asahi shinbun,* Dec. 18, 1995, p. 14.

NHK dokyumento "731 saikinsen butai" (NHK Documentary, "731 biological warfare unit"). *Asahi shinbun,* Apr. 13, 1992, evening edition, p. 19.

Nomonhan jiken ni "saikinsen" no shōgen (Testimony of "biological warfare" at the Nomonhan Incident). *Asahi shinbun,* Aug. 24, 1989, p. 3.

Nozaki, Yoshiko, and Hiromitsu Inokuchi. 2000. Japanese Education, Nationalism, and Ienaga's Textbook Lawsuits. In Hein and Selden: 96–126.

"Pesuto mōi" to hōkoku (Report on the "violence of the plague"). *Asahi shinbun,* Aug. 14, 1993, p. 27.

Powell, John W. 1980. Japan's Germ Warfare: The U.S. Cover-up of a War Crime. *Bulletin of Concerned Asian Scholars,* vol. 12, no. 4: 2–17.

———. 1981. Japan's Biological Weapons, 1930–45. *Bulletin of Atomic Scientists,* vol. 37, no. 8.

Saar, John. 1976. Japan Accused of WW II Germ Deaths. *Washington Post,* Nov. 19, 1976, pp. 1, 19.

Saikin butai moto taiin ga jitsuroku (True account of a former member of the biological warfare unit). *Asahi shinbun,* Aug. 13, 1983, evening edition, p. 9.

Saikinsen butai o tsuikyū suru Mizutani Naoko san (Ms. Naoko Mizutani, who is investigating the biological warfare unit). *Asahi shinbun,* July 12, 1996, p. 3.

Saikinsen 731 butai no katsudō (Activities of biological warfare Unit 731), *Asahi shinbun,* June 22, 1989, evening edition, p. 3.

Sanger, David. 1990. Skulls Found: Japan Doesn't Want to Know Whose. *New York Times,* Aug. 13, 1990, pp. 1, 5.

Seitai jikken o mokei de saigen (Reproducing Experiments on Live Subjects through Models). *Asahi shinbun,* July 11, 1993, p. 24.

Shimamura, Kyō. 1967. *Sanzennin no seitai jikken: Nihongun "saikin butai" no zaigō* (Three thousand human experiments: The sinful life of the Japanese military's "biological warfare unit"). Tokyo: Hara shobō.

Shishashitsu: Akuma no 731 butai (Viewing room: The Devil's unit 731). *Asahi shinbun,* Aug. 10, 1975, p. 20.

Shishashitsu: Soko ga shiritai, akuma no 731 butai (Viewing room: This is what I'd like to know, the Devil's Unit 731). *Asahi shinbun,* June 29, 1982, p. 24.

Shishashitsu: Zoku akuma no 731 butai (Viewing Room: The Devil's Unit 731 Supplement). *Asahi shinbun,* Aug. 15, 1976, p. 20.

Swearingen, Rodger, and Paul Langer. 1968. *Red Flag in Japan: International Communism in Action 1919–1951.* New York: Greenwood Press.

Takitani, Jirō. 1989. *Satsuriku kōjō: 731 butai* (Slaughter factory: Unit 731). Tokyo: Shinshin shobō.

Tekishutsu shita zōki, suketchi shita (I sketched the extracted organs). *Asahi shinbun,* Nov. 20, 1995, p. 14.

Tsuneishi, Kei-ichi. 1981. *Kieta saikinsen butai: Kantōgun 731* (The biological warfare unit that disappeared: Guandong Army 731). Tokyo: Kaisōsha.

———. 1982. *Saikinsen butai to jiketsu shita futari no igakusha* (The biological warfare unit and two physicians who committed suicide). Tokyo: Shinchōsha.

Wakamiya, Yoshibumi, 1999. *Postwar Conservative View of Asia: How the Political Right Has Delayed Japan's Coming to Terms with Its History of Aggression in Asia.* Tokyo: LTCB International Library Foundation.

Williams, Peter, and David Wallace. 1989a. *Unit 731: Japan's Secret Biological Warfare in World War II.* New York: Free Press.

———. 1989b. *Unit 731: The Japanese Army's Secret of Secrets.* London: Hodder and Stoughton.

Yamada, Seizaburō. 1974. *Saikinsen gunji saiban: Kiroku shōsetsu* (Military tribunal on biological warfare: A documentary novel). Tokyo: Tōhō shuppansha.

Yonezawa, Nobuyoshi. 1996. Saitama no kōkōsei, "731 butai" shirabeta (Saitama High Schoolers Research "Unit 731"). *Asahi shinbun,* Aug. 1, 1996, p. 31.

Yoshimi, Yoshiaki, and Toshiya Ikō. 1995. *731 butai to tennō, rikugun chūō* (Unit 731, the emperor, and Army Central). Tokyo: Iwanami shoten.

8 Biological Weapons: The United States and the Korean War

G. Cameron Hurst III

The advent of the "War on Terror" during the presidency of George W. Bush has brought to the forefront the specter of "weapons of mass destruction." The phrase was not particularly new, but in the past several years it has become ubiquitous in the media; in the abbreviated form WMD, it has become well known across the United States.

The use of this term in the United States is somewhat disingenuous. That is, the official American concern with WMD is solely that other nations or organizations might direct them against a blameless American nation. This ignores the fact that few countries possess the WMD arsenal of the United States. Except for the ICBM-mounted nuclear weapons covered under the U.S.–Soviet arms control agreements, Americans do not know how many nuclear weapons they possess, and the government refuses to allow independent inspection of U.S. chemical, biological, and nuclear stockpiles. Moreover, no nation has used WMD to the extent the United States has. Instead, in the post-9/11 world, the scenario of WMD has been one in which "axis of evil" nations or terrorist networks might employ WMD against innocent American civilians.

Indeed, the Bush administration policy of "preventive strike," a departure from past U.S. experience that flaunts international law, was formulated to justify an American attack against societies and/or organizations that are construed as threats to the U.S. The American invasion of Iraq, cleverly pitched to the American people by the White House as "Operation Iraqi Freedom," was predicated upon unsubstantiated reports of Iraqi WMD. The Bush administration also attempted to associate the Saddam Hussein regime with al-Qaeda and the 9/11 terrorist attacks, with no proof and despite the fact that the terrorists were primarily citizens of an ally, Saudi Arabia, and included not one Iraqi. Long after the invasion of Iraq, when it is generally acknowledged that there was no connection between Iraq and the 9/11 terrorists, Democratic presidential hopeful Senator John Kerry was unable to use that information convincingly enough to unseat President Bush. Such are the current fears of WMD in the wake of 9/11.

But if we shift our gaze back just sixty years, we are presented with an entirely different picture. Of course, World War II in the Pacific was concluded with the most extensive reliance upon WMD in history, the atomic bombings of Hiroshima and Nagasaki. Moreover, carpet bombings of German and Japanese cities that killed hundreds of thousands of civilians, while not involving radioactivity, were nonetheless instances of applying WMD. In the unfolding of the Cold War, furthermore, the United States became deeply involved in the development, stockpiling, and possible use of WMD. Indeed, the U.S. is not only the largest military force in the world but also the nation with the largest arsenal of weapons of mass destruction. This history and current status makes more than a bit hypocritical the Bush administration's highly moralistic condemnation of other nations as belonging to an "axis of evil" for even being suspected of some of the things of which the U.S. has been guilty.

Destroying North Korea: Bombing in the Korean War

During the Korean War of 1950–53, actual and threatened use of WMD played an important part in America's attempt, first, to halt the invasion of the southern part of the peninsula by the armies of the north; second, to unify the entire peninsula under southern president Syngman Rhee; and, finally, in the wake of the Chinese intervention, to salvage as much of the original Republic of Korea (ROK) territory as it could. UN commanding general Douglas MacArthur threatened to resort to atomic bombs in Korea within the first few weeks of the war, when ROK troops were on the run and the fate of the peninsula appeared to be in jeopardy. Later, following the massive intervention of Chinese forces, which he assured President Truman wouldn't happen, MacArthur threatened to drop "thirty to fifty atomic bombs . . . strung across the neck of Manchuria, (which would) spread behind us . . . a belt of radioactive cobalt" (Halliday and Cumings 1988, 128).

Both presidents Harry S. Truman and Dwight D. Eisenhower threatened nuclear warfare on the Korean peninsula, and Truman moved bombs to an aircraft carrier in the sea off Korea and took other steps to ready American bases in Okinawa for possible atomic bombings of Korea. In September and October of 1951, the U.S. even dispatched B-29 bombers that dropped fake atomic bombs over North Korea, either dummies or ones containing TNT. As Bruce Cumings notes: "One may imagine the steel nerves required of leaders in Pyongyang, observing on radar a lone B-29 simulating the attack lines that had resulted in the devastation of Hiroshima and Nagasaki just six years earlier, each time unsure whether the bomb was real or a dummy" (Cumings 2004, 26).

Insofar as nuclear weapons are concerned, the United States stopped short of carrying through its many threats, but seemingly not because most of the military and civilian officials shied away from their use. Rather the decision not to use nuclear weapons seems to have been based largely upon a decision to avoid escalating the conflict to a World War III level (i.e., inviting Soviet entry into the war and even greater Chinese involvement); the opposition of American allies, especially Great Britain, to use of the bomb; and the fact that North Korea had few urban targets requiring nuclear destruction. Morality seems to have played a minor role.

But despite the fact that the U.S. did not resort to atomic warfare, it used everything in its arsenal to destroy most of North Korea, with bombing that reached a total of 17,000 tons and more than half obliterated eighteen of the twenty-two major cities (Crane 2000, 168). As the architect of the air war, General Curtis LeMay, so graphically noted, "over a period of three years or so . . . we burned down *every* [*sic*] town in North Korea and South Korea too" (Halliday and Cumings 1988, 118). Just as the U.S. introduced the MOAB ("mother of all bombs") before liberating the Iraqis, it developed the huge (12,000-pound) new "Tarzan" bombs for Korea. Carpet bombing with incendiary bombs was common, and napalm, developed just at the end of World War II, was employed with devastating effect on Korean villages, towns, and cities, incinerating thousands and leaving many horribly scarred for life.

Undoubtedly the most controversial aspect of the air war against North Koreans, which Cumings among others refers to as "genocidal," was the bombing of dams and power plants in the last year of the war, during the torturous negotiations with the People's Republic of China (PRC) and the Democratic People's Republic of Korea (DPRK). In June 1952, the United States launched the biggest air raid of the war, as over five hundred planes attacked four dams along the Yalu River, including the huge Supong Dam that supplied 90 percent of North Korea's power. For the rest of the war, the DPRK was virtually without electrical power.[1] Almost a year later, American planes also bombed five dams close by P'yongyang, causing widespread flooding and "tremendous destruction of the rice crop," according to a U.S. Air Force study (Halliday and Cumings 1988, 195–96). The bombing was intended to have a psychologically crushing effect on the populace, since it came just at the end of the rice-planting season before the plants had taken root. It is unlikely that many remember that similar actions by the Nazis in Holland were condemned at Nuremberg as war crimes.

The death and destruction in the North was appalling. Even if we do not apply the term WMD to the weapons the U.S. employed in this narrow peninsula, it was by no means for Koreans the "limited" war that the Truman administration talked of waging. For them, war was total. An accurate counting of those killed in the war is still not available,[2] but one estimate of the number of North Korean civilians killed by the U.S. exceeds two million (Tucker 2000, 200). It is clear that for P'yongyang, the Korean War is not a "forgotten war" as it is sometimes called in the U.S.; indeed, maintaining vivid memories of American actions in the Korean War among the populace represents a major part of its anti-American campaign.

Biological Weapons and Their Use in Recent History

One of the greatest American concerns about WMD today is the fear that members of the "axis of evil" or another anti-American group will employ biological or chemical weapons against it; we already had a foreshadowing of that in several anthrax scares. As Condoleezza Rice was going to say in the speech she never gave on 9/11, "we need to worry about the . . . vial of sarin released in the subway." There is a legitimate fear that air, water, and food supplies could be infected, or that a virulent disease could be intentionally spread among the populace. The (then) new Department of Homeland Security's own website noted:

> One of the most important missions we have as a Nation is to be prepared for the threat of biological terrorism—the deliberate use of disease as a weapon. An effective biodefense will require a long-term strategy and significant new investment in the U.S. health care system. The President is taking steps now that will significantly improve the Nation's ability to protect its citizens against the threat of bioterrorism. The President's Budget for 2003 proposes $5.9 billion to defending against biological terrorism, an increase of $4.5 billion—or 319 percent—from the 2002 level.

Notice that there is a full new vocabulary for the world we now live in. The term "biological terrorism" is defined as "the deliberate use of disease as a weapon." The unspoken assumption about the term is that Americans would not resort to such acts nor condone them, but other people, less ethical than Americans are, would likely employ disease this way. "Terrorism" is itself a slippery term, but clearly it is a term that officially applies only to acts of others.

But in fact, during World War II and the Korean War, the United States actively developed offensive biological weapons. High-ranking U.S. military and civilian officials urged the use of disease to win the war; in the Korean case, the U.S. was accused by the Chinese and North Koreans of what the White House today would call bioterrorism (although they did not have that word then), a claim that was upheld by an international commission that investigated the charges. The remainder of this discussion will be devoted to a considering whether those accusations were true or not.

Biological Warfare in Korea: The Enemy's Accusations

Although the PRC and DPRK foreign ministers complained to the United Nations in the spring of 1951 that the U.S. had employed biological warfare (BW) against them, that charge was brushed off and soon forgotten. But early in 1952 the North Koreans and Chinese began to encounter health problems that they at first could not explain, but that later were to become the basis of charges leveled against the United States. In several locations in North Korea, Chinese and North Korean military personnel began to report American planes dropping unusual materials, such as chicken feathers and various kinds of insects (New China News Agency, Feb. 29, 1952, quoted in Endicott and Hagerman 1998, 5 and 208n11.).[3] Meanwhile, in several widely separated places across the Yalu River in Manchuria, Chinese authorities were puzzled by the deaths of a number of people from anthrax bacillus or encephalitis, because these diseases were either rare or nonexistent in the area. At first the medical authorities sent to investigate the deaths were puzzled and unable to put together sufficient reasons for the deaths, since, as they noted, "in the past this kind of encephalitis was never seen in the northeast region" (Endicott and Hagerman 1998, 5).[4]

As the number of deaths began to increase, the Chinese noticed that there was something that tied these seemingly disparate cases together: the observation that American planes had flown over the area and dropped bombs. Investigation of the sites showed the kinds of strange materials noted above, as well as boxes and unexploded bombs, but more importantly, a variety of insects, unusual for the area or for the season or in such numbers. The Chinese medical teams reached the conclusion that the American planes had been dropping these insects in order to infect the local population. The Chinese government formed a committee for epidemic control headed by Zhou Enlai with People's Liberation Army (PLA) chief of staff Nie Rongzhen and Chinese Academy of Science president Guo Moro serving as vice chairs. They telegraphed widely to provincial and local governments and army units in mid-March:

> Since January 28 the enemy has furiously employed continuous bacterial warfare in Korea and in our Northeast and Qingdao areas. Dropping flies, mosquitoes, spiders, ants, fleas . . . thirty-odd species of bacteria-carryings insects. . . . They were dropped in a very wide area. . . . Examination confirms that the pathogenic micro-organisms involved are plague bacillus, cholera, meningitis, paratyphoid, salmonella, relapsing fever, spirochaeta bacteria, typhus rickettsia, etc. . . . Now that the weather is turning warm, contagious disease and animal vectors will be active without restraint, and serious epidemic diseases from enemy bacterial war can easily occur unless we immediately intensify nationwide work on the prevention of epidemic disease. (Endicott and Hagerman 1998, 11)

In Korea as well, North Korean medical teams investigated fleas, flies, and spiders that they claimed American warplanes had dropped in DPRK territory, and in some of these insects they detected cholera, a very rare occurrence, unknown in Korea for almost sixty years (Endicott and Hagerman 1998, 8). The North Koreans as well found evidence that the United States had dropped bombs with infected insects in several areas across the DPRK. In other words, according to both the PRC and DPRK authorities, the U.S. had been engaged in biological warfare. Stephen Endicott and Edward Hagerman, the two researchers who have exhaustively studied this issue, interviewed several of the surviving Chinese doctors almost a half-century after the events. They remain as clear today as they were then that the United States had in fact released infected insects in northeastern China.

In late winter of 1952, when information about these unusual findings in northeast China and outbreaks of rare diseases (respiratory anthrax, encephalitis, etc.) was circulated, medical research teams of Chinese doctors were dispatched to examine the situation on the spot. (These are the same doctors that were interviewed a half-century later by Endicott and Hagerman.) Likewise, the North Koreans sent a Commission of the Medical Headquarters of the Korean People's Army at the end of January to investigate a strange occurrence of a variety of insects found by soldiers of the Chinese People's Volunteers in and around P'yongyang, Chorwon, and Kumhwa. In both the Chinese and Korean cases, the medical authorities could not explain the presence of the unusual materials and insects. (For example, in Korea the temperature was far too cold for such flies, spiders, and ticks to have reproduced naturally. Moreover, several types of the flies were said not be native to Korea; the ticks too "belonged to a type unknown in Korea but capable of conveying 'spring and summer recurrent fever' and encephalitis" [Endicott and Hagerman 1998]).[5] In all these cases, the doctors attributed the appearance of the unusual and disease-bearing insects to their having been dropped by American airplanes.

The information about these diseased insects was passed on to Chairman Mao Zedong by the worried general Nie Rongzhen (chief of staff of the PLA), whose immediate concern was epidemic prevention among his soldiers. Mao put Premier Zhou Enlai in charge of the situation, and he put together a six-point plan for dealing with both the potential medical problem and the political issue of calling the Americans to task for engaging in germ warfare (Endicott and Hagerman 1998, 8). Zhou's report was followed up with discussions at the highest level on this matter between the PRC and DPRK governments, and finally, on February 22, 1952, the DPRK foreign minister Bak Hun Yung issued a charge against the United States for having dropped various insects in order to spread contagious diseases (Goulden 1982, 601). Only a few days later, Premier Zhou "followed with a statement about how sixty-eight formations of American aircraft had made no less than 448 sorties over areas of northeastern China, scattering germ-bearing insects" (Goulden 1982, 601).

Retired general Yang Dezhi recalled at length in his 1987 memoirs that, after being warned via circulars in late January 1952 that the enemy had been dropping three kinds of insects:

> On February 11, four enemy airplanes flew over our headquarters, and a milky mucus was dropped on the sleeve of my uniform. Subsequently, a report arrived from Sokbyon-ri: batches of flies, milky mucus stuck on paper sheets, and graphic cards had been found in Songnydong [*sic*] and the surrounding area. . . . Tests by medical officers showed that those insects were carrying cholera and other types of germs. . . . We encountered many obstacles in the early stage of dealing with germ warfare. (Li, Millett, and Yu 2001, chap. 7, especially 157–60)

More than half a century later, the reports still appear highly suspect; since they are unsupported by, for example, any direct reports of American planes having crashed, in which either the Chinese or the North Koreans found infected insects or half-exploded bombs containing such evidence. Despite precise "statistical exactitude" as recounted above,[6] the reports do not really ring true to most who have read them. However—unlike earlier charges of germ and chemical warfare that various Communist front organizations had mounted in 1951 and that were quickly dismissed due to lack of any evidence—this time the Chinese and North Koreans had what struck many as much better proof: a number of American pilots who had "confessed" to having participated in germ warfare bombings.

The Pilots and Their "Confessions"

The whole of the Korean War is overshadowed by the first real experience by Americans of the politicization of prisoners of war, an experience with which the U.S. was unprepared to deal. While there were many prisoners of war on all sides in World War II, agreed-upon rules of international war were generally followed in the West. Thus, while no one can imagine that German prisoner-of-war camps were any picnic, Allied prisoners were generally treated well enough. Indeed, there was a proliferation in the U.S. during and after the war of exciting, and even comic, prison camp movies that concentrated upon such plots as Allied servicemen attempting to escape or German attempts to infiltrate and learn military secrets from the Allied officers, but little attention was devoted to abusive treatment or politicization of the POWs. The Asian case was quite different: Japanese prisoner-of-war camps were often brutal, with nutritional and medical deprivation, forced labor, and a high rate of death among the prisoners. Accordingly, U.S. war films emphasized these aspects.

The Korean POW experience, however, introduced a new and frightening phenomenon, and this was also reflected in the popular film of the time. The 1962 movie *Manchurian Candidate,* directed by John Frankenheimer, revolves around a war hero returned from the Korean War, who, responding to a buried hypnotic suggestion given him while a POW, tries to assassinate an American presidential candidate. The film captures well the unrealistic but strong fears that Americans had of the alien notion of "brainwashing," even though it was largely dismissed by experts after the war. Although a number of American prisoners of war did in fact "collaborate" with their Communist captors, and twenty-one remained behind in China and North Korea after the war, there was nothing like the involuntary, subconscious "brainwashing" of the popular imagination. Nor was collaboration as extensive in the Korean War as was often claimed in the popular press. As in most wars, a few collaborated and some steadfastly resisted in the face of uncommon brutality (2,701 out of around 7,140 POWs died in captivity). But the majority "simply tried to survive under the most intolerable of conditions" (Carlson 2002, xiii). Nonetheless, the POWs were politicized upon their return to the States; and many commentators, social analysts, and even psychiatrists castigated the POWs for their weakness, even going so far as to blame their mothers for lax child-rearing practices.[7]

At any rate, POWs were one of the biggest stumbling blocks to ending the Korean War, mainly because the United States refused any forced repatriation of DPRK and Chinese POWs—which extended the negotiations and the death rate immeasurably. The fate of the POWs became a political football between the two sides; and the final year of the war saw horrific casualty rates among all combatants, as the negotiators bickered over the POWs and soldiers slaughtered one another to gain control of barren granite hilltops in a trench warfare reminiscent of World War I. Chinese and North Korean forces captured thousands of UN combatants, mainly Americans, many of whom were of course pilots whose planes were shot down or crashed. Statements admitting that the United States was engaged in "germ warfare" were made to the Chinese by thirty-six pilots, and twenty-five of these are still available in United Nations documents.

The first to come to world attention via "propaganda films" was the confession at the end of March 1952 by Lieutenant Kenneth Enoch that he had participated in germ warfare. His comrade Lieutenant John Quinn made a confession a few days later, claiming that he was forced by the U.S. military to "be a tool of these warmongers, made to drop germ bombs, and do this awful crime against the people of Korea and the Chinese Volunteers" (Toland 1991, 537). Several more followed, provoking a good deal of reaction worldwide, including many demonstrations by largely Communist supporters in a number of countries. Indeed, not only Communists accepted these confessions at face value: the Dean of Canterbury, Dr. Hewlett Johnson, returned from China to state that "the facts about germ warfare are conclusive and irrefutable" (Toland 1991, 538).

These remaining confessions are extremely detailed, providing an astounding amount of information including many specific names, dates, and places. According to what the Chinese claim to have been able to piece together from the confessions, the Joint Chiefs of Staff in December of 1950 ordered the Research and Development section to "complete preparations for the use of biological weapons by the end of 1951" (Endicott and Hagerman 1998, 163). They went on to chronicle the implementation of the plan, implicating Air Force chief of staff General Hoyt Vandenberg and Far East commanding general Matthew Ridgway, and naming the various units and bases in Korea to which the infected insects were sent before being dropped in North Korea and China. They claimed that the bombings began in January 1952. Among the reasons that the Chinese claim the American pilots gave for the use of biological warfare were "to shorten the war and save American lives," to cause an epidemic and disturb the morale of the Chinese and North Korean troops, and to help disrupt the Chinese supply lines (which wasn't being affected despite heavy bombing) (Endicott and Hagerman 1998, 165).

In this short chapter, it is impossible to provide a real sense of the degree of detail that the Chinese provided regarding the U.S. biological war plans as extracted from these pilots, but it was impressive. Perhaps the summary of Endicott and Hagerman's research best captures it:

> From these officers, the Chinese acquired information about U.S. high command decisions on bacteriological warfare, why the U.S. resorted to this type of warfare, where the germ weapons were manufactured, the type of weapons used, the kinds of diseases spread, how the missions were conducted, the content of lectures given to servicemen on the history and development of and the training for biological warfare, the phases of the U.S. germ warfare program, security precautions, and the assessment of results of germ warfare by the U.S. military. (Endicott and Hagerman 1998, 163)

While these "confessions" were dismissed as so much propaganda in the United States, people in many countries accepted them at face value, and the U.S. suffered some loss of prestige. Still, most accounts of the Korean War tend to dismiss the claims as Communist propaganda, or "the big lie," as David Rees labeled it (Rees 1970, 338; see also Tucker 2000, 1:77–78). Immediately after repatriation, however, these pilots were isolated by the U.S. military and subjected to a form of "reverse brainwashing." There was a "frantic effort to prevent further impairment of U.S. prestige" (Rees 1970, 167). The pilots were put under tremendous pressure to recant their confessions, and ultimately they all did. A public statement by Attorney General Herbert Brownell that "United States prisoners of war who collaborated with their Communist captors in Korea may face charges of treason" could hardly have escaped their attention.

The recanted confessions were collected by the military, and in a dramatic gesture, U.S. chief delegate to the United Nations Henry Cabot Lodge Jr. handed over ten of these to the General Assembly's Political and Security Committee, denouncing the extraction of American confessions as "a record of unparalleled and diabolical mendacity." Reading the refutations today, in light of how much more we know about the extent of U.S. preparations for biological warfare, including information received from the infamous Japanese Unit 731 after World War II, one can detect a number of inconsistencies and errors in the flyers' statements. The primary poster boy for the recanting pilots, Colonel Walker M. Mahurin, noted in retracting his confession that statements he made to the Chinese about infected insects and activities involving biological warfare at Maryland's Fort Detrick were all made up, and were on the face of it "completely ridiculous" and "absurd." But Endicott and Hagerman argue that in fact the "absurd" statements that Ambassador Lodge tried to paint as "diabolical Chinese lies turned out to be entirely workable methods for the U.S. armed forces to use in conducting germ warfare" (Rees 1970, 171–72). But at the time, amidst relief that the disastrous war was at last concluded, the confessions were largely dismissed as so much Communist propaganda, coerced from the captive flyers. That is certainly less clear in hindsight.

The International Scientific Commission's Investigation

Undoubtedly, the best way to have got to the bottom of Chinese and Korean charges of germ warfare would have been for a distinguished medical research team to go to the sites where the Chinese claimed that biological warfare had been waged and examine places, people, and remains thoroughly. The claimants, however, were unwilling to do that, and for several months would not agree to allow International Red Cross or World Health Organization teams to investigate their charges. The PRC and DPRK considered these groups biased—they were, after all, at war with the United Nations—and their unwillingness to allow examination certainly raised a red flag of suspicion.

But ultimately an international investigation was conducted, a report filed, and the Chinese charges vindicated. Unfortunately for Beijing and P'yongyang, most of the world chose to disbelieve the report. The so-called International Scientific Commission for the Investigation of the Facts Concerning Bacterial Warfare in Korea and China was formed, went to China to investigate the situation, and issued a formal report in September 1952. Often referred to as a "700-page report," it was in fact a rather terse report of about 60 pages, with 600 more pages of charts, tables, and graphs. In the United States, the ISC has usually been considered a Communist front organization (see, e.g., Sandler 1999, 209), and today its findings are still regarded as highly suspect. The commission was, however, neither a sham nor a group staffed by persons with no credentials.[8] Composed of six members, all prominent scientists, from Brazil, France, Sweden, Italy, Great Britain, and the U.S.S.R., it was headed by Dr. Joseph Needham, a British biochemist and a distinguished scholar of Chinese science and medicine. Needham was president of the British-Chinese Friendship Association and a noted Sinologist, who, it must be admitted, was clearly supportive of the Chinese revolution. Nevertheless, only one member of the ISC represented a Communist nation, Dr. N. N. Zhukov-Verezhnikov, vice president of the Soviet Academy of Medicine. Interestingly, however, the Soviet bacteriologist had considerable experience in the field, having been involved in the earlier Khabarovsk trial of the Japanese accused of biological warfare in World War II.

Even before commencing its work, the commission felt that actually proving the charge against the United States would be almost impossible. However, after months of traveling throughout China and Korea to observe sites, read reports, and interrogate witnesses, the members of the ISC Commission reached the unanimous conclusion that China and North Korea had been subjected to biological warfare by the United States. Many other readers of the report, then as now, were unwilling to accept the evidence as so compelling. In fact, many felt that it was not on the evidence that the ISC members based their judgment but rather on a misguided willingness to accept at face value the statements of the Chinese hosts who had accompanied them on their mission. The Swedish member, Dr. Andrea Andreen, noted on her return, for example, that "we felt so sure of the integrity of our Chinese hosts that we entirely trusted statements which they made regarding the American use of germ warfare" (Rees 1970, 360). Dr. Needham himself concurred: "We accepted the word of the Chinese scientists. It is possible to maintain that the whole thing was a kind of patriotic conspiracy. I prefer to believe that the Chinese were not acting parts" (Rees 1970, 360). Indeed, Needham says the ISC was reluctant to reach the conclusions they did "because its members had not been disposed to believe that such an inhuman technique could have been put into execution in the face of its universal condemnation by the peoples of the nations."

Although the charges leveled by the Chinese and Koreans, and substantiated by the ISC, were given credence in the Eastern bloc and by those predisposed to think ill of the United States, charges that the U.S. had conducted biological warfare were dismissed as mere propaganda by the United States and its Western allies. At the United Nations they made little headway. Infected insects in freezing weather, chicken feathers, and anthrax did not convince many. Indeed, it is still widely believed that whatever outbreaks of various forms of infectious disease may have occurred in China and North Korea, these were probably due to the poor state of public health. Thus the standard accounts hold that "These epidemics were traced to poor sanitation and health conditions stemming from the war and a lack of effective medical care for the populace. However, Communist leaders used these epidemics as a propaganda tool and as a means to hide the inadequacies of their health care system" (Tucker 2000, 1:77).[9]

No one can deny this possibility, although the magnitude of mounting such a hoax seems out of proportion to the potential advantage that might accrue to the PRC for embarrassing the United States. Indeed, if the medical state of China was so miserable, the strength of the government's reaction to the initial outbreak of epidemics—sending out medical teams to inoculate millions of people against the potential infectious diseases that they claimed were the result of American bacteriological warfare—was very surprising. The Chinese military authorities sent three million doses of plague vaccine to the front in Korea, "and on 28 February (1952), although as yet there had been no recorded cases of army personnel affected by plague, the Chinese army in Korea began inoculating its troops against the plague" (Endicott and Hagerman 1998, 9, quoting the military memoirs of General Nie Rongzhen). They followed that up with inoculations, again in the millions, for cholera. More than a million Koreans were also inoculated, and a "massive health campaign got underway, with an emphasis on catching mice, exterminating insects, and sanitizing living quarters" (Endicott and Hagerman 1998, 9). The campaign was really enormous, focusing on the entire Chinese Northeast as a potential epidemic center, with efforts to protect water sources, sanitize toilets, and protect food sources, and to catch, kill, and burn vermin and insects. The recently opened Liaoning archives suggest that the "preventive health campaign achieved much" (Endicott and Hagerman 1998, 9).

This massive Chinese response to the outbreak, and feared outbreak, of infectious diseases may indeed be an indication that the state of Chinese public health was not as good as it might have been in 1951–52; indeed, given the protracted war against the Japanese, the civil war between the Kuomintang and Chinese Communist forces, and now the Korean War, it would be amazing if medical facilities, equipment, and staff had been in top shape. Nevertheless, that does not mean that plague, encephalitis, and respiratory anthrax were all locally generated and not the result of outside forces. As Endicott and Hagerman note:

> Though there is little question that everyone from Mao and Zhou on down used the threat of germ warfare to whip up support and volunteers for the public health effort against epidemic disease, there is also little question that the evidence convinced those in the field and Mao and Zhou Enlai that the Americans were experimenting with biological warfare, targeting armies in the field, the population, and the communications system. (Endicott and Hagerman 1998, 20–21)

American BW Capacity

There would appear, then, to be at least a good deal of circumstantial evidence that the U.S. military might have used biological warfare against its Communist enemies in northeast China and North Korea: Chinese medical reports, an international scientific investigation, and the confessions of a number of pilots. And although these were considered none too decisive at the time, there is still much in them that should be examined. Far more information is available on the Chinese side now to which some scholars give credence. But at the time, the focus was more on the American side and the assumed lack of evidence. Few knew anything about American military and civilian research involving biological warfare, and there was also an assumption, as there is today, that such forms of weapons were morally repugnant and thus beneath the United States. But there is considerable evidence that many people, both civilian and military, were not averse to using such WMD. But, first, did the United States have the capacity to deliver the kind of BW that the Communists accused it of in 1951?

The answer is an unequivocal yes. There is now plenty of evidence in government documents, and some solid secondary accounts by Sheldon Harris, Jonathan Moreno, and a host of other scholars, to show that during World War II, the United States developed a sizable biological warfare capability. The primary facility was located near Frederick, Maryland, at Camp (later Fort) Detrick, where construction began in April 1942 (see Covert 1993; see also Harris 2002, especially chap. 11, 201–15). The site ultimately housed nearly four thousand people, mostly military personnel, who were working on research projects under the direction of the U.S. Army Chemical Warfare Service (CWS). There were other facilities as well, in Mississippi, Indiana, and most importantly at Granite Peak, Utah, an isolated facility ideal for BW testing.

At Fort Detrick, the staff was engaged in wide-ranging research projects that concentrated first on anthrax—which military planners expected to use extensively until Hiroshima and Nagasaki made it irrelevant—and included the very kinds of things that the Japanese were working on in World War II and that would be at the core of Chinese accusations less than a decade later. As George Merck, of the chemical company of the same name, who was also head of the War Reserve Service (WRS), which coordinated BW, put it: "All possible living agents, or their toxic products, which were pathogenic for man, animals, and plants were considered" (Harris 2002, 210). Funding was ample, and BW was second only to the Manhattan Project in importance, number of people involved, and budget.

At the end of the war, as tensions with the Soviet Union led to the Cold War, Fort Detrick continued to be an important site for BW research, continuing the same types of projects that had been developed for use against the Axis Powers, only now this was enhanced by access to research that the United States received from the extensive work of Lt. Gen. Shirō Ishii and the staff of Unit 731, done in China. Since the Japanese had carried out extensive testing of various diseases on human subjects, American BW researchers now had a treasure trove of information at their disposal. The chapter in this volume by Dr. Kei-ichi Tsuneishi, Japan's leading authority on Unit 731, makes it unnecessary for me to do anything but summarize the outcome in Sheldon Harris's words: "Anxious to acquire Japan's BW and CW secrets, scientists at Fort Detrick waived all ethical considerations in their discussions with their Japanese counterparts as early as October 1945" (Harris 2002, 345). The result was that Japanese scientists were not tried as war criminals for their horrific experiments on human subjects, useful information from those experiments was obtained by American researchers at Fort Detrick, and the U.S. and Japanese governments knowingly participated in a cover-up of these activities. For that reason, relatively few Japanese outside academic circles know about—or perhaps it is more accurate to say, care to know about—human experimentation by Japanese scientists on POWs in China in World War II.

The Will to Use Biological and Chemical Warfare

It seems that, now that many documents have been declassified and many researchers have assiduously rolled back the layers of obfuscation that have hidden so much from view, we can say that the United States did have the capacity to carry out what was called at the time "germ warfare" (today's "bioterrorism") against the Chinese and North Koreans. But did the United States have the intention and will? In so many of the works on BW/CW (chemical warfare) by Americans, there is an underlying sense of national morality that finds such warfare repugnant; and indeed, while U.S. scientists may have been interested in knowing the results of experiments on humans by researchers in Unit 731, they did not conduct similar experiments. It may well be that the Pentagon has foresworn the possession or use of biological weapons since its announcement of such an intention in 1988. But what of the 1950s?

There seems little doubt that many in both military and civilian life were not opposed to the use of BW or CW, neither in World War II nor in the case of the Korean War. Certainly U.S. scientists were not averse to assisting in developing weapons of war that we today condemn as WMD. As Dr. Jonathan Moreno so nicely puts it, in a slightly different context, "At the risk of tarnishing American honor, moral compromises were viewed as necessary for survival in a new and bitterly divided postwar world. The hunger for forbidden fruit proved hard to quell as American scientists and defense officials placed on the drawing boards still more innovative weapons that created unknown and often undue risk for their handlers" (Moreno 2001, 117).

Many quotations from various civilian and military officials justifying the use of offensive biological weapons and tests on human subjects can be marshaled to prove that U.S. authorities clearly would have used BW in the early Cold War, when it appeared that the very doors of the liberal democratic Western political system were being beaten down by a rising tide of Communist revolution. And just as there has long been the assumption by many that the atomic bomb was deployed against the Japanese for racist reasons, certainly in the Korean war the Koreans and Chinese had been racially stereotyped and dismissed as "Gooks" and "Chinks," not to mention having been lumped together as "Godless Communists." There is little reason to believe that U.S. authorities would not have resorted to BW to save the situation in Korea. Certainly President Harry "The Buck Stops Here" Truman had not flinched from using the atomic bomb before. Indeed, he was piqued that so many scientists wrung their hands over the issue when it was after all he who had made the decision. There seems little doubt but that Truman would have employed these weapons of mass destruction as well. But there is no evidence that he did.

Conclusions

While it is true that we do not actually have a "smoking gun" or an unchallenged confession, the weight of circumstantial evidence against the United States is substantial. In the words of detective novels, the United States had motive, means, and opportunity.

The motive was to end the war. As the war was going against the United States, especially after the entry of the Chinese into the war, despite MacArthur's professed belief to the contrary, America needed everything it had to get back to even. And once the U.S. had made the negotiations even more difficult by introducing the idea of no forced repatriation, Washington was hard pressed to keep the Chinese and the North Koreans talking. American servicemen were dying at an alarming rate, and the only way to settle the war—and not allow it to escalate into World War III by involving the Soviet Union—was to make the peace negotiations with the Chinese and the North Koreans succeed. The U.S. adopted a scorched-earth policy, destroying everything in its path to force its enemies to negotiate. There were few people opposing biological means.

The means were there before the war, because the United States had already been planning for biological and chemical warfare against the Japanese. Now it had considerably more information about various forms of BW and CW, thanks to the deal struck with Ishii and other members of the notorious Unit 731. The Army, the Navy, the Air Force, and the CIA were all in the business of developing biological and chemical weapons, both at home in Fort Detrick and in Utah, and of course north of Tokyo as well, in the Far East Medical Section's 406 Medical General Laboratory and, from the spring of 1952, the 8003 Far East Medical Research Laboratory (see Endicott and Hagerman 1998, 143–52).

In Japan, both American and Japanese researchers, some of whom had been involved in biological warfare experiments during World War II, were deeply involved in biological warfare research, especially insect and mosquito vectors. Moreover, the Air Force was busy developing capability in biological warfare under the U.S. Air Force Psychological Warfare Division and its operational arm, the 581st ARC (Air Resupply and Communications Service), which provided several forms of support for CIA covert operations behind the lines in North Korea and China. So the opportunity was there as well.

But as most everyone has concluded, there is no "smoking gun," no incontrovertible paper trail that shows that American military authorities actually ordered the dropping of infected insects on Chinese and North Korean territory to in some fashion interrupt or stop their ability to wage war against UN forces. The evidence remains tantalizingly strong but circumstantial nonetheless: the U.S. had the technological wherewithal to have delivered various forms of infectious diseases; the budget for U.S. biological warfare during the Korean War rose from just over $5 billion to $345 billion; captured U.S. servicemen were discovered to have been inoculated against plague; captured U.S. pilots seem to have been given lectures on biological warfare; Korean agents trained by the CIA were captured behind enemy lines supposedly with the mission to investigate the effects of BW among Chinese and Korean troops; reputable Western scientists investigated the claims of BW and found them credible. The list is very long. Merely circumstantial evidence, but weighty nonetheless. I do not subscribe to the technological imperativist view that if you make it, you must use it. But some do.

The Korean War was fought in a totally different environment than the U.S. has known for the past forty years. For one thing, it was the last war before widespread television coverage. Telecommunications were such that, unlike the wars from Vietnam up to the current war in Iraq, Americans did not experience the Korean War so viscerally, watching it from around the dinner table. Americans read of the Korean War in the newspapers and magazines and heard reports on the radio, but had to go to the movies to see Pathé News strips showing what "our boys" were doing over there. There were no embedded journalists, and no one interviewed Kim Il Sung on the nightly news just before the invasion.

And there were no massive protests against the waging of the Korean War as there would be against the war in Vietnam. As a result, there was less distrust of what the American government told the public. Here the issue seemed clear: Communists and their sympathizers claimed that the United States had used BW and CW, weapons of mass destruction, against the enemy. But the American government denied it. And there it still rests.

Notes

1. The Supung dam also supplied electric power to northeast China, and the British were especially displeased that they were not apprised of this attack (Halliday and Cumings 1988, 188).

2. For a discussion of the statistical problems, see Tucker 2000, 1:98–101 ("Casualties" entry).

3. At this time, Endicott and Hagerman is far and away the most authoritative work on the subject, and I have endeavored to summarize this extensive work in this brief

chapter. I have not been able to access most of the Chinese primary sources on which much of their work is based; therefore, my conclusions must be tentative.

4. This is a translation of a report from a medical research team in Fushun led by Dr. Li Peilin.

5. The authors are here citing Chinese documents from the Liaoning archives.

6. Goulden dismisses this "exactitude" as "a device propagandists use to give credence to otherwise unprovable allegations" (Goulden 1982, 601). Of course, if they were vague, they would likely have been dismissed precisely because they lacked such exactitude.

7. For a good discussion of the history of the analysis of the Korean war POWs, see Carlson 2002, 1–21.

8. I am indebted to my student David Leaf for his investigation into the commission's report. His research has been an invaluable aid in the preparation of this article.

9. "Traced" may not be quite accurate here; "attributed" is more appropriate, since no research team investigated the sites and produced a contradictory report.

References

Carlson, Lewis H. 2002. *Remembered Prisoners of a Forgotten War: An Oral History of Korean War POWs.* New York: St. Martin's.

Covert, Norman M. 1993. *Cutting Edge: A History of Fort Detrick, Maryland, 1943–1993.* Fort Detrick, Md.

Crane, Conrad C. 2000. *American Airpower Strategy in Korea, 1950–1953.* Lawrence: University Press of Kansas.

Cumings, Bruce. 2004. *North Korea: Another Country.* New York: New Press.

Endicott, Stephen, and Edward Hagerman. 1998. *The United States and Biological Warfare: Secrets from the Early Cold War and Korea.* Bloomington: Indiana University Press.

Goulden, Joseph C. 1982. *Korea: The Untold Story of the War.* New York: Times Books.

Halliday, Jon, and Bruce Cumings. 1988. *Korea: The Unknown War.* New York: Pantheon Books.

Harris, Sheldon. 2002. *Factories of Death: Japanese Biological Warfare, 1932–1945, and the American Cover-up.* New York: Routledge.

Li, Xiaobing, Allan R. Millett, and Bin Yu, eds. and trans. 2001. *Mao's Generals Remember Korea.* Lawrence: University Press of Kansas.

Moreno, Jonathan. 2001. *Undue Risk: Secret State Experiments on Humans.* New York: Routledge.

New China News Agency. 1952. US Aircraft Again Drop Bacteria-Laden Insects. *Survey of China Mainland Press* (Hong Kong), Feb. 29, 1952, no. 285, pp. 2–3.

Rees, David. 1970. *Korea: The Limited War.* Baltimore: Penguin Books.

Sandler, Stanley. 1999. *The Korean War: No Victors, No Vanquished.* Lexington: University Press of Kentucky.

Toland, John. 1991. *In Mortal Combat: Korea, 1950–1953.* New York: Quill/William Morrow.

Tucker, Spencer C., ed. 2000. *Encyclopedia of the Korean War: A Political, Social, and Military History.* Santa Barbara: ABC-Clio Inc.

9 Experimental Injury: Wound Ballistics and Aviation Medicine in Mid-century America

Susan Lindee

> High speed motion pictures (2,000–2,800 frames/second) show that the abdomen of a cat swells greatly immediately after the passage of a high velocity steel sphere. . . . The general effect is that of an explosion within the abdomen.
>
> —from a manuscript for publication, W. O. Puckett, W. D. McElroy, and E. Newton Harvey, January 1945. Box W–Z, Harvey Papers

I begin by conjuring for you the image of an explosion within the abdomen of an injured cat, shot in a wartime laboratory as part of a project to develop more effective bullets. My paper focuses on experimental injury, and on the ways that, as Donna Haraway suggests, "animals hail us to account for the regimes in which they and we must live" (Haraway 2003). One of the most powerful regimes we occupy in the twenty-first century operates at the intersection of war and technical knowledge.

Over the last hundred years, biologists, physicists, engineers, psychologists, and other scientific experts have become critical to the practice of war. Indeed, war arguably has become the dominant scientific enterprise in the industrialized world, absorbing more funding, time, and personnel than any other single technically driven domain. Nuclear, biological, and chemical weapons, now feared for their potential use by terrorists, are all products of scientific expertise. Meteorology became a science in response to the demands of air power (Jonasson 1958); ornithologists played a role in Pacific weapons testing (see range of essays in MacLeod 2000); the shape of modern bullets reflects laboratory research in wound ballistics (Prokosch 1995, 1–29; Harvey 1948); nuclear missiles use advanced computing technologies (MacKenzie 2000, 1–94); and the high quality of care now available in an urban emergency room reflects medical experience with battlefield trauma (see Cooter, Harrison, and Sturdy 1999). War, science, and the healing arts of medicine are bound up tightly together in twentieth-century history.

"Public health in reverse" is a term usually used to refer to biological weapons, but I want to expand the meaning and suggest that other technical realms devoted to producing human injury were versions of public health in reverse (see Balmer 2002). They involved the application of the sophisticated mathematical and experimental arsenal of Western science to the production of greater, more efficient, more reliable bodily damage. As Larry Owens has suggested, ballistics has been the quintessential science, linking Galileo and the Aberdeen Proving Ground in a single arc of technical knowledge geared to the needs of the sovereign state (Owens 2004; see also Prokosch 1995, 1–29).

In this article, I track some elements of this convergence of technical expertise and the state's monopoly on violence, focusing on two scientific enterprises as they evolved in the United States during and immediately after the 1939–45 war. Wound ballistics and aviation medicine both involved the creation of controlled, experimental wounds. Aviation medicine had its origins in studies in the 1880s and later of the biomedical consequences of high-altitude climbing and travel by hot-air balloon; wound ballistics began in studies in the 1840s of the effects of rifled firearms. Terminal ballistics, the study of the general physical effects of projectiles, has a long history stretching back to the scientific revolution, but wound ballistics reflected battlefield experience with weapons that damaged flesh in unexpected ways. Both enterprises are still underway—with specialized journals, international conferences, and so on. These two research programs during World War II and the Cold War were linked by their relevance to national security and by their embeddedness in the familiar networks of mid-century techno-scientific mobilization in the United States. They were also linked sociologically, centering around a group of researchers at Yale and Princeton universities, some of whom worked on both topics.

In twentieth-century scientific research, human and animal bodies were experimentally starved, shelled, drowned, dropped from high places, shot through the abdomen, irradiated, or subjected to decompression or blunt trauma. Animals were surrogate humans in this military research. Their bodies were damaged in order to improve weapons technology. Technical experts in the United States studied bodies wounded in the lab and wounded on the battlefield. They studied body armor and radiation effects at high altitudes. They mapped the soldier's cartography in configurations that reflected not function or structure, but relative vulnerability to missiles. Diagrams depicted, for example, a soldier's body divided into segments that are more or less likely to be the sites of fatal wounds, or the anatomic location of 6,003 hits on 850 people killed in action in Italy (both from Coates and Beyer 1962). Such maps could reveal patterns, showing where a wound was more likely to produce death, with the surface of the body presented in terms of organs differentially relevant to incapacity and death. Similarly, when the Yale physiologist John Fulton was helping to plan a wound ballistics program, he described the brain to a colleague as "a semi-fluid substance, suspended by fairly inelastic attachments in the cerebro-spinal fluid in a rigid box." This was a way of seeing the brain as a target for a bullet: Fulton selected those properties of the brain relevant to its demolition by firearms (Fulton to Harvey, September 29, 1943, Harvey Papers).

In such enterprises, technical knowledge could function simultaneously to facilitate both healing and injuring. Pilots were made nauseated experimentally in order to discover techniques that would prevent such nausea and permit them to continue bombing runs. And cats were shot in order both to develop more destructive projectiles and to determine better healing methods. Technological and scientific innovations that produced injury in some people were commonly construed as protecting others: all increases in the effectiveness of weapons enhance their capacity to injure enemies and therefore protect allies. And innovations that protected or healed were commonly intended to allow those healed to injure others. So, for example, we have Malcolm C. Grow, a Philadelphia physician who fought in World War I and became a leading researcher in aviation medicine during World War II. He developed body armor for pilots, electrically warmed clothing for flight crews, fire-resistant neck protection, and special combat rations for long flights. In other words, Grow played a critical role in enhancing the survival of pilots and crews on bombing runs and thereby enabling them to continue to drop bombs. In a related manner, economists helped guide World War II bombing runs: if you knew how economies worked, you also knew how to undermine them.[1] Urban fire control experts, who knew how to prevent cities from burning, also knew how to make them burn faster (see Eden 2004); and psychiatrists who understood mental health planned dirty tricks, propaganda campaigns, and psychological torture strategies (see Gilmore 1998).

The fact that those injured, in these cases, would be persons identified as enemies of the United States has no particular bearing on the problem. The quandary is that science, possibly the most impressive and promising expression of the human mind, has facilitated the infliction of as much damage to people all over the world as any of the psyche's less savory capabilities. It has done so, furthermore, even in the acts of protecting, shielding, and healing. The late French theorist Michel Foucault once said that knowledge was not made for understanding, it was made for cutting (Foucault and Rabinow 1984, 88). In the sciences and technologies of war, understanding and cutting often function together. My work suggests that it is important to notice this, and to think critically about it, because the consequences of technical knowledge matter to us all.

Wound Ballistics

Studies of the effects of firearms on living flesh were carried out by military experts as early as 1848, when rifled firearms began to produce wounds that appeared to be the result of an "explosive effect." Injury from these wounds extended far beyond the actual path of the projectile, a phenomenon that was the subject of much speculation. The American researcher Charles Woodruff in 1898 compared the effect to that produced by moving a hand through bathwater: The "particles of fluid making way for the bullet are given a tremendous centrifugal velocity, which they impart to all surrounding particles" (Woodruff 1898, cited in Prokosch 1995, 11–13). In 1916 and 1917, U.S. Army doctor Louis

Wilson fired a gun into gelatin shot through with black threads so that he could track the movement produced by the bullets. He modeled his gelatin's density and resistance to reflect the varying degrees of softness of body tissues, and he concluded from his work that "the softer the organ or tissue the further away from the track of the missile will serious secondary results of injuries occur" (Wilson 1921, cited in Prokosch 1995, 13–14).

A few years later Army investigators at the Aberdeen Proving Ground in Maryland began shooting anesthetized pigs and goats. They carefully placed metal screens both in front of and behind the targets, so that the velocities of bullets as they entered and emerged could be measured. By this means, they could calculate how much velocity was lost. They found that there was a threshold of about 2,500 feet per second, above which the character of the wound began to change radically. This observation was to have an impact on weapons designers in the ensuing decades (see Prokosch 1995, 14–15).

After 1939, British groups began exploring the effects of high-explosive bombs as a reaction to German bombardment. A team of scientists from the anatomy department at Oxford University, including the distinguished zoologist, and later lord, Solly Zuckerman, shot animals and gelatin blocks and used "spark shadowgraphy" to photograph the external changes in the targets. They were able to document the expansion of gelatin to three to four times its original volume at the moment when the missile passed through it. "Precisely the same changes occur in human or animal tissues that are traversed by high velocity missiles," they wrote. "The distortion to which they are subjected can only be likened to that of an internal explosion" (Black, Burns, and Zuckerman 1941, cited in Prokosch 1995, 16–17). That such research might pose an ethical problem—in that it involved the production of knowledge that was both offensive and defensive at the same time—did not occur to Zuckerman. Many years later, the defense expert and pacifist scholar Eric Prokosch asked him about this dilemma, and Zuckerman replied that "the question of ethics was not one which posed itself at the time during the Second World War." (This exchange is described in Proskosch 1995, 17.)

The American wound ballistics program that began in 1943 documented the effects of missiles with unprecedented rigor and mathematical certainty. Carried out after 1943 primarily at Princeton University, under the guidance of physiologist E. Newton Harvey, it remains a touchstone of high technical quality and careful data collection in the wound ballistics community.

It began after R. H. Kent, a ballistics expert at Aberdeen Proving Ground, outlined the need for a more scientific program to "obtain knowledge of the wounding power of fragments as related to their weight and velocity." The goal was to determine the "most efficient design and use of anti-personnel missiles" (Kent 1943; for a published summary of the project and its development, see Harvey 1948). The proposal called for the production of scientifically controlled wounds that could be used to predict events on the battlefield. Ideally, Kent said, this knowledge would be correct in absolute terms, which is to say that it could be used to predict the actual number of casualties to be caused by a particular missile. In practice, of course, a numerical prediction was impossible. Due to the many variations in field conditions, estimates of absolute numbers of casualties were "likely to be subject to great error." Fortunately, however, the data could simply be comparative rather than absolute. Some kinds of projectiles would be more likely to produce more wounds than others. The ballistician and technician needed to know which kinds.[2]

The longing expressed here, for a predictable battlefield with a guaranteed number of kills from every missile, suggests some of the key threads in the deep consensus underlying these research programs. Scientific research was expected to control and rationalize the chaotic process of war. This expectation depended on the assumption that the chaos was not a fundamental property of organized, socially sanctioned violence, but an aberration, reflecting inadequate statistics, poorly standardized technologies, inappropriate rules, and so on. This is the classic perspective of modernity, as defined by Max Weber and others, with its emphasis on reason, bureaucracy, and the technical management of disorder. Weber himself made the comparison to the army: modernity was militaristic in its longing for rules that operated without regard to persons. This longing, I suggest, was manifest in particularly stark and transparent ways in the wound ballistics research program.

Harvey, who oversaw the research on wound ballistics at Princeton, also worked on aviation medicine (decompression sickness). His research before 1943 dealt with bioluminescence in Pacific organisms. He was experienced with the problems of diving, and this kind of knowledge prepared him to work on the problems of pilots. While his work in aviation medicine, then, reflected prior expertise, the work in wound ballistics involved entirely new forms of knowledge. At the request of representatives of the Committee on Medical Research, which was the medical arm of the U.S. Office of Scientific Research and Development, his laboratory became the center of the wartime and postwar wound ballistics program. The initial request came from his friend John Fulton at Yale (and Fulton was also chair of the committee on aviation medicine). Harvey's work on wound ballistics began in October 1943 and was completed in February 1946.

Most of the research was conducted in the Biological Laboratories at Princeton University, where Harvey had a team of five biologists working with him.[3] He also had ballistics and X-ray technicians. The laboratory contained a smooth-bore .30 caliber gun mounted so that it was aimed at a wooden backstop, on which the anesthetized cats were photographed as they were shot. There were several instruments for recording the velocity of the bullet, the shock wave, and the X-ray image. Westinghouse built the X-ray apparatus. The chronograph was borrowed from Aberdeen Proving Ground in Maryland. The group had an 8 mm Faxtax and a 16 mm Eastman camera. Imaging technologies, missile technologies, and organismic technologies came together in a small room in the Princeton biology labs. The wound events recorded in this laboratory became the basis of scientific papers, written by Harvey and his coworkers, that answered the question: How would it be possible to maximize the severity of wounds produced by firearms?

For the purposes of their research, it would have been preferable if both bullet and target could be "full size." An animal about the size of a human being would have provided a closer guide to battlefield wound events. But Harvey did not have room on his campus even for goats (the original species considered), and in the interests of economy, Harvey's team reduced the size of both missile and target in proportion. "A .4 gram missile moving 2,700 fps and striking a 3-kg animal represents a situation, so far as mass of missile and mass of target are concerned, analogous to those of standard army rifle ammunition and the human body" (see Harvey et al. 1962, 147; Harvey 1948). The "3-kg" animal he referred to here was the cat.[4]

This group used high-speed cameras to take pictures at a rate of 8,000 frames per second of the "changes which occur when a high-velocity bullet enters soft tissue" (Harvey et al. 1962, cited in Coates and Beyer 1962, 147). The wound occurs in a few thousandths of a second, but Harvey's team could make these rapid events visible, with high speed and X-ray photography.

In other experiments in the spring of 1945, Harvey's assistant I. M. Korr suspended tissues (frog hearts, cat guts) and living guppies in tanks through which missiles were fired, to test the indirect effects on living tissue of shots fired into liquid. In one experiment, twenty-two excised frog hearts, twelve anesthetized guppies, and the gut of a cat were all exposed to the water pressure produced by a bullet (see Korr 1945). The researchers also shot human flesh. Human skin was obtained from the abdominal regions of fresh cadavers, cut into strips, mounted, and then shot with steel spheres ranging in size from 2/32″ to 8/32″ diameter at impact velocities from 1,300 ft./sec. to 4,000 ft./sec. In some experiments a single layer of skin was used, in others multiple layers. This permitted the group to calculate the "critical velocity for skin entry": 170 ft./sec.

Different parts of the cat's bodies were shot and studied. One image in the group's 1948 paper shows an abdomen of a cat shaved and marked with a grid pattern that can make the distortion produced by the bullet visible; others show parts of cat bodies, such as a colon with an air pocket used in shooting experiments. Shooting a living cat's head caused the skull to break apart at the sutures, but an empty skull showed only an exit and entry hole, demonstrating the role of the tissue itself in the most devastating effects of these weapons (Butler, Grundfest, and Korr 1945). The energy of the bullet was transferred to the soft tissues, and they rapidly moved away from the path, thus acting like "secondary missiles." The body's own substance, set in motion by the bullet, was the agent of most of the damage.

Harvey's team wanted to quantify this damage and calculate the "law of force which retards the missile." They found that the resistance to the missile was proportional to the square of the missile's velocity. The retardation coefficient of living cat muscle measured the loss of velocity that a sphere experienced in going through the thigh. Wound events were carefully made into technical abstractions, which thereby enhanced their application to other problems. Thus Harvey proposed that it would be possible to use the equations based on their experiments to calculate "how many milligrams of TNT exploded within the body will produce a temporary cavity whose maximum volume is the same as that of a missile of a given weight striking the body with given velocity" (Harvey 1948, 197).

Surely he was not proposing that anyone planned to place carefully measured TNT in a human body and explode it. Rather, he was making a claim about the generality of his experimental wounds. His equations could capture the bodily effects on any type of tissue, of any form of energy. Cat muscle and human muscle, TNT and bullets, were circulating and equivalent entities in the calculations of wound ballistics experts.

In November of 1950, as the Korean War began, a different kind of research subject became available, and the body of the soldier, wounded or killed in the field, became a form of experimental evidence. Small casualty surveys had been carried out in World War I, and injuries and wounds in both Allied and enemy soldiers 1939–45 had been studied and catalogued late in World War II. But the work in Korea started with the outbreak of hostilities and was carried out by field researchers who tracked and catalogued wounds and mortar fragments using the methods of natural history: they classified, compared, and named the objects that they collected.

This reflected an emerging perspective on the battlefield, widely shared after 1940, in which it doubled as a laboratory, producing not just military results but also scientific ones. Battlefields increasingly came to be understood by scientists, engineers, physicians, and even generals as open-air laboratories, testing grounds for new technologies and for the production of large numbers of destroyed buildings, burned cities, and grievously wounded, gassed, traumatized, or disfigured subjects. All these damaged entities—people, cities, factories, societies—could be used to gain new technical knowledge *that could then be productively applied in civilian life.*

The scale of this battlefield experimentation is part of what I am trying to map in my larger project, but it is clear that it is much more expansive than practitioner accounts in atomized individual fields might lead us to realize. The battlefield laboratory interested many kinds of physicians and medical researchers, of course—the claim that war is "good for" medicine refers to the experimental and experiential value of the battlefield for medical experts. But the battlefield laboratory also interested chemists, psychologists, statisticians, economists, engineers, fire control experts, entomologists, biologists, and others.[5]

The Korean War, coming after the practices of the battlefield laboratory had become well established during World War II, was a particularly productive research site. New technologies and interventions were scientifically tested in Korea from the earliest days of the war, as the post hoc surveys of Italy and France were replaced by real-time field research in wound ballistics in Korea.

From November 1950 until May of 1951, Carl M. Herget, an Army Ph.D. who had been working for several years on body armor, Captain George Coe, a member of the chemical corps, and physician Major James Beyer of the Medical Corps worked together in Korea. They were the Wound Ballistics Survey of the Medical Research and Development Board of the Surgeon General's Office of the Department of Army. Their survey included studies of wound events produced on the battlefield and of body armor and its protective qualities (Herget, Coe, and Beyer 1962).

In the charts and diagrams that made up most of their final report, the team presented data on 7,773 wounds in 4,600 persons. Through their careful analysis of frontline events and soldiers' bodies, they found that much of the ammunition on the battlefield was basically wasted. Most fragments from most bombs hit no one, and, at least in Korea at this point in the war, small arms killed or wounded very few soldiers (Coates and Beyer 1962; see also Harvey et al. 1962). Only 7.5 percent of all casualties were caused by small arms, while 92 percent of casualties were the result of mortar and grenade fragments. Like geologists or ornithologists, the wound ballistics researchers collected field objects that could be placed in relationship to each other and to their natural consequences. Fragments of bombs and grenades from killed soldiers were placed in order to compare their size and shape. The diversity of the technological world of war was subsumed under the methods of natural science.

Eventually, as their fieldwork progressed, the relevant sciences came to include sociology. Without quite intending to do so, the experimenters carried out a sociological study of the impact of scarcity. This was during their field test of a form of self-defense, body armor. By early 1953, the Army had about 122,000 body armor vests in use in the field in Korea. These were fiberglass-nylon multilayer vests that weighed about six or seven pounds. The Wound Ballistics team wanted to figure out if soldiers wearing vests were more likely to survive, so they attempted to use the vests in a controlled scientific study during real battle. In other words, there were not enough vests for everyone. The controls in this experiment were very distressed, and a wounded soldier was likely to have his vest stolen from him in battle (which meant that the vest could not be tested and examined by those compiling data). This also made it more difficult for the team to figure out who had been wearing a vest when actually hit and who had not. Demand for the vest "became so acute" in one campaign that the researchers "lost control of the vest study." Soldiers were wrapping multiple vests around their heads and groins, taking vests from injured comrades and even taking vests removed from injured soldiers at the hospital (Herget, Coe, and Beyer 1962, cited in Coates and Beyer 1962, 744). The scientific field study, intended to provide reliable data on body armor and survival, was swamped by the chaotic conditions in the domain under study.

Wound ballistics thus involved both laboratory and field research, and experimental and "natural" wounding and protecting. The knowledge it produced was expected both to save soldiers' lives and to enhance their ability to kill others. Similarly, aviation medicine focused on knowledge that could both protect bomber crews and enhance injury to enemy populations on the ground.

Aviation Medicine

In aviation medicine, this equation was sometimes made explicit. So, for example, in a foreword to a 1951 conference held at Randolph Field, Texas, USAF Major General H. G. Armstrong said that the effectiveness of the Air Force was measured in terms of combat striking power, and combat striking power depended on healthy crews (Armstrong 1952). The Air Force Medical Service was therefore the maintenance division for the "human component" in an efficient man-machine complex. Pilots needed to be kept healthy and alert so that they would be able to carry out their bombing missions.

Aviation medicine was an extremely complex, multidisciplinary enterprise. By the 1960s this research involved physicians, physiologists, engineers, anthropologists, mathematicians, psychologists, and other experts, as well as pilots, technicians, divers, and military leaders. An airborne pilot was a cyborg, a human body surrounded by machine parts and atmospheric phenomena, which could be managed only by attention to all levels of the experience. Research in aviation medicine encompassed studies not only of pilots' bodies but of helmets, goggles, clothing, anti-g suits, cold chambers, and safety devices (see Report to A. N. Richards 1943).

One of the earliest historians of aviation medicine was the Yale physiologist John Fulton, who also had overseen the wound ballistics program and who founded the program in the history of medicine at Yale.[6] Fulton was also one of the leading proponents of psychosurgery, especially lobotomy, in the United States (see Pressman 1998).

Fulton tracked the origins of aviation medicine to Robert Boyle's work in the 1640s with the air-pump, inasmuch as he viewed all scientific study of oxygen as relevant to the survival of crews at high altitudes. But a more proper starting place might be the effort by French and British scientists to decipher the effects of high altitude on climbers in the nineteenth century (see Bert 1878). Mountain sickness was both a military and a colonial problem, and climbers were sometimes accompanied by medical experts who tracked the result of low oxygen on Pike's Peak, or later in the Andes, during the International High Altitude Expedition of 1935 (Barcroft et al. 1921–23).

Decompression sickness, important in diving, was not expected to be a problem in aviation in the 1930s, because it would take a long time to reach a height at which pilots would be affected. But as the war geared up in 1939, and more crews were airbound and flying at altitudes of up to 35,000 feet, reports of decompression symptoms appeared in the scientific literature in nearly all belligerent countries (Hoff and Fulton [1942] cataloged these reports).

In September 1940 the U.S. National Research Council, as a part of the general mobilization of science in the United States, appointed a Committee on Aviation Medicine, which immediately turned its attention to decompression sickness. Frederick G. Banting, at Toronto, was already using human subjects in his research at a new aeromedical laboratory, as were researchers at a diving unit run by A. R. Behnke at the National Institutes of Health in Washington, at the Mayo Clinic, and at several centers in Britain (see Boothby, Lovelace, and Benson 1939–40; Air Corps News Letter 1941; Behnke 1942; Matthews 1944).

By 1942, Carl Schmidt at the University of Pennsylvania was placing human subjects in a refrigerated decompression chamber to study the effects of low oxygen and low temperature on respiratory, cardiovascular, and visual functions; Robert Wilkins at Evans Memorial Hospital was making subjects black out by stressing their circulation systems; Wallace Fenn at the University of Rochester was placing subjects in a tank with their head protruding through a rubber collar while pressure was applied to the body to test blood pressure; and Henry Ricketts at the University of Chicago was keeping people in low-oxygen conditions for six hours each day, for six weeks, in order to test the long-term consequences of prolonged anoxia. (Actually, Ricketts was trying to do this, but not entirely succeeding: "Dr. Ricketts reports great difficulty in securing subjects to carry out his plan of using one subject at a time for a period of weeks.") (For descriptions of all these projects, see Report to A. N. Richards 1943.) This was normal science that was intended to create a controlled form of human injury and new knowledge.

At first, the machines to test the limits of bodily endurance were built by companies that also made amusement park rides. Yale scientist Harold Lamport spent half of the summer of 1942 visiting such parks, trying to find the most nauseating rides. Lamport told Fulton that the "Spitfire" and "Rolloplane" seemed promising, and the Eyerly Aircraft Company of Salem, Oregon, was willing to produce a faster laboratory version of the Rolloplane for five thousand dollars. This would reach a speed of 50 rpm in five to ten seconds. "The ready shifting of the pivoted car suggests its use for studying lateral and negative acceleration as well as the more usual positive direction," Lamport said (Lamport to Fulton, September 18, 1942, Box 105, Folder 1435, Fulton Papers; see also Fulton 1948a). He included with this letter his own sketch, from memory, of the ride. Here surely is an example of the movement of technical knowledge from outside the laboratory to inside it!

Meanwhile the Subcommittee on Decompression Sickness of the OSRD was placing undergraduates at Yale into decompression chambers to figure out whether some individuals were resistant to the bends. They found that about half of these students were able to withstand exposure to 38,000 feet for three hours without symptoms (Report to A. N. Richards 1943). Other groups were trying to decide what to do about "the anxiety state in combat flying." Captain Eugene Du Bois of the U.S. Office of Naval Research summarized the problem in a 1945 report about what was variously called "flying fatigue," "flying stress," and even "lack of moral fiber" or "cowardice." The likelihood of pilots experiencing such stresses, he proposed, followed a standard Gaussian curve (though he had not constructed such a curve based on data), and among the factors that could produce this stress were "enemy action" and the "sight of friends being killed" (Report, Fulton, January 27, 1943, point 17, Fulton Papers). Du Bois hoped that collecting data about this stress could facilitate its control.

Pilots in the new Army Air Corps were vulnerable not only to the effects of rapid changes in atmospheric pressure, but also to crash injuries specific to air travel and to the physiological effects of deceleration. A study organized by Hugh de Haven at the Cornell Medical College, and continued with the oversight of the Committee on Aviation Medicine of the National Research Council, focused on the scientific study of midrange crashes. There was no point, study organizers noted, in tracking trivial accidents, or in tracking "accidents of such severity that the plane was completely disintegrated" (Du Bois 1948, 223).They therefore studied crashes that involved serious but survivable injury, and found that most serious injuries in early crashes were to the head and the face. Minimizing those injuries would require the cooperation of the airline industry. The cockpit, as it was constructed in 1940, was filled with hazards for the pilot, including an instrument panel "bristling with projections" and poorly designed control wheels (ibid.).The "Crash Injury Conferences" that began in 1943 focused on bringing together air force, air industry, and scientists to determine how to make cockpits safer (ibid.). (The three-point safety belt originated with this research.)

At the Aeromedical Unit of the Mayo Clinic and the Aeromedical Laboratory at the University of Southern California, human centrifuges were used to expose experimental subjects to the extreme changes in speed that could be expected in flight during war. Radial and linear acceleration could produce vertigo, disorientation, nausea, and even unconsciousness if they were dramatic enough, and experimentally producing this unconsciousness could provide insight into how to control it. Film recorded the facial expressions of subjects who were brought to this physiological state of crisis by artificial means. A portable oscillographic unit developed at the University of Virginia could even be placed in an airplane and used, with a motion picture camera, to track the consequences of the transition from 1 to 5 g. The sagging of loose tissues of the face, reduction of blood content of the ear, disappearance of the ear pulse, blackout, and semiconsciousness, followed by a period of disorientation and then full return to normal functioning, provided "factual and quantitative data" of tremendous value to the Army Air Corps (Landis 1948, 242).

Aviation medicine was thus a field built around a technology that exposed human beings to unnatural conditions. Early in this enterprise the human components in planes were often seen as just as malleable as the machines they would control. A popular strategy was to attempt to change the bodies of the pilot and crew, rather than to change the airplane. So for example in 1941 and 1942, pilots were given drugs that researchers hoped would permit them to tolerate lower levels of oxygen. Later, when it became clear that night vision would be important to hitting enemy targets, crews were given high doses of vitamin A. Similarly, the inhalation of oxygen prior to flight as a method to prevent decompression pains was tried and widely adopted (Bronk, 1948, 207). Both the machine and the body of the pilot could be reshaped as a result of this biomedical research.

Biomedicine was as much a Cold War science as physics. Detlev Bronk proposed in 1948 that biologists were as important as engineers and physicists to the productive use of air power. He said physicists and engineers had developed machines that could not be used by human beings, and then, "the progress of aviation again awaited the assistance of the biologist" (Bronk 1948, 207).

At the same time, physicians and other medical experts were called on by those involved in wound ballistics to become experts not only of wounds, but of "weapons and missile identification." Every physician, one report suggested, should be trained in the recognition of mortar or grenade fragments or radiation burns because "all doctors now may anticipate military service or the responsibility for civilian populations under the fire of every conceivable weapon" (Coates and Beyer 1962, 724). The bodies to be injured in future wars could be expected to be everywhere—partly as a result of the air power capabilities that aviation medicine enhanced.

Conclusion

In 1946, thirty-four normal young men were starved in a Minnesota laboratory, given only a "European type famine diet averaging daily 1,790 calories." They lost from twenty-seven to sixty-five pounds, and they showed muscular weakness, depression, sensations of cold, and "unremitting hunger" (Summary of Reports Received . . . 1946, 776). The experimental human starvation, described in a Committee on Medical Research report, was produced in a laboratory in order to gain practical knowledge of the impact of one kind of bodily injury—the injury produced by inadequate food—on surrogate soldiers. Injuring, wounding, protecting, and starving were scientific activities, often on a rather grand scale.

In an army report on wound ballistics, published by the Office of the Surgeon General in 1962 (Coates and Beyer 1962), the photographs of cats, bullets, lung X-rays, mortar fragments, and field hospitals were joined by a series of postmortem photographs of soldiers shot or blown apart in various ways. These photographs are gruesome, but they are also technical images demonstrating what a bullet does when it pierces a helmet or enters the thorax at the third right intercostal space, or showing how a land mine produces evisceration. The pictures are informative on multiple levels. They can permit medical experts to examine the kinds of injuries that war produces, and thereby prepare them to manage those injuries. But they also provide testimony to the difficulties of turning such bodily damage into quantitative charts—the difficulties of managing the body of the soldier as a rational resource. The bodily consequences of a land mine are sufficiently chaotic to subvert the project within which the photographs are embedded. The body's testimony, here and perhaps always, can be unruly.

Much of this militarized research reflected the urge to quantify, to chart, and thereby to make the chaotic conditions of the battlefield into something that could be governed by reason. Indeed, the longing to rationalize the battlefield is a moving subtheme in the letters and reports. The wounds produced were rational themselves: cats were shot to help ballistics experts improve weapons, and subjects were nauseated to help pilots survive. These acts "make sense" in twentieth-century culture.

I will follow the early twentieth-century biologist and philosopher Ludwik Fleck in suggesting that those things seen to be neutral or rational—those things understood to be outside of the realm of emotion—are precisely the things around which crucial values and assumptions are expressed. Fleck, in his shrewd psychosocial analysis of knowledge and emotion, proposed that emotion is everywhere, in every act, and if and when emotion seems to disappear, then that point of disappearance is a point of critical consensus. It is as though Fleck construed neutrality and rationality as cultural blind spots. They were, his analysis suggested, notions around which the consensus was so thick that emotion could seem to be absent (Fleck 1979). But what was the nature of the consensus that made shooting cats or starving soldiers emotionally flat, or neutral? What were participants agreeing about exactly?

In her 1982 paper "Hand, Brain, and Heart," the feminist philosopher Hilary Rose noted that the scientific revolution in the seventeenth century was the result of the fusion of two kinds of labor that had earlier been seen as fundamentally incompatible (Rose 1983). Physical labor had long been marked as socially inferior to the labor of the mind, but the new sciences brought together the labor of the head and the hand—of thinking and doing—and the new experimentalists manipulated the material world in order to understand it. Mere thought was no longer enough; the new natural philosophy required experiment. Yet as Rose pointed out, at the same historical moment that the head and the hand came together, another kind of labor was radically excluded. Caring labor, the labor of the heart, was construed by the early architects of modern science as inimical to objectivity, reason, and truth. Just as physical labor had been associated with the lower classes, so emotional labor was associated with women, who were found by the new sciences to be unreliable knowers on multiple levels. Emotions were as suspect and threatening as women, and modern science was therefore literally concocted out of the erasure of emotion. This is part of the reason that introducing caring labor into the practice of science has been so vexed: emotion, caring, violates one of the founding narratives of modern science.

When E. Newton Harvey was first asked to participate in wound ballistics research in the fall of 1943, he responded hesitantly. He said he was not a surgeon or pathologist, and knew nothing of the human body and how it was damaged. Furthermore, he said, "I would not be interested in a casualty survey, either at the front or in hospitals in the USA, as this subject would be too distressing to me. The theoretical aspects of wound ballistics, however, are very interesting" (Harvey to Fulton, October 5, 1943, Harvey Papers). What were the theoretical aspects of wound ballistics? What theories apply here? I would suggest that perhaps Fleck's theory of rational neutrality as a product of so-cial consensus and Rose's theory of the necessary erasure of emotion are most relevant.

Like my actors, who expected that the experimental wounds they produced would have more general relevance, I want my story to provide a way of seeing the relationships between government-sponsored research and experimental wounding more generally. I propose that wound ballistics and aviation medicine can be used to pry open mid-century state science at the point at which a cat gets shot or a pilot is subjected to mechanically induced nausea. Their stories can thereby suggest the centrality of injuring to many forms of biomedical knowledge. I construct this injuring not as aberration or pathology—not as an abridgement of knowledge production as usual—but as quintessentially nor-mal, the product of a deep consensus that we are called upon as scholars to understand and elucidate.

My fragmentary and exploratory paper here does not resolve the problems. It is, however, an effort to frame some questions. It is a research map that es-tranges experimental wounding and that reflects the grand question of why and how injured bodies have been understood to instantiate political power. I sug-gest that in practice, the exact kind of evidence provided by a wound in the laboratory, the urban center, or the battlefield is not obvious, and that the ex-perimental wound may therefore be a critical starting point for the assessment of twentieth-century science.

Notes

1. There is a fascinating discussion of this in Eden 2004. See also, for a somewhat different use of economic knowledge as an aid to government policy, Perkins 2004.

2. This might be the memo that began the project. It was sent to Lewis Weed Sep-tember 6, 1943, and it was included later that month in the minutes of the first meeting of the National Research Council Division of Medical Sciences Conference on Wound Ballistics held in Washington, D.C., September 25, 1943. Minutes are in Box W–Z, Har-vey Papers.

3. Photographs of the wound ballistics laboratory are in BH262, Harvey Wound Bal-listic Typewritten Reports #5, Harvey Papers.

4. Cats were also used in research on motion sickness and aviation medicine. The flight surgeon Isaac H. Jones in the 1930s dropped cats from various heights and photo-graphed their fall, with variations: blindfolds, surgically damaged ears, and so on (Jones 1937, 114). Kittens were also used in studies of water compression—they were sub-merged up to their necks in water and subjected to compression so rapid it lasted less than 1/1000th of a second. The kittens suffered hemorrhage, fractures, and concussion. This is described in a report by J. W. Ward of Vanderbilt University (Ward 1946).

5. Steve Sturdy has suggested that chemical weapons facilitated the mingling of physiology and battlefield research after 1915. Both physiologists and military com-manders began to speak of the "theater of war itself as a vast experimental ground . . .

[with] human beings providing the material for these experiments" (the British director of Gas Services C. H. Foulkes, in Cooter, Harrison, and Sturdy 1998, 74). He suggests that both medical scientists and military thinkers were "coming to share a view of the war itself as an experimental enterprise, in which new techniques of warfare were continually being developed and tested, and in which the line of demarcation between the laboratory and the battlefield was increasingly blurred." Sturdy emphasizes the degree to which this way of thinking shaped scientific research, so that animals injured by chemicals in the lab were referred to as "casualties," and in how the community of physiologists became advisers to the Army not only in relation to chemical weapons, but also regarding nutrition, the prevention of work-related illness, and surgical shock.

6. Fulton's treatment of aviation medicine remains a critical resource; see Fulton 1948b.

References

Air Corps News Letter. 1941. Washington, D.C.

Andrus, E. C., et al., eds. 1948. *Advances in Military Medicine.* Boston: Little, Brown and Co.

Armstrong, Harry G. 1952. *Principles and Practices of Aviation Medicine.* 3rd ed. Baltimore Williams and Wilkins.

Balmer, Brian. 2002. Killing "Without the Distressing Preliminaries": Scientists' Defence of the British Biological Warfare Programme. *Minerva* 40: 57–75.

Barcroft, J., et al. 1921–23. Observations upon the Effect of High Altitude on the Physiological Process of the Human Body, Carried Out in the Peruvian Andes, Chiefly at Cerro de Pasco. *Philosophical Transactions of the Royal Society,* B, 211: 351–480.

Behnke, A. R. 1942. Physiological Studies Pertaining to Deep Sea Diving and Aviation, especially in Relation to the Fat Content and Composition of the Body. *Bulletin of the New York Academy of Medicine* 18, no. 2: 561–85.

Bert, Paul. 1878. *La Pression barometrique.* Paris: Libraire de L-Academie de Medecin.

Black, A. N., B. D. Burns, and Solly Zuckerman. 1941. An Experimental Study of the Wounding Mechanism of High-Velocity Missiles. *British Medical Journal* 20 (December): 872–74.

Boothby, W. M., W. R. Lovelace, and O. O. Benson. 1939–40. High Altitude and Its Effect on the Human Body. *Journal of Aernoautical Science* 7: 461–68.

Bronk, Detlev. 1948. Introduction: Aviation Medicine. In *Advances in Military Medicine,* ed. E. C. Andrus et al., 1:207–21. Boston: Little, Brown and Co.

Butler, E. G., Harry Grundfest, and I. M. Korr. 1945. Ballistic Studies on Human Skin. Washington Meeting Report. May 10, 1945. Typewritten Report #5. Harvey Papers.

Coates, J. B., and J. C. Beyer. 1962. *Wound Ballistics.* Washington, D.C.: Office of the Surgeon General, Department of the Army. Online at http://history.amedd.army.mil/booksdocs/wwii/woundblstcs/default.htm.

Cooter, Roger, Mark Harrison, and Steve Sturdy, eds. 1998. *War, Medicine and Modernity.* Phoenix Mill, Gloucestershire, U.K.: Sutton Publishing.

———. 1999. *Medicine and Modern Warfare.* Amsterdam: Rodopi.

Du Bois, Eugene F. 1948. The Study of Crash Injuries and Prevention of Aircraft Accidents. In E. C. Andrus et al., eds., 222–31.

Eden, Lynn. 2004. *Whole World on Fire: Organizations, Knowledge and Nuclear Weapons Devastation*. Ithaca, N.Y.: Cornell University Press.

Fleck, Ludwik. 1979. *The Genesis and Development of a Scientific Fact*. Chicago: University of Chicago Press. Originally published in German (Basel: Benno Schwabe Co., 1935).

Foucault, Michel, and Paul Rabinow. 1984. *The Foucault Reader*. New York: Random House.

Fulton, John F. 1948a. Altitude Decompression Sickness. In *Advances in Military Medicine*, ed. E. C. Andrus, et al., 1:318–30.

———. 1948b. *Aviation Medicine in Its Preventive Aspects: An Historical Survey*. London: Oxford University Press.

Fulton Papers. The Papers of John F. Fulton. Yale University Library, New Haven.

Gilmore, Allison B. 1998. *You Can't Fight Tanks with Bayonets: Psychological Warfare against the Japanese Army in the Southwest Pacific*. Lincoln: University of Nebraska Press.

Haraway, Donna. 2003. *The Companion Species Manifesto: Dogs, People, and Significant Otherness*. Chicago: Prickly Paradigm Press.

Harvey, E. Newton. 1948. Studies on Wound Ballistics. In *Advances in Military Medicine*, ed. E. C. Andrus, et al., 1:191–205. Boston: Little, Brown and Co.

Harvey, E. Newton, et al. 1962. Mechanism of Wounding. In Coates and Beyer, 143–235.

Harvey Papers. The Papers of E. Newton Harvey. American Philosophical Society, Philadelphia.

Herget, Carl M., George B. Coe, and James C. Beyer. 1962. Wound Ballistics and Body Armor in Korea. In Coates and Beyer.

Hoff, E. C., and John F. Fulton. 1942. *Bibliography of Aviation Medicine*. Springfield, Ill.: Charles C. Thomas.

Jonasson, Jonas A. 1958. Chapter 11: The AAF Weather Service. In *The Army Air Forces in World War II*, ed. Wesley Craven and James Cate, 7:311–38. Chicago: University of Chicago Press.

Jones, Isaac. 1937. *Flying Vistas: The Human Being as Seen through the Eyes of the Flight Surgeon*. Philadelphia: J. B. Lippincott.

Kent, R. H. 1943. Bulletin of the Conference on Missile Casualties, p. 7. September 6, 1943. Harvey Papers.

Korr, I. M. 1945. Indirect Injury by High-speed Missiles to Living Tissues Suspended in Aqueous Media. April 17, 1945. Typewritten report #4. Box B, H262, Harvey Papers.

Lamport to Fulton. 1942. September 18, 1942. Box 105, Folder 1435, Fulton Papers.

Landis, Eugene M. 1948. The Effects of Acceleration and Their Amelioration. In E. C. Andrus et al., eds., 232–60.

MacKenzie, Donald. 2000. *Inventing Accuracy: A Historical Sociology of Nuclear Missile Guidance*. Cambridge: MIT Press.

Matthews, B. H. C. 1944. Human Limits in Flight. *Nature* 153: 698–702.

MacLeod, Roy, ed. 2000. *Science and the Pacific War: Science and Survival in the Pacific, 1939–1945*. Dordrecht: Kluwer Academic.

Owens, Larry. 2004. The Cat and the Bullet: A Ballistic Fable. *Massachusetts Review* (Spring): 179–90.

Perkins, John. 2004. *Confessions of an Economic Hit Man*. San Francisco: Berret Koehler Publishers.

Pressman, Jack D. 1998. *Last Resort: Psychosurgery and the Limits of Medicine*. Cambridge History of Medicine. New York: Cambridge University Press.

Prokosch, Eric. 1995. *The Technology of Killing: A Military and Political History of Anti-Personnel Weapons.* New York: Zed Books.

Report to A. N. Richards. 1943. Appraisal of Projects in Aviation Medicine. Fulton Papers.

Rose, Hilary. 1983. Hand, Brain and Heart: A Feminist Epistemology for the Natural Sciences. *Signs* 9, no. 1: 73–96.

Sells, S. B., and Charles Berry, eds. 1961. *Human Factors in Jet and Space Travel: A Medical-Psychological Analysis.* New York: Ronald Press Co.

Summary of Reports Received by the Committee on Medical Research of the Office of Scientific Research and Development, from January 7 to January 12, 1946. 776, Box BH262.p, Committee #2, Harvey Papers.

Ward, J. W. 1946. January 14–26 Bulletin of the Committee on Medical Research, OSRD. Harvey Papers.

Wilson, Louis B. 1921. Dispersion of Bullet Energy in Relation to Wound Effects. *Military Surgeon* 49, no. 3: 241–51.

Woodruff, Charles E. 1898. The Causes of the Explosive Effect of Modern Small Caliber Bullets. *New York Medical Journal* 67, no. 30: 593–601.

10 Stumbling Toward Bioethics: Human Experiments Policy and the Early Cold War

Jonathan D. Moreno

Despite a burgeoning literature on bioethics and the history of bioethics, little has been written about the relationship between the origins of modern bioethics in the later 1960s and the human-experiment policies and practices of U.S. national security agencies during the preceding decades. A notable exception was the work of the President's Advisory Committee on Human Radiation Experiments (ACHRE) in 1994–95, which operated under a pair of executive orders to review much previously secret material on government-sponsored experiments involving ionizing radiation and to assess the ethical status of those experiments. Much of the information gathered by ACHRE was also relevant to biological and chemical warfare experiments (ACHRE 1996).

In the decade since ACHRE, for which I was a senior staff member, I have attempted to build on that foundation by developing a general account of the history and ethics of human experiments by national security organizations during the Cold War. My principle effort in this regard was *Undue Risk: Secret State Experiments on Humans* (Moreno 2001), as well as a number of papers. As the following discussion will show, that account continues to develop with new revelations about the period. Moreover, following the September 11, 2001, events and the later anthrax attacks, there has been new impetus for human experiments that raise issues reminiscent of the early Cold War era and cannot be understood without that perspective.

The present discussion concentrates on what I consider to be the critical period in the development of Cold War human research ethics policies in the national security establishment, 1947 to 1953. The beginning of that time saw the first articulation of the term "informed consent," and the last year included both the Pentagon's adoption of the Nuremberg Code and several notable deaths. One of the fatalities, of a young Royal Air Force engineer in a sarin gas experiment, is finally being fully investigated in a London inquest as I write this, and it sheds light on the shadowy cooperation of the Western allies on the human effects of unconventional weapons.

Setting the Stage: Nazi and Imperial Japanese Experiments

Three common misconceptions about the concentration camp experiments are that the experimenters were crackpots, that the experiments were junk science, and that they were all about racist eugenics. In fact, a number of those who either conducted or authorized the experiments were distinguished scientists, in some cases with international reputations. At least two of the experiments, on hypothermia and explosive decompression, yielded useful medical information that is now part of the scientific canon. And in a number of instances the sponsoring entity was the Luftwaffe, the Nazi German air force, which was interested in improving the battlefield performance of its surgeons. The experiments were indeed heartless and murderous, but if that had been all they were, and besides performed by simple sadists, they would not have the historic importance they have, nor would they have attracted the intense interest of the U.S. military-legal community after the war.

A similar story can be told about the Imperial Japanese army's biological and chemical weapons experimental establishment in Manchuria during the war. Important military doctors and scientists conducted horrific studies that might even have exceeded the Nazis' in their sheer sadism, including routine live dissections so that the effects of various agents on organs could be more directly examined. The investment made by the Japanese government in an attempt to perfect biological and chemical weapons seems to have dwarfed the German efforts in this area (see "Deals with Devils" in Moreno 2001). But unlike the case of the Nazi doctors, the United States did not conduct a war crimes trial of the leaders of the Japanese experiments, a fact that has led to decades of speculation that the Americans preferred to keep the Japanese advance in the field to itself. What is certainly the case is that U.S. spending on biological and chemical weapons increased dramatically in the early 1950s, though there is no conclusive evidence that they were used in the Korean conflict, in spite of North Korean and Chinese charges.

The Nazi doctors' trial resulted in the famous Nuremberg Code, a ten-point code of ethics written by the three American judges as part of a decision in which fifteen of the defendants were found guilty, seven later hanged (*U.S. v. Karl Brand et al.*, cited in Moreno 2001, 80). One motivation for this historic document, which emphasizes that the human subject's "voluntary consent" must be obtained, that laboratory and animal work must precede human experiments, and that the experimenter must be thoroughly competent, was the defense lawyers' argument that the Allies had engaged in similar experiments with prisoners and other vulnerable populations. Although these experiments were not designed to tolerate the deaths of subjects, as were those done by the Germans, the fact that they were done threatened the moral standing of the prosecution. Finally the judges properly rejected any moral equivalence, but they were struck by the lack of recognized international standards for human experiments.

However, the prosecution of the Germans did not run a smooth course. The Nazi defense lawyers were able to demonstrate that the World War II Allied forces had themselves conducted experiments on people who might well be regarded as vulnerable to coercion. This refutation was surprisingly effective. For example, the defense introduced into evidence a *Life* magazine article from June 1945, which depicted a United States malaria experiment conducted with eight hundred federal prisoners who claimed to have volunteered for the experiment. Although (unlike the Nazi experiments) no one died of malaria and, in my view, these were genuine volunteers who were not facing subhuman conditions and the likelihood of extermination, it became clear that universally recognized rules of human experimentation did not exist. If there were no guidelines and if the Allies had conducted similar experiments on imprisoned persons, the Germans' lawyers argued, how could the Nazis be held to a higher standard?

Using this logic, the German lawyers forestalled conviction of the Nazi officials until, in the end, guilty verdicts were based upon the grounds of murder, conspiracy to commit murder, and the new charge of crimes against humanity. The Nazis were *not* found guilty based on the Nuremberg Code, for this would have been ex post facto justice. The Nazi defense of human experimentation succeeded in slowing the proceedings, and they also effectively raised the pressing question of human experimentation and coercion. Indeed, the issue of human experimentation was not lost on the three judges, all of whom were American. They understood that international medical ethics standards urgently required articulation. Hence they devoted a portion of their ruling to the ten-point statement that has come to be known as the Nuremberg Code. In the ensuing decades the principles expressed in the code have come to dominate moral conventions about human experiments. Meanwhile, in the absence of any public accounting following the war, the main legacy of the Japanese experiments seems to be a body of knowledge about biological and chemical weapons that was the foundation for both the U.S. and Soviet offensive programs through at least the early 1970s. Then the United States ended its offensive programs and destroyed its stockpile in accord with international agreements. However, the Soviet Union secretly continued and expanded its program through the end of the Cold War. Today, of course, interest in defending against these weapons has become a high priority once again, as have human experiments. I will return to this point at the end of the paper.

Postwar Human-Experiments Policies in the U.S. National Security Establishment

The only government entity ever to have adopted the Nuremberg Code as a whole and verbatim was the U.S. Department of Defense in 1953. This turn of events followed a roughly six-year process in which both the Pentagon and the new Atomic Energy Commission (AEC) struggled with the problem of human experiments in an atmosphere highly sensitized by the Nazi doctors' trial.

The first phase appears to have taken place early in 1947, when the AEC learned of a highly classified experiment in which seventeen hospitalized patients were injected with plutonium. The injections were motivated by a desire to learn more about plutonium as an internal emitter so as to help protect the young scientists who were working with the material in the atomic bomb project. The AEC decided not to release the information, and its medical officials and advisors developed special rules to govern the use of radioisotopes in medical experiments, a responsibility that fell to the fledgling agency as it was the world's only source of nuclear material at that time. The nation's atomic energy policy also encouraged the creation of constructive and peaceful ways to use radioactive energy, including particularly new medical treatments, partly to counter the image of atomic power's association with nuclear war.

Reacting to the plutonium injection information, in 1947 the AEC specified that any experiments involving radioactive material would have to have the volunteers' "informed consent in writing."[1] The meager record strongly suggests that the AEC administrators had to be careful not to offend the physicians by implicitly suggesting that they could not be trusted with their patients. Nonetheless, this was the first time that the phrase "informed consent" is known to have appeared in any written document. But the agency's bureaucracy appears to have forgotten the policy only a few years later. For example, within several years of the statement requiring informed consent, the AEC, the Massachusetts Institute of Technology, and the Quaker Oats Company implemented a study at the Fernald School in Massachusetts. The Fernald School was a residential institution for young people with a range of objectionable behaviors. The purpose of the study was to determine that the healthful quality of the cereal was as advertised and, additionally, that this brand of cereal was superior to its competitors. The methods of the experiment were highly problematic: radiolabeled nutrients were placed in the students' breakfast cereal. Although permission was sought from the parents, the relevant documents mentioned only that the children had been selected for a "science club" with certain special privileges (Moreno 2001). The experimenters neglected to mention the trace levels of radiation in the children's breakfast cereal. Throughout the 1950s the AEC participated in a number of other radiation experiments that at the very least do not seem to have been compatible with the 1947 directives. Not only sloppy bureaucratic practices but also the insistence on professional autonomy among scientific workers characterized resistance to novel ideas about research volunteer self-determination for the next several decades.

As the 1940s drew to a close, the AEC had to deal with another complex problem involving human experiments, as it worked with the Pentagon on a project to develop a nuclear-energy-powered aircraft. A difficulty was determining how much lead shielding would be required to protect the crew from the energy source. An experiment was proposed to gather human data to determine how much exposure would be too great, but immediately the problem of identifying research subjects came up. The idea of using soldiers was quickly rejected as too politically sensitive. Those opposed to human experimentation had a difficult time refuting the claim that human experimentation carried any risk different from that of normal military service, though some maintained that "it's not very long since we got through trying Germans for doing exactly the same thing [i.e., human experimentation]" (ACHRE, cited in Moreno 2001, 148).

Advocates of using long-term prisoners argued that such persons were traditionally utilized as research subjects and that the work could be done in a manner consistent with the requirements of the Nuremberg Code. In the end, however, the joint panel was unable to agree on recruiting prisoners or any other healthy volunteers. Instead, starting in the early 1950s, research grants were given to important cancer research centers where cancer patients were receiving radiation therapy and their psychomotor skills could be tested. Data from these sick patients was presumably not ideal for military applications.

Also in the early 1950s, defense planners feared that the Soviet Union was on course to surpass the United States in atomic, biological, and chemical weapons, or ABC warfare. Once again, human experiments would be needed as animal studies provided only limited information. But the Pentagon had no policy that set out the conditions for such activities. To address this lacuna in policy, President Truman's defense secretary asked several Pentagon advisory committees to make recommendations. After months of deliberation the advisors largely opposed creation of a new policy, fearing legal consequences. In contrast, the department's general counsel's office apparently was more concerned about the consequences of a lack of policy, and recommended the adoption of the Nuremberg Code. The proposal proved controversial, and it remained for President Eisenhower's defense secretary to sign off on the memorandum that had been prepared by the agency's lawyers, on February 26, 1953.

This entire discussion was deemed sensitive, and the memorandum itself was classified "top secret." In the weeks and months following the signing, efforts were made by the uniformed services to disseminate the policy that required written consent for all experiments on defense against atomic, biological, and chemical weapons. These efforts appear to have met with mixed success, partly due to continued professional resistance among scientists and officers, and partly due to confusion about what sorts of activities came within the policy's rubric. For example, the vast majority of the more than two hundred thousand soldiers assigned to train in the presence of atomic bomb tests from 1953 to 1972 were not asked to give written consent, but a small number of those men who participated in psychological testing did sign forms. Apart from the variable of certain activities being directly supervised by a physician, it is hard to discern a rationale for when the policy was actually applied and the participants considered as research subjects.

What Counts as a Medical Experiment?

The problem of when it is acceptable to expose soldiers, sailors, or airmen to experimental conditions continues to the present day. An interesting example of this problem that only came to light years after the ACHRE final report is Project SHAD, or "Shipboard Hazard and Defense." These 1960s exercises were revealed following persistent complaints by veterans in the late 1990s. A preliminary investigation by the Pentagon in 2002 confirmed that dozens of these tests took place.

Experts in this field had long known that environmental tests of biological and chemical simulants took place during the Cold War in the airspace above major cities and in the New York City subway system. However, the Project SHAD revelations pointed to exercises on the oceans in which sailors were exposed to aerosols from tugboats mounted with biological disseminators. In many instances the exposure was accomplished from spray tanks mounted on attack aircraft towers. The purpose of these trials was to assess the vulnerability of naval ships to chemical and biological agents.

For many years it was thought that the substances to which the sailors were exposed were inert simulants, but in its investigation the Pentagon found that sometimes actual nerve agents were used. On these occasions, such as a 1964 Pacific Ocean test called Flower Drum, the Department of Defense found that extensive protective measures were used, including masks (Department of Defense 2002).

The men exposed in the course of the SHAD trials seem to have known that they were part of an experiment, but there was no consent process, and the details sufficient to satisfy Nuremberg standards were absent (Deployment Health Support 2002). In June 2003 the Pentagon released what it considered to be a final set of reports on these exercises that might have exposed 5,842 people to chemical or biological weapons, while members of Congress insist that further investigation is warranted (*New York Times* 2003). The Department of Defense investigation has not reported any adverse medical findings, though as this is being written an Institute of Medicine panel is engaged in a review of SHAD's long-term health effects (Institute of Medicine of the National Academies 2002).

Was SHAD a human experiment or a field trial? Again, the problem turns on the question of what counts as a human experiment. In a different kind of case, since the 1991 Gulf War many servicemen and women have objected to orders to be vaccinated for anthrax with a vaccine preparation that was not approved for prevention of inhalational anthrax and whose production quality has been suspect. Some also took other medications that were hoped to provide protection against nerve gas and biological agents, though they were not approved by the Food and Drug Administration for these purposes and have subsequently been alleged to contribute to Gulf War syndrome. Were these soldiers participants in uncontrolled human experiments? Again, there are serious definitional problems.

1953: A Pivotal Year

The signing of the Pentagon policy based on the Nuremberg Code and requiring written subject consent was only one of several important events in

1953. The others were three deaths in military-sponsored experiments, two in the U.S. and one in the United Kingdom that may partly have been under American auspices. At least the broad outlines of these incidents have been known for some time. The third, the one in the United Kingdom, has recently been reopened in an inquest. Enough information is becoming available that the beginnings of a nexus among the three can be established.

In January 1953, a New York City tennis pro named Harold Blaur died in a mescaline-derivative study at the New York Psychiatric Institute, where he was being treated for clinical depression (see Moreno 2001, 195–99). The study was sponsored by the Army Chemical Corps, which participated in a cover-up with New York State. The details were revealed only as part of a Congressional investigation in the late 1970s. News about the death of a human subject must surely have reached the highest levels of the Pentagon and reinforced the conviction among advocates of the Nuremberg Code–based policy proposal that rules were badly needed.

The year 1953 also saw the beginning of the CIA's infamous MKULTRA project, one of a number of activities intended to apply biological and chemical agents to undercover espionage and sabotage. One aspect of the project was an extensive network of financial support for LSD and behavioral experiments, often using "front" foundations and corporate entities to distribute funding. One victim of the project was a CIA scientist assigned to Fort Detrick in Maryland, Frank Olson, whose expertise was anthrax. Olson died in November 1953 when he tumbled from a New York City hotel room window. He had been taken to New York to be seen by a CIA-cleared physician after being dosed with LSD. When MKULTRA was revealed in the mid-1970s by Congress, the government stated that his death was a psychotic episode brought on by the LSD dosing. However, some continue to suspect that the full story has not been told. Family members report that Olson was disturbed by things he had seen in the months prior to his death, though he refused to talk to his wife about the details. Forensic evidence from Olson's remains indicates a blow to the head separate from his mortal injuries. That and other peculiarities about the case (such as the fact that the hotel room window was closed and the shades drawn when Olson allegedly jumped), have left serious doubts in the minds of many.

On May 6, 1953, about ten weeks after the top secret Pentagon memo was signed, 200 mg. of liquid sarin was poured onto a double layer of uniform clothing that was tied on the arm of Aircraftsman Ronald Maddison, a British Royal Air Force engineer. Within half an hour the twenty-year-old Maddison lost consciousness. He died later that day. The experiment took place at Porton Down, the United Kingdom's military research and development facility. Following an internal Ministry of Defence investigation the actual circumstances of the death were attributed to a "misadventure" that resulted in Maddison choking to death, but continued complaints about experiments at the site and allegations of dozens of other experiment-related deaths led to a police investigation that began in the late 1990s. Finally in May 2004, fifty-one years after his death, a new inquest began in a London court, the original Ministry of Defence investigation having been ruled inadequate. Never before has an inquest been conducted so long after the fact (*London Telegraph* 2004).

In 2002 the United States acknowledged that Porton Down was part of Project SHAD, one of the sites at which nerve agents were sprayed by air to assess the effects of environmental factors on the gases. The Porton experiments in which Maddison took part were apparently commissioned by the Tripartite Conference (the U.S., U.K., and Canada), which had met since March 1947 and which was established to engage in cooperative research projects, including those in atomic, biological, and chemical weapons.

The three deaths in 1953 point at least to a high level of activity concerning novel weaponry and their effects on the human body. The Blaur death may have increased pressure to establish a written policy in the Department of Defense, as I have suggested, but Olson's death resulted from a CIA operation. If the Porton Down sarin gas experiment later in the year was conducted under the auspices of the three closely allied governments, it raises the question whether the new U.S. policy should have applied, and if so, whether it was adequately communicated to the British site.

Stumbling toward Bioethics

The importance of the Nazi concentration camp experiments in the history of human research ethics is widely understood, and the Imperial Japanese atrocities are gradually becoming a part of the grim pantheon that has given rise to modern attention to biomedical ethics. More complex and subtle is the relationship between the early Cold War national security policy discussions and events that I have described and the field of bioethics as we know it today. For all the inadequacies of U.S. policies and their application, they were far ahead of the civilian world in the same period, where there was little interest in these questions and would not be until the mid-1960s.

Yet there are suggestive connections between the world of national security policies and human experiments and that of the incipient field of bioethics in the academic world. A source of a substantial portion of the Nuremberg Code was the American Medical Association's expert witness, Andrew Ivy. Ivy was one of America's most influential physicians and vice president of health sciences at the University of Illinois. He ensured that the American Medical Association adopted and published in its *Journal* several ethical principles in December 1946, just before he was to travel to Nuremberg to give his testimony in the Nazi doctors' trial. Ivy thus established academia's contribution to a code that would later govern military experiments, at least in theory.

Still more striking were the roles of distinguished academic scientists such as Henry Beecher and Louis Lasagna who became important early voices in the emerging field of bioethics in the 1960s. Both conducted secret research on hallucinogens supported by U.S. Army contracts in the early 1950s. Lasagna, interviewed by the ACHRE forty years later, said that he reflected "not with pride" on his participation (ACHRE 1996, 79). Clearly, these experiences influenced the thinking of at least some important scientists who became interested in ethical issues in later years.

What does seem clear is that the standard "origins story" of bioethics—that it came about virtually de novo in the late 1960s as the result of concern among a handful of thinkers about medical experiments, organ transplantation, artificial organs, genetics, and other issues—must be supplemented with a far more sophisticated understanding of institutional interactions and cultural vectors over the preceding decades. Such an account would also make clear that bioethics can justifiably speak to our current situation, in which human experiments for various national security purposes are once again being proposed. These include both new and more effective treatments for disease entities such as anthrax and smallpox and "non-lethal weapons" programs to disrupt terrorist operations. In the face of such a future and with awareness of the past, the Hegelian philosophy of historical cycles seems anything but far-fetched.

Note

1. The full statement reads: "(a) that a reasonable hope exists that the administration of such a substance will improve the condition of the patient, (b) that the patient give his complete and informed consent in writing, and (c) that the responsible next of kin give in writing a similarly complete and informed consent, revocable at any time during the course of such treatment." Cited in Moreno 2001, 141.

References

ACHRE (Advisory Committee on Human Radiation Experiments). 1996. *The Human Radiation Experiments*. New York: Oxford University Press.

Department of Defense. 2002. Fact Sheet on Project Shipboard Hazard and Defense (SHAD). http://deploymentlink.osd.mil/pdfs/flower_drum_phase_i.pdf (accessed July 2, 2003).

Deployment Health Support. 2002. *DeploymentLINK*. DoD Releases Information on 1960 tests. http://deploymentlink.osd.mil/news/jan02/news_10402_001.shtml (accessed June 28, 2003).

Institute of Medicine of the National Academies. 2002. Long-term Health Effects of Participation in Project SHAD. http://www.iom.edu/project.asp?ID=4909 (accessed June 28, 2003).

London Telegraph. 2004. Fifty-One Years On, Sister Hears How Sarin Airman Died. May 6, 2004. http://wwww.telegraph.co.uk/news/main.jhtml?xml=/news/2004/05/06/nport06.xml (accessed May 23, 2004).

Moreno, J. D. 2001. *Undue Risk: Secret State Experiments with Humans*. New York: Routledge.

New York Times. 2003. Investigations of Chemicals Will Continue. July 12, 2003, p. A8.

Part Two: The Conflicted Present and the Worrisome Future

11 Toward an Ethics of Iatrogenesis

Renée C. Fox

"Iatrogenesis" is a term with Greek roots that literally means "doctor-originated." It is customarily applied to the negative side effects of the actions that physicians take in their one-on-one care of individual patients. However, the concept is also applicable to the adverse effects that medical or public health interventions can have on groups of individuals—both on persons for whom these measures were destined and those on whom they have a more indirect, ramifying impact.

The phenomenon of iatrogenesis is intrinsic to medicine and medical action in all of its forms. Although Hippocrates' ancient injunction "do no harm" is still a primary moral commandment under which modern physicians practice medicine, they continually violate this proscription in carrying out their mandated professional responsibilities. No matter how competent, scrupulous, prescient, or humane they may be, physicians cannot totally avoid doing harm as well as good through the preventive, diagnostic, therapeutic, and prognostic actions that they undertake on behalf of the persons for whom they care. The fact that the term "iatrogenesis" is part of the nomenclature of medicine indicates that it is formally recognized as a recurrent happening in the practice of medicine.[1] Nevertheless, its origins, manifestations, and import have not been extensively or deeply explored. In the medical literature, the attention accorded to iatrogenesis has tended to focus on the potential "routine" and "idiosyncratic," "predictable" and "unpredictable," "tolerable" and "dangerous" toxic effects and allergic side reactions of medically prescribed and administered drugs—often collectively termed "adverse drug events." In bioethical as well as medical publications, iatrogenesis is frequently conflated with medical errors and mistakes, with which there is much more overt preoccupation. There is also evidence that many patients do not clearly distinguish between medical errors and "nonpreventable adverse events" (Gallagher et al. 2003). Rarely has iatrogenesis been linked with the concerned reflection on the types and problems of medical uncertainty that pervade medical and medical sociological writings. And there is virtually no discussion of how physicians think and feel about the harm that can accompany or ensue from actions that they intended to be therapeutic or ameliorative, or about how they actually handle, or should try to manage, these infelicitous events.

In this article, I would like to take some preliminary steps toward providing a conceptual framework within which more serious consideration can be accorded to the experiential and ethical implications of iatrogenesis for physicians and the practice of medicine, and to the relationship between iatrogenesis, medical uncertainty, and medical error. I approach this task with a number of underlying, more-than-medical assumptions: that unintended consequences are inherent, general properties of human action and interaction; that many actions have multifarious outcomes, some "good," some "bad," some anticipatable, some not, some immediate, some delayed, some ephemeral, some lingering or enduring; that not all of the unwanted and undesirable effects of action are avoidable; and that while some mishaps or mistakes are potentially blameworthy, many are not. Seen in a larger philosophical perspective, these attributes of human action and their repercussions bring in their wake troubling, often dilemma-ridden encounters with the ambiguous boundaries and the complex interplay between doing good and doing harm, in a vast array of endeavors—including those as diverse as writing a novel or providing humanitarian aid:

> When a surgeon operates on a young girl, he isn't saying, "I'm going to make an incision on this young lady's stomach that not only is going to scar her but will affect her sex life to some degree for the next thirty years." He just says, "Scalpel, nurse," and does it. The surgeon is focused on the act, not its reverberations.
>
> As a novelist you are engaged in something analogous. . . . [Novelists] are sensitive and insensitive. Full of heart and heartless. You have to be full of heart to feel what other people are feeling. On the other hand, if you start thinking of all the damage you are going to do, you can't write the book—not if you're reasonably decent. . . . The point is that you are facing a real problem. Either you produce a book that doesn't approach what really interests you or, if you go to the root with all you've got, there is no way that you won't injure family, friends, and innocent bystanders. (Mailer 2002, 76)
>
> * * *
>
> Unfortunately, in the parts of the world where we work, there are no harm-free choices. In most cases there is no luxurious choice of doing no harm, but rather choosing what is the lesser evil. . . . I would assume that there are very, very few interventions in conflict settings that do not have negative consequences. Forget the dream of a harm-free intervention. . . . You have to be aware of the consequences of what you do and the harms you cause and choose the lesser ones. (Anderson 1998, 137)
>
> * * *
>
> Although the occurrence of negative consequences from positively intended action may not be unique to medicine, the distinctive nature of medical work augments the significance and the potential gravity of the harmful side effects that it continually engenders. Health and illness, medicine and medical care are palpably connected with "some of the most basic and the most transcendent aspects of the human condition": with intimate aspects of the human body, psyche, and story; with the entire life cycle, from conception and birth, through aging and death; with pain and suffering, accident and injury; and with the ultimate inevitability of human mortality. These are involved and at stake in the care that physicians deliver—and in the sequellae, impact, and outcome of that care. (Fox 1980)

Doing Harm to Do Good

"Medical care is about our life and death . . . [and] the liberties taken [are] tremendous," surgeon Atul Gawande has written. "We drug people, put needles and tubes in them, manipulate their chemistry, biology, and physics, lay them unconscious and open their bodies up to the world" (Gawande 2002, 4, 46). The responsibility that physicians carry for dealing with the illnesses and injuries of patients, and their travail, allows and obliges them to probe the inner chambers of patients' bodies and also of their minds in ways not only that break cultural taboos, but that expose them to risk and subject them to harm. A major origin of iatrogenesis lies in the paradoxical fact that many of the medical actions that physicians undertake for the purpose of treating and benefiting patients are helpful partly because they are harmful.

An archetypical example of a deliberate way in which physicians "wound" patients in order to diagnose, deter, or remedy their ailments is the performance of surgery—which has been described by Gawande as an act of "calculated violence," carried out with a "righteous faith that it [is] somehow good for the [patient]" (Gawande 2002, 16). Organ transplantation from a living donor is an especially audacious form of surgically harming a person with the intent of doing therapeutic good, because the procedure that the donor undergoes is not executed for his or her benefit. Rather, it is done to sustain the life of someone else. With the consent of the healthy live donor, a surgical team removes one of his/her vital organs—usually a kidney—and another team transplants the organ into the body of a waiting recipient, who is a patient with an end-stage disease. In the case of the transplantation of the right lobe of a liver from a living adult donor into an adult recipient, there is a substantial risk that the donor will experience harmful difficulties. Out of 449 such transplants performed in the United States between 1997 and 2000, 3 donor deaths occurred, and as many as 65 (14.5%) of the donors had one or more complications—especially biliary complications (Brown et al. 2003).

What Nicholas Christakis has termed this "two-edged feature of medical care" is not confined to surgery. It pervades medicine. It is implicated, for example, in cancer chemotherapy, in which the drugs utilized kill healthy cells in the course of killing the cancerous ones, and which can subject patients to such physically and psychologically painful and damaging effects as fever, infection, anemia, severe fatigue, hair loss, incontinence, impotence, premature menopause, and memory and concentration problems (sometimes referred to by patients as "chemo brain" or "chemo fog"). In addition, as the instance of cancer chemotherapy illustrates, the more powerful the medical intervention, the more likely it is to have significant negative as well as positive consequences. One of the more poignant instances of the emergent and protracted damage that aggressive and effective therapy for cancer can cause is to be found in the treatment of childhood leukemia. As a result of the administration of chemotherapy and radiation early in life to children afflicted with this most common malignancy of childhood, what was formerly a 90 percent chance that a child suffering from this disease would die from it has been transformed into an 80 percent chance that he or she will survive and that the leukemia will be cured. Nevertheless, physicians have gradually been discovering that what has justifiably been called this "medical marvel," has serious, long-term side effects, including stunted growth, low thyroid function, kidney problems, heart and lung disorders, infertility, posttraumatic stress, learning disorders, and even the development of new cancers (Duenwald and Grady 2003).

Doing Good That Causes Harm

The converse of this pattern of "doing-harm-in-order-to-do-good"—that is, "doing-good-that-causes-harm"—also permeates medicine, and is probably the most frequent source and manifestation of iatrogenesis. It is particularly salient and recurrent in connection with the use of drugs for the treatment of patients' disorders. No "all-therapeutic" drug exists that is devoid of side effects. Furthermore, in spite of the impressive pharmacological progress that has accompanied the advance of biomedicine, an encompassing, deterministic understanding of drug action does not exist, which means that clinical pharmacology is essentially empirical. This makes it hard for physicians to forecast how a specific individual will respond to a prescribed medication—especially to predict whether that person will experience any of the known, adverse effects of a drug (which ones, and with what severity), or a dangerous idiosyncratic reaction to it (such as anaphylactic shock in response to penicillin). The best indicators available to physicians in this regard are whatever clinical data exist that describe how a particular patient has previously responded to being treated with the drug in question, including the patient's own oral testimony about his/her prior toxic, allergic, or other unfavorable reactions.

A new field of inquiry known as pharmacogenetics is developing around the study of the role that individual inheritance plays in the individual variation in drug response. It is premised on the suppositions that "clinically important inherited variations in drug metabolism" are "common" and that along with "the effects of age, sex, disease, or drug interactions, genetic factors . . . influence both the efficacy of a drug and the likelihood of an adverse reaction" (Weinshilboum 2003). But the potentiality that pharmacogenetics has to elucidate the inherited determination of drug effects and to apply this knowledge to how physicians select medications and drug doses for individual patients is still only a promise—and one that is fraught with "formidable" genomic issues and problems (Evans and McLeod 2003, 547).

Further complicating the situation is the fact that many persons who have chronic diseases or disorders are treated with an intricate, long-term battery of drugs that even with careful and artful balancing by a skilled physician trigger problematic drug interactions along with numerous adverse effects. The high pill burden, onerous medication schedule, and disturbing side effects make it difficult for many patients to faithfully and precisely adhere to the prescribed course of treatment necessary for the optimal management of their condition, and may eventuate in their taking the drugs intermittently or totally discontinuing them. In the case of the treatment of infectious diseases—notably HIV/AIDS and tuberculosis—this not only has deleterious consequences for such "nonadhering" patients, but also has contributed to the mutation of the pathogens that cause these diseases into drug-resistant strains, with grave public health implications for controlling their epidemic spread. Even when "treatment noncompliance" is not involved, physicians' continuous, relatively nonselective use of certain groups of drugs to treat infections and infectious diseases may lead to widespread resistance to them. This has conspicuously and problematically come to pass as a result of the "overuse" of antibiotics.

So-called nosocomial, or hospital-acquired, infections—which are "by far the most common complications affecting hospitalized patients," and "the most common type of adverse events in health care"—are "due in large part to indiscriminate use of antibiotics" (Burke 2002, 651). They consist primarily of four kinds: urinary tract infections (usually catheter-associated), surgical-site infections, bloodstream infections (most often associated with the use of an intravascular device), and pneumonia (generally ventilator-associated). "One fourth of nosocomial infections involve patients in intensive care units, and nearly 70 percent are due to microorganisms that are resistant to one or more antibiotics.... [They] affect approximately 2 million patients each year in the United States [and] result in some 90,000 deaths" (ibid.).

On the other hand, succeeding in eradicating certain pathogens from the environment may also have negative consequences. According to the so-called hygiene hypothesis in the emerging field of dermo-epidemiology, there is an inverse relationship between exposure to microbes and parasites, on the one hand, and the development of allergies, on the other. This hypothesis is partly based on the observation that allergies are less common in large families of lower social class status. It appears that chronic viral and bacterial infections, together with infestations of endoparasitic disease, act as important protectors against atopic dermatitis/eczema and other forms of allergy. Therefore, eliminating these infections may have the undesirable effect of promoting allergy development (Flohr 2002).

One of the most significant and serious current examples of the harm that can be set in motion by eliminating a disease-bearing pathogen from the human environment is associated with the present status of smallpox. The twenty-three-year-long global eradication of smallpox that has been achieved is a public health and medical triumph of the late twentieth century. However, the freedom attained from this infectious and contagious disease and the suspension of smallpox vaccination that it has made possible have rendered the world population highly vulnerable to the intentional or unintentional release of the variola virus that causes smallpox. This has heightened the anxiety that now exists about the threat of biological warfare and terrorism and the possibility that the smallpox variola might be used as a weapon. In the United States, the government has responded with a plan to reintroduce smallpox vaccination, beginning with the vaccination of members of the military, hospital workers and health professionals, and firefighters and police, who, in the instance of a biological warfare attack, would be most likely to have "frontline" contact with persons who have diagnosed or undiagnosed smallpox. This plan has ignited debate about how many and which persons to vaccinate, about the risk of the adverse effects that will result from vaccination (ranging in gravity from diffuse skin eruptions to brain damage and death), and about how to monitor and minimize them.

It is known that the adverse consequences of the resumption of smallpox vaccination will be of two sorts: those that will occur among vaccine recipients and those that will result from the secondary transmission of vaccinia virus from a recently vaccinated person to a susceptible host. Although retrospective analysis of secondary transmission in the past indicates that it was "remarkably infrequent," experts agree that at present, there is reason to be especially concerned about secondary transmission within hospitals, through the intermediary of health-care personnel who, in this era, are susceptible both to smallpox and vaccinia. The danger is augmented by the fact that the "composition of hospitalized patients in the 21st century is dramatically different from that in the mid-20th century." Many hospital inpatients are "immunocompromised" (have reduced immunity), because of the cancer chemotherapy they undergo, the corticosteroids they receive for conditions such as rheumatoid arthritis or asthma, or the regimen of immunosuppressive drugs they must continuously take to prevent a rejection reaction following organ transplantation, or because they have contracted HIV/AIDS. In addition, patients in medical, surgical, or neonatal intensive care units make up a sizable proportion of today's hospital populations. All these groups of patients would be insufficiently defended against smallpox if they came into contact with newly vaccinated health workers or other recently vaccinated people. And it is considered highly inadvisable for such unresistant patients to be vaccinated (Sepkowitz 2003, 439, 443, 445).

The U.S. government is formulating its smallpox policy and vaccination plan, in part, on mathematical modeling of smallpox attack scenarios (Bozzette et al. 2003). But the more people who are vaccinated, the more there are likely to be serious complications. And "no statistical model can predict the thoughts of a terrorist . . . [or] tell how individuals or countries will act in times of crisis." "As in clinical medicine," two physician-coauthors declare, "one always wants to ensure the best outcome, but at times one is forced to make a decision that merely averts the worst." In the case of the plans for a U.S. vaccination program against smallpox, they conclude, "we will know whether our decisions are right or wrong only on the basis of the eventual outcome" (Schraeder and Campion 2003, 382).

Iatrogenesis and Medical Uncertainty

Underlying and contributing to the phenomenon of iatrogenesis, the numerous forms that it takes, and its frequency is the prevalence of uncertainty in medicine and medical practice. Uncertainty, along with iatrogenesis, is inherent to medicine. "Scientific, technological, and clinical advances change the content of medical uncertainty and alter its contours; but they do not drive it away. Furthermore, although medical progress dispels some uncertainties, it uncovers others that were not formerly recognized, and it may even create new areas of uncertainty that did not previously exist" (Fox 2000, 409). Thus, to a degree that is fluctuating, but essentially irreducible, medicine is fraught with uncertainty. As they go about their diagnostic and therapeutic, preventive and prognostic work, physicians are confronted with three fundamental types of uncertainties that may complicate or curtail their ability to anticipate adverse consequences of their actions, to forestall them, or to mitigate them if and when they happen.

> These are the uncertainties that originate in the impossibility of commanding all the vast knowledge and complex skills of continually advancing modern medicine; the uncertainties that stem from the many gaps in medical knowledge and limitations in medical understanding and effectiveness that nonetheless exist; and the uncertainties connected with distinguishing between personal ignorance and ineptitude, and the lacunae and incapacities of the field of medicine itself. (Fox 2000, 410)

Gawande has vividly described the omnipresence of these uncertainties in the realm of surgery:

> Every day surgeons are faced with uncertainties. Information is inadequate; the science is ambiguous; one's knowledge and abilities are never perfect. Even with the simplest operation, it cannot be taken for granted that a patient will come through better off—even alive. Standing at the [operating] table my first time, I wondered how the surgeon knew that he would do this patient good, that all the steps would go as planned, that bleeding would be controlled and infections would not take hold and organs would not be injured. He didn't, of course. But still he cut. (Gawande 2002, 15–16)

A difficult discernment to make is whether and when physicians are responsible for the uncertainty surrounding their medical actions and the deleterious consequences of that uncertainty. "Is it my fault, or the fault of the field?" is the way a medical student once posed the question. Is it an exculpable, albeit regrettable, "maloccurrence," or is it "malpractice?" is the distinction that an experienced obstetrician-gynecologist of my acquaintance uses when he grapples with this issue (Weinstein 2003). And under what circumstances is it necessary, sagacious, commendatory, or blameful for physicians to proceed in the face of uncertainty, even though this may augment the possibility that their interventions may result in harm to the patient? The failure of a physician to command and deploy available knowledge that might have averted the occurrence of a harmful event could be considered an iatrogenic error, both of omission and of commission. But how culpable is the physician for such a breach in knowledge?

In *Forgive and Remember*, sociologist Charles Bosk's classic, firsthand study of "managing medical failure" in the context of the training and socialization of young surgeons, he sets forth an enlightening typology that distinguishes between "technical" and "judgmental" errors, which are considered by senior surgeons in that setting to be "blameless," and "normative" and "quasi-normative" errors, which they regard as "blameworthy" (Bosk 1979, 36–70). However, Bosk does not deal with a deep-structure dilemma emanating from the uncertainties surrounding virtually everything that physicians do. Although it may seem ideal for physicians to be watchfully aware of the medical uncertainties that are always present and vigilantly responsive to them, they must also have enough confidence in the knowledge and techniques of their field, and in their own knowledge and competence, to believe that the medical action they take is judicious, and likely to benefit the patient. Too much consciousness of uncertainty, and "Hamlet-like" doubting and self-doubting in response to it, can impede physicians' ability to act decisively, with enough clear-mindedness to avert harmful errors that irresolution or excessive "uncertainty about uncertainty" can cause.

Probabilistic Reasoning, Individual Variability, and Iatrogenesis

It is not without irony that some of the indwelling cognitive characteristics of modern Western medical knowledge, and the mode of thought on which its application is premised, are fundamental sources of medical uncertainty, iatrogenesis, and the relationship between them. Physicians care for patients as individuals; but the knowledge that they draw upon to do so is amassed and organized on an aggregate basis, and is brought to bear on the problems of particular patients through a probabilistic mode of reasoning that is systematically speculative. Because this is so, as a thoughtful primary care physician explains, although "[m]aking judgments about complex individual circumstances in the context of different degrees of uncertainty" that is called for "in the routine reality of . . . medical practice" is "grounded in clinical experience . . . [and] knowledge of scientific findings," it is "not a simple . . . input [of] information . . . output [of] decisions" process (Hurwitz 1997). It is often hard for a physician to foresee how a specific person under his or her care will respond to a given treatment, and where on the spectrum of known reactions and results the outcome for *this* patient will fall. Such clinical predictions are made all the more difficult by the way that the biological, psychological, and social variability of human beings may affect their responses. The influence that individual variability and probabilistic reasoning from aggregates has on the phenomenon of iatrogenesis is especially apparent in the prescription of medications. Drugs that work effectively for most patients may fail to work in others, and whether efficacious or not, they will be harmful to certain of the patients for whom they are prescribed. As previously discussed, foretelling precisely which patients will experience adverse effects or failures and proactively protecting them against these eventualities are not easily accomplished.

One of the ways in which physicians deal with such negative reactions is to prescribe medications that have been developed to treat the adverse effects of other drugs—such as anti-emetics for the nausea and vomiting induced by cancer chemotherapy or, as recently reported, sildenafil citrate (Viagra) to offset the sexual dysfunction in men associated with the antidepressant medication they are receiving. However, since no drug is entirely free of side effects, this may trigger a cascade of side effects—those emanating from the "remedial" drug, superimposed upon the ones that it is intended to counteract.

The Ethos of Modern Western Medicine and Iatrogenesis

Some of the social attitudes and values that undergird modern Western medicine are also conducive to iatrogenic occurrences. The belief in scientific and technological progress—in their dynamic capacity to continuously bring forth better means to understand, prevent, and treat illness, to prolong life, and to fend off death; the optimistic hope of developing new "wonder" drugs; the dauntless and bellicose commitment to "conquering" and eliminating major diseases that afflict humankind; and the conviction that taking vigorous, even aggressive action to deal with disease, illness, and injury is salutary—all sustain modern medicine, give it momentum, and have galvanized the impressive advances that have been made in medical science, care, and health under its auspices. However, these same attributes of the ethos of modern Western medicine can also generate harm, through excessive fervor, insufficient recognition of limits and limitation, underestimation of risk, and reluctance to rigorously distinguish patients who can benefit most from an enthusiastically espoused procedure or medication from those who can benefit least. When physicians are caring for desperately ill patients under circumstances of high medical uncertainty, their tendency to behave with such relentless activism, accentuate-the-positive tenacity, and "we shall overcome" indomitableness may be reinforced.

This was the disquieting situation that historian Judith P. Swazey and I found to be characteristic of organ replacement (the transplantation of solid organs and the development of an artificial heart) in the United States, and that led us in the 1990s, after twenty-three years of joint, frontline research in this area, to "leave the field." As we wrote at the time:

> [W]e have come to believe that the missionary-like ardor about organ replacement that now exists, the over idealization of the quality and duration of life that can ensue, and the seemingly limitless attempts to procure and implant organs that are currently taking place have gotten out of hand. In the words of a transplant-nurse specialist, "perhaps the most important issue in a critical examination of transplantation involves the need and criteria for responsible decisions about when to stop, when to say 'enough is enough' to the transplant process." (Park 1989, 30)
>
> In the final analysis, our departure from the field . . . is not only impelled by our need to distance ourselves . . . emotionally. It is also a value statement on our part. By our leave-taking we are intentionally separating ourselves from what we believe has become an overly zealous . . . commitment to the endless perpetuation of life and to repairing and rebuilding people through organ replacement—and from the human suffering and the social, cultural, and spiritual harm we believe

such unexamined excess can, and already has, brought in its wake. (Fox and Swazey 1992, 204, 209–10)

Thus far, the ongoing history of gene therapy has dramatically, and in several instances tragically, epitomized the impasses, disappointments, and damage, more than the achievements, that can emanate from fervid belief in the curative power of energetically applying frontier science to clinical medicine and patient care. The hundreds of clinical trials that have taken place in the fledging field of gene therapy, supported by millions of dollars, have occurred in an atmosphere of exuberant expectations about how the explosion of molecular biological knowledge set off by the "biological revolution," and the mapping and sequencing of the genes in the human body accomplished by the Human Genome Project, will fundamentally change and improve the practice of medicine by illuminating the etiology and mechanisms of human diseases and providing the basis for more potent and rational therapy. And yet, in spite of all that has been scientifically, technically, financially, and emotionally invested in them, only one set of gene therapy trials has been successful: the treatment by a team of physicians and geneticists associated with the Necker Hospital for Sick Children in Paris of eleven children with "X-linked" severe combined immunodeficiency (SCID), an extremely rare disease that affects males and often causes the children afflicted with it to die from infection before they are one year old. Like numerous other gene therapy trials, these involved the use of a modified retrovirus to insert a "corrective" gene into the host genome—in these cases, into the children's blood-forming stem cells—and then return these "corrected," "healthy" cells to the patients. What appeared to be the full and sustained restoration of immune function in nine of the children treated this way resulted from the procedure.

Clinical investigators have not been oblivious to the dangers that might be associated with the deployment of retroviruses. "Because retroviral vectors are thought to insert themselves at random positions in the host genome, insertional mutagenesis as a potential risk of retroviral gene therapy has been debated for some years" (Noguchi 2003, 193). Such a risk was considered to be very low in humans—an assumption that has been reinforced by the climate of zeal, audacity, high expectations, and hoped-for success that has surrounded gene therapy. However, in September 2002, at a routine checkup of the fourth patient on whom supposedly successful gene therapy for X-linked SCID had been performed (a boy who had reached the age of three), the Necker team discovered that what they termed "a serious adverse event" had occurred. The child had developed a leukemia-like disorder that was interpreted as "the consequence of [an] insertional mutagenesis event." Apparently, the gene inserted inside the boy's stem cells had landed on, and activated, a cancer-producing gene (oncogene) called LMO-2, which can cause leukemia (Pollack 2003b). The team quickly proposed to French regulatory authorities the halting of their gene therapy trials until "further evaluation of the causes of this adverse event," a "careful reassessment of the risks and benefits of continuing gene-therapy trials for severe combined immunodeficiency," and a "thorough reassessment of the potential risk of retrovirally mediated gene therapy," more generally, were carried out (Hacein-Bey-Abina et al. 2003). In the United States, the Food and Drug Administration (FDA) "put three similar gene-therapy trials on hold . . . [a]s a precaution." Subsequently its Biological Response Modifiers Advisory Committee met and "recommended that gene transfer trials for severe combined immunodeficiency in the United States be allowed to proceed, but with careful attention to inclusion and exclusion criteria, so as to provide the best ratio of benefit to risk, relative to other therapies" (Noguchi 2003, 193). "That an instance of insertional mutagenesis first happened in humans during a clinical trial surprised some," commented Philip Noguchi, acting director of the FDA's office of cellular, tissue, and gene therapies, "but not those of us who regulate biologic products such as gene therapy":

> We take to heart the words of Robert Ingersoll: "In nature there are no rewards or punishments; there are consequences." Gene therapies are constructs derived from nature; they are not of nature. The manipulations needed to create genetic therapy add enormous complexity to considerations of safety and preclinical toxicity testing, and for every intended consequence of a complex biologic product, there are unintended consequences. (Noguchi 2003, 193–94)

In December 2002, a second child among the eleven with SCID who had been treated with this form of gene therapy in France was found to have the same leukemia-like disease, seemingly induced by the boy's stem cells landing near enough to the LMO-2 oncogene to switch it on (Pollack 2003b). After a month of studying the situation, on January 14, 2003, the FDA announced that as a precautionary measure it was suspending twenty-seven gene therapy trials, involving several hundred patients, that entailed using retroviruses to insert genes into blood stem cells, regardless of the disease being treated. In the United Kingdom, an X-SCID trial was halted as well. And the U.S. National Institute of Health's Recombinant DNA Advisory Committee (RAC) urged some ninety other retroviral trials targeting blood cells to consider a pause.

"The exciting thing was that it was working," commented Dr. Joseph C. Glorioso, president of the American Society of Gene Therapy and chairman of Molecular Genetics and Biochemistry at the University of Pittsburgh. "The horrible thing is that a shadow has been cast over the success." But, he added, "I don't think it will kill the field. I think it will cause us to work harder and engineer our way out of the problem" (Pollack 2003a).

At an emergency meeting of RAC that was convoked in early February 2003, the principal investigator of the French trial, Alain Fischer, and his chief collaborator in the United States, Christof von Kalle (at the Cincinnati Children's Hospital Medical), reported that a third child now had T cells with the same gene insertion near LMO-2, and that it was possible more patients would be found to have this insertion (Kaiser 2003). The denouement of these once-acclaimed trials has not yet occurred.[2]

Toward an Ethics of Iatrogenesis

It would be beyond my competence as a sociologist to forge a set of precepts that might constitute the building blocks of an ethics of iatrogenesis. There is only one foundational statement that I feel qualified to make in this connection—namely, that because it would be utopian to suppose that means can be found to eliminate all elements of unpredictability and inadvertence from medical action, or to ensure the felicity of all outcomes, thinking and acting in ways that are directed toward minimizing harm and maximizing good constitute the highest level of ethicality in this sphere to which physicians can aspire. This is the pragmatic, bluntly stated ethical advice that economist Mary B. Anderson, president of the Collaborative for Development Action and director of the Local Capacities for Peace Project, gave to humanitarian workers, which I quoted earlier. "Forget the dream of a harm-free intervention," she declared. "You have to be aware of the consequences of what you do and the harms you cause and choose the lesser ones" (Anderson 1998, 137). In a more pensive tone, the physicians weighing the risks and benefits of resuming smallpox vaccination, whom I previously cited, expressed the same opinion: "in clinical medicine, one always wants to ensure the best outcome, but sometimes, one is forced to make a decision that merely averts the worse" (Schraeder and Campion 2003).

In the way of a conclusion to the medical sociological reflections on the phenomenon of iatrogenesis that I have presented, I would like to make a few suggestions that might contribute to the moral, philosophical, and medical professional processes of consideration through which more refined and detailed ethical insights could be elaborated.

To begin with, I share the conviction of anthropologist Clifford Geertz that it is fruitful to approach what he calls "philosophical investigation" of ethical matters that involve values and beliefs with "an empirical base" and a "conceptual framework" that "give . . . attention [to] how . . . actual people in actual societies living in terms of actual cultures . . . define situations and how they go about coming to terms with them." The role of this kind of analysis of values, he takes care to state, is "not to replace philosophical investigation . . . by descriptive ethics, but . . . to make it more relevant" (Geertz 1973, 141). In this regard, as I mentioned at the outset of my discussion, I have the impression that in medical, philosophical, and social science literature, there is very little of such "empirically oriented" and "theoretically sophisticated" (ibid.) discussion of how physicians individually, and as members of the culture of medicine, define, experience, interpret, and respond to iatrogenesis, its perennial occurrence, and its multiple manifestations, in the various medical contexts and social settings in which they work. In fact, the term "iatrogenesis" is rarely invoked—not even in connection with the adverse side effects of drugs about which there is such abundant discussion in medical publications.

My first recommendation, then, as a stepping-stone to the development of an effective, reality-grounded ethical approach to iatrogenesis, is to call for systematic empirical research on how, when, where, why, and in what forms it occurs in medical practice; how physicians think about it; what they do to try to deter it; and how they cope with the harmful concomitants and consequences of their beneficently intended actions. Within the framework of such an inquiry, exploring on the one hand, why there appears to be relatively little attention given to the intrinsic relationship of iatrogenesis and its unintended consequences to all forms of medical care, and on the other, why iatrogenesis is frequently not distinguished from medical error, might be revealing in an ethically pertinent way. Here I offer a counterintuitive hypothesis: Is it possible that physicians find it more difficult to deal with the adverse consequences of their actions that are *not* caused by mistakes than those that are, because it confronts them with situations inherent to medicine for which readily available means of explanation and rectification do not exist and that make the limitations in their control over doing no harm starkly apparent to them? In this connection, S. Ryan Gregory has proposed a correlative idea: It might be easier for doctors to accept their own fallibility, he has suggested, than the fallibility of medical science, which physicians regard not only as the bedrock of their knowledge and skill, but also as a counterweight to their imperfections, and a "remedy" for them.[3]

It would also be both edifying and useful to have more knowledge of what medical students and house staff are taught and learn about iatrogenesis, intellectually and attitudinally, explicitly and implicitly, in what courses and clinical contexts, through the intermediary of which teachers and medical happenings. I have already intimated that the participant observation I have done in American medical school and academic hospital settings has given me the impression that a great part of whatever training U.S. physicians receive to enable them to recognize and deal with iatrogenesis is centered around the adverse secondary effects of drugs. How functionally specific this learning remains, or whether general insights and principles derived from it are connected with other sources and patterns of iatrogenesis, is unclear to me.

Finally, I think that there would be some value in examining the underlying premises and subtexts of the various means and methods that have been proposed or advocated for making the practice of medicine more effective and less injurious, including the following:

- "benefit-risk ratio" reasoning;
- the conduct of so-called evidence-based medicine (that is, the integration of individual clinical expertise with the best "external clinical evidence" derived from basic medical sciences, clinical research conducted via large, randomized, controlled clinical trials, and meta-analysis of disparate published clinical studies) (Sackett et al. 1997);

- the position taken by the U.S. Institute of Medicine in its report *To Err Is Human*, that problems of health care quality and safety have more to do with poorly designed "outmoded systems of work" than with the individual actions of individual physicians (Committee on Quality of Health Care in America 2000, 4).

Although they do not directly refer to iatrogenesis or invoke it by name, the underlying assumptions on which these approaches rest are germane to how the medical profession views, or is being advised to view, the etiology and prevention of adverse medical events. These assumptions would have to be taken into account in the formulation and fostering of an "ethics of iatrogenesis."

* * *

I hope that this discussion will increase interest in the phenomenon of iatrogenesis, persuade readers that it merits more consideration than it has been given, and help to identify its relation to medical error and medical uncertainty, while showing that it is not synonymous with medical mistakes.

Notes

This paper owes much to a manuscript on "social iatrogenesis" and the "unanticipated consequences of medical intervention" on which physician-sociologist Nicholas A. Christakis and I are currently working.

1. Preliminary research by student physician-historian S. Ryan Gregory suggests that the term "iatrogenic disease" began to be broadly used in the medical literature during the decades following World War II. Although the concept itself was not new, entries using the terms "iatrogenic disease," "iatrogenesis," or "iatrogenic" did not appear in American catalogues of the medical literature before that time. How and why these terms became prominent at this historical juncture remains to be studied.

In the 1960s, when the American catalogue known as *Index Medicus* had gained its current status as an international reference guide to the medical literature, works cited under the entry "iatrogenic disease" were plentiful. The authors of these articles, who came from diverse national backgrounds, used the terms "iatrogenic disease," "iatrogenic," and "iatrogenesis" to apply to a wide range of phenomena that included adverse drug reactions, surgical mistakes, and physician-initiated epidemics.

2. The chief investigators of these gene therapy trials for X-linked SCID deserve commendation for the rapidity, honesty, and openness with which they have continuously reported on the adverse developments that have taken place and the alacrity with which they called a moratorium on the trials when these unfortunate events happened.

3. In a face-to-face discussion with S. Ryan Gregory about an earlier draft of this paper (which he kindly read), he told me that he saw a connection between what I have called my "counterintuitive hypothesis" in the text above and the inclination of late nineteenth- and early-twentieth-century American physicians of the caliber of Richard Cabot to believe that "human fallibility in medicine" could be "redeemed by . . . the supposed infallibility of science" and that "the new scientific practice of medicine" had the "potential to transcend human error." Gregory has developed these ideas more fully in

an unpublished working paper entitled, "Human Mistakes: Richard Cabot and the Study of Medical Errors, 1880–1915."

References

Anderson, Mary B. 1998. "You Save My Life Today, but for What Tomorrow?" Some Moral Dilemmas of Humanitarian Aid. In *Hard Choices: Moral Dilemmas in Humanitarian Intervention,* ed. Jonathan Moore, 137–56. Lanham, Md.: Rowland and Littlefield Publishers.

Bosk, Charles L. 1979. *Forgive and Remember: Managing Medical Failure.* Chicago: University of Chicago Press.

Bozzette, Samuel A., et al. 2003. A Model for a Smallpox-Vaccination Policy. *New England Journal of Medicine* 348, no. 5: 416–25.

Brown, Robert S., et al. 2003. A Survey of Liver Transplantation from Living Adult Donors in the United States. *New England Journal of Medicine* 348, no. 9: 818–25.

Burke, John P. 2002. Infection Control—A Problem for Patient Safety. *New England Journal of Medicine* 348, no. 7: 652–56.

Committee on Quality of Health Care in America, Institute of Medicine. 2000. *To Err is Human: Building a Safer Health System.* Washington, D.C.: National Academy Press.

Duenwald, Mary, and Denise Grady. 2003. Young Survivors of Cancer Battle Effects of Treatment. *New York Times,* January 8, 2003, pp. A1, A20.

Evans, William E., and Howard L. McLeod. 2003. Pharmacogenomics—Drug Disposition, Drug Targets, and Side Effects. *New England Journal of Medicine* 348, no. 6: 538–49.

Flohr, Carsten. 2002. Personal communication, December 15.

Fox, Renée C. 1980. The Human Condition of Health Professionals. In *Essays in Medical Sociology: Journeys into the Field,* 572–87. New Brunswick, N.J.: Transaction Books.

———. 2000. Medical Uncertainty Revisited. In *The Handbook of Social Studies in Health and Medicine,* ed. Gary L. Albrecht, Ray Fitzpatrick, and Susan C. Scrimshaw, 409–25. London: Sage Publications.

Fox, Renée C., and Judith P. Swazey. 1992. *Spare Parts: Organ Replacement in American Society.* New York: Oxford University Press.

Gallagher, Thomas H., et al. 1992. *Spare Parts: Organ Replacement in American Society.* New York: Oxford University Press.

———. 2003. Patients' and Physicians' Attitudes Regarding the Disclosure of Medical Errors. *Journal of the American Medical Association* 289, no. 8: 1001–1005.

Gawande, Atul. 2002. *Complications: A Surgeon's Notes on an Imperfect Science.* New York: Henry Holt and Company.

Geertz, Clifford. 1973. Ethos, World View, and the Analysis of Sacred Symbols. In *The Interpretation of Cultures: Selected Essays,* 126–41. New York: Basic Books.

Hacein-Bey-Abina, Salima, et al. 2003. A Serious Adverse Event after Successful Gene Therapy for X-Linked Severe Combined Immunodeficiency (Correspondence). *New England Journal of Medicine* 348, no. 3: 255–56.

Hurwitz, Brian. 1997. Clinical Guidelines: Philosophical, Legal, Emotional and Political Considerations. Draft paper commissioned by the *British Medical Journal.*

Kaiser, Jocelyn. 2003. RAC Hears a Plea for Resuming Trials, Despite Cancer Risk. *Science* 299, no. 5609: 991.

Mailer, Norman. 2002. Birds and Lions: Writing from the Inside Out. *New Yorker,* December 23 and 30, 2003, pp. 76–84.

Noguchi, Philip. 2003. Risks and Benefits of Gene Therapy (Perspective). *New England Journal of Medicine* 348, no. 3: 193–94.

Park, Patricia M. 1989. The Transplant Odyssey. *Second Opinion* 12 (November): 27–32.

Pollack, Andrew 2003a. F.D.A. Halts 27 Gene Therapy Trials after Illness: Leukemia-like Cases in 2 Children in France Prompt the Action. *New York Times,* January 15, 2003, pp. A1, A17.

———. 2003b. 2nd Cancer Is Attributed to Gene Used in F.D.A. Test. *New York Times,* January 17, 2003, p. A24.

Sackett, David L., et al. 1997. *Evidence-Based Medicine: How to Practice & Teach EBM.* London: Churchill Livingston.

Schraeder, Terry L., and Edward W. Campion. 2003. Smallpox Vaccination—The Call to Arms. *New England Journal of Medicine* 348, no. 5: 381–82.

Sepkowitz, Kent A. 2003. How Contagious Is Vaccinia? *New England Journal of Medicine* 348, no. 5: 439–46.

Weinshilboum, Richard. 2003. Inheritance and Drug Response. *New England Journal of Medicine* 348, no. 6: 529–37.

Weinstein, Robert S. 2003. Personal communication, January 6.

12 Strategies for Survival versus Accepting Impermanence: Rationalizing Brain Death and Organ Transplantation Today

Tetsuo Yamaori

In Japan today, through what might be called "reckless medicine"—specifically, research on human cloning and the use of embryonic stem cells—there has come into being a frenzied effort, inhumane and excessively optimistic, to reconstruct what is fundamentally human. Why has this "reckless medicine" emerged in Japan? Our urgent task is to investigate the meaning of this development in both the past and the present, and at the same time to explore countermeasures and decide the direction that should be taken in the future. We must begin by probing the historical and social background of these matters and by drawing lessons from what we find. In other words, we must look once more into our own history and in this way pursue the kind of bioethics that is critically needed in our new century. Here I will put forth a proposal based on what I understand to be the central and critical issue.

The Divine Face and the Demonic Face of Medical Science: Unit 731 and Aum Shinrikyō

When considering Japan's own history of reckless medical science, the first example that comes to mind is the biological warfare unit known as Unit 731. Formed in the 1930s, Unit 731 continued to conduct inhumane experiments until the end of World War II in order to develop bacterial warfare. It was a secret research organization based in Manchuria, and it conducted horrendous experiments on living Chinese prisoners of war, persons referred to as "*maruta*," or logs. Many prominent physicians, such as Dr. Shirō Ishii, were responsible for the development of this unit and its inhumane activities.[1]

It was Colonel Ishii who first proposed the idea of a special unit devoted to investigating bacterial warfare, and he was given the task of forming it. Upon graduating from Kyoto Imperial University's Faculty of Medicine in 1920, he served as a probationary officer in the Imperial Infantry 3rd Regiment and later at the First Kyoto Infantry Hospital and Fushimi Infantry Hospital. In 1927 he entered the Graduate School of the Kyoto Imperial University's Faculty of Medicine and became a doctor of medicine. From 1928 until 1930 he traveled in Germany for research, and in 1931 he started work at the Epidemic Prevention Laboratory in the Military Medical School in Tokyo.

There are three main ways to disperse biological weapons. One way is to scatter pathogens from aircraft, a second is to utilize bombs, and a third is through means of sabotage. In other words, this third way involved introducing pathogens into foodstuffs or water wells, thereby creating an epidemic of things such as the plague, cholera, or typhoid fever.

Even though much information about the military's inhumane medical experimentation conducted by Ishii and his unit has come to light, the actual circumstances surrounding what happened have not been adequately investigated. So many aspects of their activities defy belief, leaving one to wonder what on earth would prompt anyone even to conceive such projects. Although, because I am not an expert in this particular field of research, I will avoid going into depth concerning Unit 731, I wish to note that this entire subject strikes me as having similarities with the Aum Shinrikyō cult's sarin gas attacks in Tokyo in 1995. Many innocent people fell victim to this act of terrorism, and a number of the perpetrators within the Aum group were capable young scientists and physicians, persons who had received their education at some of Japan's most prominent science universities. Recently, Shōkō Asahara, the leader of the Aum cult, was given the death sentence for his part in that crime. Nevertheless, despite the number of years that have passed since the crime itself, there still remains considerable mystery about how such a heinous group act came to be conceived and carried out.

Over half a century separated the days of Unit 731's crimes and those of the sarin gas attacks by the Aum cult. Differences exist in the nature of crimes committed by the military in one case and a religious group in the other. Of course, even in spite of the differences, we cannot deny the similarities, especially that both involved reckless medical experimentation. There are two points in particular that I wish to explore in regard to both crimes. The first concerns the problem of "evil" that is inherent in both medical science and religion. My second point relates to the essence of medical science and religion and their inevitable constructs to ensure survival. I think that these two points are closely linked to contemporary medical science, to bioethics, and to what we are here calling "reckless medicine." In looking at these we confront some very thorny issues.

Taking up the first point, I note that the Expert's Panel on Bioethics of Japan's Council for Science and Technology published an interim report, *Research Guidelines for Embryonic Stem Cells*, on December 26, 2003. Following the cloning of Dolly the sheep in February of 1997, the Japanese government passed new legislation concerning cloning technology. In this legislation rules governing research using embryos and the treatment of human zygotes through successful growth of human embryonic stem cells were spelled out. This report took into consideration all of the most up-to-date information to provide guidelines that address the related ethical issues.

The consensus concerning research into the hotly debated subject of regenerative medicine was that, for the time being, human zygotes would not be used in regenerative medicine, although human embryonic stem (ES) cells could possibly be used for clinical application in the future. Basically, it is not permissible to use human zygotes in regenerative medicine, but the use of human ES cells was condoned. This means that research and experiments utilizing human zygotes are prohibited, but experiments using human embryo clones and human embryonic stem cells are permissible. The reasons given were that the latter were "not deemed to be undermining human dignity" and that research into ES cells has the potential to advance many areas of regenerative medicine in the future. The authors of the report even went so far as to say that "it has the potential to contribute greatly to the development of fundamental research into the life sciences" (Expert's Panel on Bioethics 22). Although the report also expresses concern about dangers in research using human ES cells, without question the overall tone of the report reflects great expectations and highlights the great potential of research using human ES cells. Here we are faced with a difficult problem. It shows up in the interim report's way of drawing a line to divide what is considered tolerable from what is considered unacceptable in research and treatment. Supposedly drawn by persons with special expertise, this line becomes a kind of law that regards tolerable research as "good" and its contrary, unacceptable research, as "evil." The prestige of "expertise" too is placed on a rather arbitrary distinction between research that does not undermine "human dignity" and actions that supposedly do. This gives rise to a concept that radically divides things into two directions: a life science that is evil and another that is good. Treatments too become one or the other, evil or good.

We must, however, be skeptical about that line separating the good from the evil: Is it accurate and is it so absolute? Who is to be given the ultimate task of being objective enough to decide what exactly undermines human dignity, and how can the objectivity of those so deciding be guaranteed? Surely we know that standards have continuously evolved with the passage of time and in accord with advances in medicine and the life sciences.

Here is where I wish to assert that this split-directional mode of construing good and evil kinds of medical treatment must be exposed as having reached its own stage of fully exhausted viability. Thus, an important point here is that we must refrain from any longer trying to develop and refine this approach. This would also mean we need to realize that both good and evil are intrinsic within medical research and treatment. It is virtually impossible to separate them. Perhaps now we should become skeptical about the usual dualism and tackle the possibility that both a divine face and a demonic face show up within the world of medical research. If we refuse to make a basic reevaluation of these matters, we could very well run the risk of giving help to persons conducting research not unlike the patently criminal research carried out by the Nazi experimenters and Japan's Unit 731.

Especially on this point, an incident such as Aum Shinrikyō's sarin gas attack in Tokyo in 1995 encourages me to think again about how recklessly medical science can be used. In the aftermath of those attacks, religious authorities, the media, and various experts were unanimous in their opinion that Aum Shinrikyō's actions were beyond the pale of the comprehensible to the minds of ordinary people and obviously were understood only by the perpetrators themselves in their own closed, antisocial world. In other words, religions also divide into two: good religions and evil religions. Aum Shinrikyō provided a perfect model of the latter, with adherents who are surely hell-bound. Here, too, we see the same two-directional pattern. The world divides into the sane and insane, good versus evil, God in opposition to the devil. Historical examples of religious warfare such as the Crusades in the West or the *Ikkō-ikki* in medieval Japan were not taken up for consideration within this simplistic interpretative dualism. It is, I claim, the same narrow-minded and ego-centered approach that refuses to recognize that there are both good and evil characteristics in the life sciences and in all medical research.

Next, in connection with another comment about the crimes of Aum Shinrikyō, I wish to introduce my second point, which concerns strategies for "survival." It is good to recall that both science and religion have been very closely bound to human projects for ensuring survival. Human history is virtually a story of efforts by humans to secure their own survival. In science we see the latest technologies trying to do that—through organ transplantation and in the various forms of regenerative medicine. Survival is their goal. But the deluded people in Aum Shinrikyō, even if it became a terrorist organization and caused the death of innocents, were attempting to secure their own salvation—their own *survival*—beyond an anticipated and impending Armageddon. Surely this was a selfish act based on delirious fantasy, but it was oriented to ensure their "survival." Warped notions of superiority and of deserving to survive while others perish are imbedded in such thinking.

The Choice: Orientation to Survival Theory or to Impermanence

We must also recognize certain differences in historical contexts in which Eastern and Western civilizations devised their strategies for survival. If we were confronted today with a catastrophic crisis such as the great, world-destroying flood described in the Old Testament, what would we do? I believe that we basically would have two alternatives. One alternative is symbolized by the story of Noah and his ark. God, angered by human depravity, sent a cataclysmic flood, but Noah was able to survive with his wife and children by building an ark. This is a tale of only a select few surviving a crisis of human extinction. This myth of survival is in some ways the parent of what might be called the "survival principle." It is something that pervades the history of Jewish and Christian societies, giving rise to such concepts as a "chosen people" and even to certain versions of evolution theory. Moreover, it may be said to have formed the basis of later philosophical and ethical assumptions about how a person should live, and even to have provided foundational ideas in contemporary political and economic theory.

For a modern example I point to the tragedy of the sinking of the *Titanic,* one of the world's greatest nautical disasters. It occurred in April 1912, but remains today deeply engraved in our memory because of the 1,500 out of 2,200 passengers and crew who shared the fate of the ship. This spectacular modern version of the story of Noah's Ark presents a stark division of life and death, the saved and the unsaved. Needless to say, this same "strategy of survival" is also at work in the arena of contemporary medicine. I refer, for instance, to the life-manipulating technology that involves having one person die by brain death but another be selected to survive by getting the other's organs. Another example on a global scale is the proposal for "sustainable development" taken up at the United Nations Earth Summit in Rio de Janeiro, Brazil, in 1992. It constituted a strategy for maintaining and extending economic development by selecting certain regions and resources for that purpose. It seems clear, therefore, that the theory of survival continues to exert an enormous and consequence-filled influence today.

There is an alternative. It is the decision, if humanity were to be assailed by a calamity like Noah's flood, to die. And that decision is made upon realization that the vast majority cannot evade dying. This alternative expresses a view of life in which being part of a small minority to survive personally is rejected. It involves the decision to stand with the majority and to share their deaths in every way. Such a decision, I believe, arises most readily in a context where a Buddhist view of impermanence is foundational. It embraces the fact that nothing in the world is permanent and unchanging; all things inevitably perish. Thus, no living thing can escape death. Put succinctly, this was the Buddha's view of impermanence. Within this position, what is moral flows from clearly recognizing that any "survival" will be only a limited survival. In contrast to the "theory of survival," this approach may be called a "theory of impermanence."

Although I refer here to the Buddhist view of impermanence, the formulation of this belief is not uniform. For example, the impermanence expounded by the Buddha is a dry, unemotional awareness, while the understanding of it in Japan reveals a rather different quality. The *Tales of the Heike* of medieval Japan open with oft-quoted lines: "The bronze bell of the Jeta grove monastery reverberates and sounds out the impermanence of all things." The tone of this communicates a sense of transiency that involves tears and the pathos of sorrow. There is, then, a difference between in one case early Buddhism's philosophical and objective grasp of the nature of things, and in the other an emotional comprehension, one in which tears are shed in boundless sympathy for all those who are perishing. When one visits the parched regions in India where the Buddha carried on his activities, one senses a qualitative difference between ideas of impermanence there and what appears in the *Tales of the Heike*, wherein the nobles of the Heike clan sink into the waters of Dannoura. In that scene they, one after another, meet with reality of impermanence, but they do so convulsed with pain and perceptible sorrow.

By contrast, we can take note of a haiku by Ryōkan, a Zen monk who lived from 1758 to 1831:

Showing their backs,	*ura o mise*
showing their fronts—	*omote o misete*
the scattering red leaves	*chiru momiji*

Here we find notes arising from a crystal-clear awareness of impermanence, one in which the speaker, in anticipating death, delights in a return to nature. This sense of impermanence could even be called a bright one. This is why I suggest that there is no uniformity in how impermanence is grasped.

Our problem today is that we seem destined to face the following dilemma. We envision the massive wave of globalization beginning to pour down upon us, and, even in resisting it, we glimpse a picture of ourselves trying *to survive—* we are ironically bound to the very "survival theory" we are trying to resist. However, is it not the case that just when we seem to be bending under the immense pressures of the times, we find from the depths of our own consciousness emanating strains of the principle of impermanence? Will these two different, even opposing, melodies—one grasping for survival and the other accepting impermanence—ever be able to be harmonized into a duet? Or will each of them just continue, like automated dolls awkwardly trying to keep up with a frenzied rhythm? I think our century is the one that has to decide on one or the other of these alternatives.

Body-Spirit Dualism and Cannibalism

If a Japanese of the ancient Man'yō period (seventh–eighth centuries) were to come back to life today, I suspect that person would agree to the program of organ transplantation. Such a person would freely and affirmatively offer his own organs to others, because the people of the Man'yō era did not have strong attachments to their own bodies. When we look, for example, at the elegies (*banka*) in the *Man'yōshū*, the collected poetry of that age, we find a expression of the belief that at death the spirits of the dead separate from the corpse and ascend to high places, mountains for instance. And there is no interest whatsoever in the body that would have been left behind. This is to say that, after death, the corpse is merely the cast-off husk of the spirit. What was of concern to the Man'yō people was the destination of the spirit, not the body. The latter, in fact, might be left to be devoured by dogs or birds. Thus, if a wandering monk or a beggar slit open the chest and drew out organs, making some use of them, people then would not have shrieked with alarm or raised protests.

In other words, the Man'yō era people differentiated the physical body and the spirit, themselves taking the stance of unambiguous dualism. This is why I can imagine that they, even if confronted with the phenomenon of organ transplantation, would not have been greatly shocked. This attitude has always been present in Japanese society. It persists in the folklore-embodied notion that what is important is the spirit, and that the bodily remains are no more than a kind of sacred debris. They are to be exposed and reduced to bones. Between the Japanese of that era and the ethos of modern organ transplantation, therefore, there was this point of similarity. Further similarities would be impossible to demonstrate since, for example, today's transplant surgeons focus on trying to determine the precise point of "brain death," whereas the Manyō people gave no thought to an attempt to determine the instant of death.

To the Man'yō people a person was not deemed dead simply because consciousness had been lost or breathing had stopped. Rather, such conditions were thought to indicate that the spirit had departed temporarily from the body. It was believed that that spirit might return, and therefore the lifeless body was left to lie undisturbed for a period of time. This was called *mogari*, a time that could extend from several days to several weeks. During it the survivors sought to beckon the spirit back to the body. It might be called a period of "near-death experience," and the rituals conducted were known as "spirit calling" (*tama-yobai*). During *mogari* the person was not considered dead, for the spirit was only journeying in other realms, inclusive of hells or heavens. There would gradually come a time, however, when the expectation that the spirit would return had to be relinquished. When the odor of putrefaction arose from the corpse, the survivors came to accept that the rituals of spirit calling had been ineffective, and at that point death was socially recognized.[2]

We could say that the failure of the calls to the spirit to return, as indicated by the odor of putrefaction, corresponds to our notification of brain death. Unfortunately, of course, once decomposition of the body has begun, the organs are useless. In most of human history most practices of putting the organs or body parts of the dead to "use" were related to cannibalism. This practice was widely distributed among peoples of the world, especially when they were facing death through starvation. During times of war and famine, the impulse to find a *survival* strategy by eating the flesh of the dead was almost unavoidable. We see it taking place among starving soldiers during World War II, as narrated in Shōhei Ōoka's novel *Nobi* (translated as *Fire on the Plains*), and also depicted in the scene of the shipwreck in Taijun Takeda's *Hikarigoke* (Luminous moss). It occurred during the Cultural Revolution period in China and among victims of a plane crash in the Andes mountains in 1972. Needless to say, if one searches back into history, many such examples might be found. The Christian sacrament of Holy Communion, with bread and wine for Christ's body and blood, may also be said to reflect the practice of cannibalism. Within Japan, the outbreaks of eating human flesh during the famines of the Tenmei era (1781–89) in the Nanbu province in the northeast have been transmitted through vivid accounts.

When cannibalism occurs during times of war or famine, the point of death of a person on the verge of dying will surely vary according to the conditions of those making the determination. Some would decide to cannibalize a body already when it seemed that the spirit had left the corpse, but others would not remove the organs until the last possible point before the odor of putrefaction arose. Some might eat the flesh raw, whereas others might roast or smoke the organs to preserve them. These are what I have called strategies for survival, and with them people seek, through the effective utilization of another's organs or other body parts, somehow to extricate themselves from crisis.

We may even say that the ways in which bodies were treated in traditional folk societies have, in effect, been adopted into the arena of modern medicine. The hospital room scene in which an artificial respirator has been introduced to revive a dying patient seems to overlap with the ancient rituals for recalling the spirit. The figure of the physician who announces the death of the heart may be superimposed over the ancient shaman who declared that the spirit had departed for good. Behind the medical specialists anxiously awaiting the moment of brain death, we see the shadowy figures of persons in the past plotting an effective utilization, through consumption, of body parts. When we make ourselves aware of our human history, it becomes very difficult for us, especially when we are seeking to grant survival to our own lives through transplanted organs, not to be reminded of the cannibalism widely recognized in folk societies.

Exchanging Hearts and Heart Contemplation: Two Narratives

In 1999 a transplantation procedure, inclusive of the heart, was performed by a medical team at Osaka University. This occurred after a moratorium on such transplantations had meant that thirty-one years elapsed since the first such heart transfer had taken place. This was in 1968, when a heart had been transplanted by Dr. Jurō Wada in Sapporo, Japan. Wada was subsequently vilified, and the long moratorium began. The "secretive" nature of Wada's operation was criticized in the media, by Japan's medical community, and in general society. He was made the object of blame, perhaps even becoming a scapegoat. By contrast, the transplantation performed at Osaka University in 1999 was celebrated widely as a success and bathed in media spotlights that made it look like a heroic episode, one introducing a wonderful new age. The old and easily comprehended story of good contrasted to evil appeared: the "tale" of organ transplantation in modern Japan now could be told, with Dr. Wada as its villain and the Osaka team as its hero.

Constructing such events as stories is nothing new—across both East and West. The heart organ has often been at their center. The grand Sacré Coeur Cathedral rises from the hills of Montmartre in Paris. Sacré Coeur—"sacred heart"—appears in the names of many Catholic churches, even in Japan. Seishin (Sacred Heart) Women's University, so respected that even the current empress of Japan is a graduate, is an example. But how did this name originate? The tale is instructive. We are taken back to the seventeenth century and to a country village near Florence, Italy. An abnormal condition arose in the body of Benedetta Carlini, the abbess of a convent in that area. One night Jesus Christ appeared as a beautiful youth with long hair and approached the bed of the abbess. Declaring "I have come to take your heart," the young man pulled up his sleeves and drew her heart from the abbess's body, placing it in his own breast. He then left.

For three days thereafter, Benedetta lived without a heart. Then, in the middle of the night, Christ again appeared with a host of saints. He held aloft a large heart bound with a sash of gold. It was heart of Jesus himself. He ordered that Benedetta's robe be removed, and into her exposed side he inserted his own heart. As was the case of lovers who appear in the medieval tales of chivalry, here also the two became one in body and heart. Afterward, Benedetta was tried as a heretic by the Church and spent thirty-five years in confinement, finally dying at the age of seventy-one. Gradually, however, this incident became the object of discussion concerning the fusion of physical and spiritual love. It eventually gave rise to worship of the "sacred heart." Moreover, in the eighteenth century, it came to be recognized officially by the Church. This is a Western narrative of the exchange of sacred hearts. I myself, however, find the image of the abbess Benedetta receiving Christ's heart somehow coalescing with that of Dr. Wada transferring a heart from one person to another.

I am also reminded of the technique of heart contemplation found in Indian esotericism. There is an ancient method of meditation called "heart-disc contemplation." In it the heart is seen in the form of the moon (*gachirin-kan* in its Japanese version), and this is thought to be held within the breast of what Japanese refer to as Dainichi Nyorai, the central focus of spiritual attention in esoteric Buddhism. But it is also thought to lie in the breast of someone engaged in this meditative practice. This heart is envisioned as burning with a flaming crimson color and is contemplated as a lunar disc at rest on a lotus blossom. Of course, in addition to the heart as object, there are contemplative techniques focused on the five organs and six viscera that were developed in esoteric practice. The meditation on the heart, however, was given particular attention. Through it, practitioners pursued the actualization of the experience of mystical union with Dainichi Nyorai, which is the cosmos itself.

It was Kūkai (774–835) who adapted this form of meditation to Japan, giving it a new and distinctive interpretation. At the site of contemplative practice, a personalized Dainichi approaches the meditator and the latter approaches Dainichi. Kūkai describes this process as "[Buddha] entering self / the self entering [Buddha]" (*nyūga ganyū*). Important here is the mutual approach and coalescing of the two hearts. When they have come together, a single cosmic lunar disc is visualized. This corresponds to what Kūkai explained as an "attainment of Buddhahood with this very body" (*sokushin jōbutsu*).

I find it fascinating that within the Christian world we find the mystical experience of the "Sacred Heart" and in the Buddhist world the "heart-disc contemplation." Whereas in the Christian context an *exchange of hearts* between the divine and the human being is envisioned, in the Japanese Buddhist context it is the *fusion in body and mind* of Dainichi Buddha and a human that is taken as the final, ecstatic goal. These two narratives, one from the West and the other from the East, may perhaps be said to be reflected even today in how we conceive of certain medical procedures.

The Etiquette of Dying and the Depiction of the Buddha's Self-Sacrifice

Ever since the matters of brain death and organ transplants came to be widely discussed in society I have been concerned that the *etiquette of dying* would be meeting its own end.[3] It seemed inevitable that the act of dying, which over centuries and through generations had its own etiquette and ritual, by which is expressed an essential respect for human beings, would lose its dignity. If we look, for example, at the meticulous legal and medical procedures involved in determining brain death, we wonder about the family of the dying person at that time. Where are they? What are they doing? What *can* they do? How do they pass that time apart from the one who has so long been a part of themselves? Why are they themselves not caring for the dying one? Such core questions about what is changing at this critical junction in life are completely neglected. What matters is being kept in the dark and left without discussion. What one hears instead is the rather flippant reference to the deceased's family need for "privacy," or their desire to avoid publicity. To me these shallow expressions seem no more than unconvincing abstractions that run roughshod over the actual feelings of dying persons and those who, close to them through life, wish to be with them at their deaths.

What once were extensive and meaningful rituals in connection with dying seem now about to be reduced to the "ritual" of signing an organ-donation card. But does this not amount to little more than putting a circle or a check on a piece of paper in a context that euphemizes it all as "altruism"? Rituals are reduced to a series of decisions—whether the corpse will be cremated or buried and whether the ashes will be scattered and whether the body will be donated for research. But is this real ritual? Just as the disposition of the deceased's material property is unrelated to the ritual or etiquette of dying, so too the declaration concerning one's organs on a donor card, supposedly as just another kind of "property," seems divorced from meaningful rituals of dying.

At present there is much public talk about "death education." Because dying has increasingly been confined to hospitals, the opportunity to witness the dying process in the home and in the context of the family has been lost. Dying in hospitals separates dying from ordinary life and conceals its actuality from the family. For this reason, "death education," scarcely necessary in the past, is said now to be something needed by younger generations. What dying is is to be "taught" from elementary school on, and school children are said to need to be brought to the bedsides of the dying so that they can have personalized "experience" of death.

At first glance, such an approach to the problem may seem reasonable, but is it not rather just another case of idealizing something that had already become too abstract and separated from life? Is it really possible to *teach* death? When I was a child in school, I witnessed my eighty-year-old grandfather's death at home: his weakening, becoming bedridden, and then dying in pain. At that time, I saw only that the living gradually grow feeble, emit odors of decay, and then perish; I did not grasp "dying" or the meaning of a human death. I thought that my grandfather died much like a cat or dog or other small animal. Notions of the dignity of a human being did not occur to me. I looked on my grandfather's death as similar to the biological death of an animal.

Why was this? I wonder if it was not because I could not sense or perceive my grandfather's "etiquette of death." What was most important in the scene was not visible to a school child. I believe my grandfather indeed had his own way of dying, and had his own etiquette of death. Perhaps he uttered the *nenbutsu* prayer, unknown to others. Perhaps he imparted in some form an expression of the meaning of his life. Such rituals of death, however, were not clearly perceived by the family. It must be said that in our family life in the late 1930s, the tradition of giving dying its own etiquette had already begun to vanish into the twilight. I now recognize this with great regret. Through the spread of the notion of brain death and organ transplantation, this trend toward the loss of contextualized ritual is only bound to deepen.

Dying without an appropriate etiquette is very much a departure from what in the past was referred to as a "great death," one involving rebirth in the Pure Land (*dai-ōjō*). To die without such a context of etiquette is little different from the way in which a cat or dog might die. It reinforces a sense that the bodily remains may be nothing more than refuse, to be disposed of like the body of an animal. This analogizing of humans to animals may be connected to how easily some greet a technology that would use the organs of animals to ensure the survival of persons whose own organs were threatening to fail. Xenotransplantation technologies would, it is assumed, allow for the organs of pigs or monkeys to replace defective ones in humans. Once that takes place, I suspect, the strategy of survival, technologically implemented, will have completely smothered what may still be left of the rituals and etiquette of dying.

I have one more topic I wish to discuss. It has to do with what in Buddhism is a teaching about the need to make offerings as an expression of selfless giving (*dāna* in Sanskrit; *fuse* in Japanese). Some feel that organ transplantation should be condoned as acts that manifest that spirit of selfless giving, simply because in this way new life is given through the sacrifice of one's own organs. In this interpretation, although brain death and organ transplantation are advanced technologies given birth in the modern West, the spirit behind them can match what is present also in Buddhist thought. Traditionally "giving" in the Buddhist tradition primarily involved bestowing goods such as clothing or food or, alternatively, more spiritual gifts such as the dharma itself. When pushed to the extreme, it might also involve the notion that one might want to sacrifice one's own body and life for the sake of others. If one takes such an attitude to its extreme, it leads to the notion of sacrificing one's body to bestow it on others. Organ donation then would be its logical outcome.

On the surface, although such thinking may appear reasonable, I do not find it so. I hold that it is erroneous to connect the spirit of selfless giving in the Buddhist tradition so directly to the notion of brain death and the practice of organ transplantation. And here I put forth my reasons. There is a well-known tale of the Buddha "casting away his body to feed hungry tigers." According to this legend the Buddha in a previous life threw his body from a cliff so that starving tigers might feed on his flesh. In Japan this story is known especially through its depiction on a celebrated altar case in the Hōryūji constructed in the seventh century. Noteworthy, however, is the fact that in later periods of Japanese history there were almost no allusions to this tale. It appears that its details were too brutal, too overtly graphic to gain much favor. Pictorial representations of this tale traditionally consisted of three frames. The uppermost frame shows the Buddha, as a prince who has seen a starving tigress and her cubs, removing his garments. The middle frame is the scene in which the graceful, refined body of the prince is falling from the cliff to the ground below. The lower frame depicts a close-up of the tigers tearing and devouring the fallen body. The upper two frames beautifully describe the bodhisattva-prince's decision to sacrifice himself. The lower frame, however, brings into view a transformation of everything—so that what had been beautiful and noble has turned into a scene of what is grisly and ugly. It becomes something from which we would want to turn our eyes.

This narrative of the Buddha's self-sacrifice appears in Jataka tales and some sutra literature in India, and it received pictorial depiction in Central Asia and China. While examples are few, it is also seen among the cave wall paintings at Qizil and Dun-huang. Five years ago I visited Dun-huang expressly in order to see the paintings of this tale with my own eyes. I also took that opportunity to speak with the director of the research institute there. I still remember clearly his explaining that, in spite of the fame of this tale, graphic representations of it are disproportionately rare. He seemed to glance off into space when telling me this.

I had checked on some of the facts before my journey and knew how rare were such paintings. Moreover, in some cases, the lower frame alone has been defaced with mud—and not just once or twice. I was led to wonder whether the Buddhists of Central Asia and China had, like the Japanese, found uncomfortable the scene of the devouring of the young man's body. I suspect that they, too, felt it was deeply disturbing.

Early on I had begun to wonder whether perhaps Christian themes of sacrifice had been incorporated into this tale and its representations. The act of throwing one's body to tigers depicted seemed like it might have come via contact with the narrative of the sacrifice of Jesus on the cross. By the time of the formation of the tale of the sacrifice to tigers, it is not impossible that, with the transmission of Greco-Roman culture into Gandhara, aspects of the Christian tradition might possibly have reached India. So I wondered whether this might have been a catalyst for the narrative of the Buddha's self-sacrifice for the sake of hungry tigers. Had the concept of sacrifice in Christian teachings been appended to the Buddhist spirit of selfless giving? I wondered if this relatively late story had been born out of these conflated images of giving and sacrifice.

That remains possible. There is, however, another way of understanding the depictions of the Buddha's sacrifice of his body, and it is this one that I find more plausible. It takes into account the possibility of influence from the hunting culture of northern nomadic tribes. In such societies animals are hunted, bred, domesticated, and slaughtered. Every part of an animal, including its organs, is used to sustain daily life. Waste is not permitted. The range of animals so used extends all the way from the gentler species of deer and rabbit to the more ferocious ones of lion and tiger. When the more dangerous ones are hunted, the result may be either that the animal is killed and consumed or that the hunter himself is killed and devoured. Humans who have not been alert or are overcome by drowsiness may become the food for their own prey. That is, humans have their place in the food chain of the natural world. This is the struggle for survival. Perhaps then this reality is what has been depicted in the final scene of the tale of the young prince being so devoured by starving tigers. If so, we are forced to seek the concept underlying the prince's self-sacrifice not in a transmission of the Christian principle of sacrifice or in Buddhist practices of selfless giving, but in the influence of the consciousness present in hunting societies.

I am attracted to this explanation and suspect that it reflects the truth of the matter. In the third frame of the pictorial representations of the tale, we see that, just as humans dismember and consume animals, so animals may dismember and consume humans. It shows a form of culture that lies outside concepts of sacrifice and, instead, highlights the harshness of life that is impervious to the religious humanism of "selfless giving." This severity, in a word, indicates that human beings carried on their lives within the food chain in which they ate or were eaten—surely the code of hunting societies.

Is it not the case, however, that being themselves a consumed part of the food chain was for human beings something shed when the development of agriculture and animal domestication created a new socio-ecological order? By being liberated from this aspect of the food chain, human beings became able to establish human-centered principles. A new ethics of the human order was created in which, although animals might still be slaughtered, it was no longer necessary for humans themselves to be consumed. The point I wish to make here, however, is that it is an error to put forth the tale of the Buddha's sacrifice in feeding tigers as an example within the Buddhist tradition used to rationalize the practice of organ transplantation based on the notion of brain death. There is something self-serving in the effort to use this minor narrative within the Buddhist tradition to justify this modern practice. I think it wrong, even arrogant, to twist the major emphases of our Buddhist tradition in order to elevate this minor motif into a grand rationalization for a modern medical technique that is otherwise ethically problematic.

I plan, at the end of my own life, to fast and then die. Of course, if I meet with an accident or with sudden death, there will not be time for an extended fast. But should I be blessed with a natural death or death by illness, it is my plan to fast to the end. For this reason, I have no impulse to want to receive the organs of others should my own organs fail. No one need carry an organ-donation card on my behalf. I want no life-prolonging treatment, and I want to avoid having someone determine by technology that my brain has died. Consequently, I have no inclination to donate my organs. This is because I believe that fasting can serve as a starting point in giving dying its proper etiquette. Should I be so fortunate, I hope to be able to pass through a rich and fruitful period between the entrance into the fast and my death. I do not know what words may leave my lips during that time. Perhaps it will be a hymn or a popular song or, perhaps, the voicing of the *nenbutsu*. Perhaps it will be a death cry. I may be bereft of words and end in utter silence. Whatever the outcome, I have no concern. I believe, however, that fasting will be the best ceremony of death left to me. Exactly what form this ritual of death will take is my great uncertainty, but it is something to which I look forward with great anticipation and pleasure. It is not that I am resigned to death or have awakened to death. Rather, it is simply that I believe that meeting the end in such a way signifies ending life in a distinctively human manner.

If a starving tiger should approach my dying body, I would naturally be terrorized by it. Selfless giving would not be my impulse. But my preference is, in fact, to bring to mind a totally different scene from the Buddhist tradition of dying. It is of the *parinirvana*, the death of the Buddha. Often painted, it portrays him lying in the middle of the scene, surrounded by his disciples. But there too are animals of all kinds, quietly watching and awaiting his peaceful end. When I note that I prefer to face my own death with that scene in mind, it is not because I presume to be able to follow the Buddha's manner of dying to that degree. What I like in this scene is how it portrays dying as possible without others, humans or animals, looking on to see how they themselves might profit from that death. In the scene of the *parinirvana* the animals are not there with the hope of getting and consuming some organs or parts of the body. They are there to be present and watchful at the time of another's death.

I realize full well that we cannot know exactly how we will die. And I, in fact, very suddenly may lose consciousness or be taken into a hospital to die. When I waken, I may find intravenous equipment attached to both arms and tubes running through my nostrils and mouth. I may even be tied down to prevent movement. It is not impossible that, failing to fulfill my cherished hope to fast my way into death, these mechanized procedures, too much like the features of hell, will overcome me. At that time, it will all be over.

Notes

1. My sources for this are primarily Akiyama 1956, Gunji 1982, and Tsuneishi 1995.
2. This is treated in more detail in Yamaori 2004.
3. This is a topic dealt with in Yamaori 2002.

References

Akiyama, Hiroshi. 1956. *Tokushu butai*. Tokyo: San'ichi shobō.
Expert's Panel on Bioethics. 2003. Committee of Japan's Council for Science and Technology. *Research Guidelines for Embryonic Stem Cells*. An interim report, published December 26, 2003.
Gunji, Yōko. 1982. *Nana-san-ichi Ishii butai*. Tokyo: Tokuma shoten.
Tsuneishi, Kei-ichi. 1995. *Nana-san-ichi butai*. Tokyo; Kōdansha.
Yamaori, Tetsuo. 2002. *Kokoro no sahō*. Tokyo: Chūkō shinsho.
———. 2004. *Wandering Spirits and Temporary Corpses: Studies in the History of Japanese Religious Traditions*. Ed. and trans. Dennis Hirota. Kyoto: International Research Center for Japanese Studies.

13 The Age of a "Revolutionized Human Body" and the Right to Die

Yoshihiko Komatsu

Entering a New Era

Over the last twenty-five years the most active front in scientific and technological advancement was no longer in the physical sciences but in the biological ones. Among these advances, those within the field of medicine—a field intimately bound up with being born, being ill, aging, and dying—have rapidly increased the pace of their development, beginning with the complete mapping of the human genome at the turn of the century and the establishment of human embryonic stem cells. Tailor-made medical pharmacogenomics and regenerative medicines have been heralded worldwide as "the medicine of our dreams," and, accordingly, nations and corporations have been investing exorbitant sums into their research and development. Not only is it clear that "biotechnology" has already become the central focus of twenty-first-century science and technology, but we have entered into what can be called, I suggest, an era of "corporeal revolution."[1]

The main characteristic of this corporeal revolution is that the human has become not merely the *subject* in this revolution but its *object* as well. In other words, we, the actors in this revolution, have made the human body its direct target by taking our own bodies as the material for research and development. This certainly has not been a characteristic of any of our other, earlier, "revolutions." Today, while there is a tendency to emphasize the silver lining of such technology, it should also be realized that revolutionizing the human body and the way we exist in this world essentially is something that has the power to decide the fate of all civilization and culture.

This new revolution may be the biggest development since the theories of Copernicus and Darwin. However, it must be pointed out that the changes in the world brought about by biological science are on a *qualitatively* different level from those in the past. In contrast to the problems of Copernican and Darwinian theory, which involved realizing truths in nature that lay beyond man's ability to alter them, the problems of biological science today involve intervention into, manipulation of, and control over both nature and the human body.

Our reach now extends all the way to the genetic level, touching the most fundamental elements of the human body. At such a crucial moment in human history, it seems that while there has certainly been some debate, much of it has been limited in both scope and depth. Our discussion has been unable to reach the crux of this issue. Discussing things in terms of the "dignity of life" or according to the principle of a "right to self-determination" (or "autonomy") has become almost pointless. As citizens of a global community, we owe it to ourselves to expand the horizons of this debate. With that in mind, I offer a few personal observations and reflections, critically examining past debates and assessing the coming corporeal revolution.

From the "Dignity of Life" to the "Dignity of the Human Body"

The Unassailability of "Bio-Manipulation"

Shock waves circled the globe when Dr. Severino Antinori, an Italian, announced in April 2002 that a cloned human would be born within the year. Although there is probably a need to examine thoroughly the real reason why, out of all the various aspects of the "corporeal revolution," we have a particularly strong aversion to cloning human beings, it is a fact that the idea of cloning humans is repugnant to most people.[2] We need to point out, however, that by focusing so intently on the prospect of a cloned human, we risk overlooking something terribly important.

This is that cloning's putative value will lie not merely in the creation of a cloned human but, more importantly, in the creation of a cloned human embryo (Kayukawa 2003). Such an embryo (made by replacing the genetic code of a human embryo with the genetic code of a patient to create embryonic stem cells that might then be induced to differentiate into a necessary organ) will make it possible, in theory, to replace "organ transplantation" with "regenerative medicine." Some claim that even immuno-rejection can thus be avoided. Importantly, though, the decisive difference between the traditional method of organ transplantation and the cloned-embryo method lies in the vast profit potential of the latter. This is precisely the reason why corporations and governments are investing enormous sums in it. Put bluntly, cloning technology is intimately tied up, to an unprecedented degree, with corporate profits and national interests. Furthermore, because in most countries the general rule is for there to be no remuneration for pre-implantation eggs donated for the making of a cloned embryo, the later financial profits, which may be huge, will not benefit the original donors of the ova. Naturally, the same type of structure applies to other forms of regenerative medicine and tailor-made therapies. In sum, the corporeal revolution does not merely refer to the manipulation of life. It consists of the radical change that occurs by transforming the human body into a resource, making it into a commodity, and putting it and/or its parts on the market. This is at the very heart of what it means to revolutionize the human body, and we must thoroughly consider what these aspects of this revolution really mean.[3]

The reality is, however, that current debates almost never confront the core issue. Our aversion to the use of the human body in both research and industry appears to be, by comparison, far weaker than our aversion to the outright cloning of whole humans. This is so despite the fact that, whereas only *unfertilized* eggs are used in the creation of cloned human embryos, when it comes to the creation of embryonic stem cells, not only unfertilized eggs but also fertilized eggs and fertilized embryos are used.

We clearly have not grasped what is fundamental in this. I suggest that one reason for this is that, until now, our debates have pivoted around the concept of "the dignity of life." However, on the concrete level this stated concern has very easily been diverted into the question "Is this *human* life or not?" If we answer this in the negative, the door, ironically, actually gets opened for the use of human bodies for research and commercial purposes.

For instance, in the United Kingdom and Japan, the use of human fertilized eggs in research is permitted until the *primitive streak*[4] develops, approximately fourteen days after fertilization. But this is merely the result of groping around to locate a time period during which an embryo can be considered merely a "thing." That is, when the "dignity of life" seems to fetter the use of embryos in research and industry, one merely needs to find a time period to which the "dignity of life" does not apply. If prior to the development of a nervous system—that is, when distinctively *human* features are thought not yet to inhere—one can say that "human dignity" will not be involved, the matter is taken to be a nonissue, and obstacles to usage are removed. This is why I claim that the notion of "dignity of life" is largely ineffective. And the only reason we think there is something unusually weird about cloning is because of the hold on us of the notion of a distinct "human personhood" handed down to us by John Locke and others.

In contrast to this, I will here delineate a concept I have called "reverberating death," one first proposed in a 1996 book with that title in Japanese (Komatsu 1996). No matter whether death is viewed as a discrete moment or as a process that occurs over time, most physicians and bioethicists invariably take it to be an event (or physiological state) that involves an *individual*. The phrase I use to describe that way of conceptualizing things is "death hermetically contained within the individual." However, even though death certainly affects the dying individual in a special way, each death also radiates out, or reverberates, beyond that individual, penetrating the lives and feelings of the bereaved, triggering a range of emotions from joy to sorrow, from pain to relief. I suggest that "death" reverberates. Both sides are affected: the dying and those who watch him or her die, the one who has died and those who have been deeply affected by it.[5]

If death reverberates in this way, the same can be said about being born. When she learns of her pregnancy, a woman often struggles with conflicting feelings of joy and anxiety. And when she feels the fetus move, she may begin to talk to the yet-unseen fetus. This too creates a ripple effect, affecting those around the expectant mother. In the same way as death, birth occurs within a matrix of human relationships and reverberates among them.

Nevertheless, even persons concerned about the use of fertilized embryos often find themselves ensnared in the premises of the proponents of such use— premises that understand human life only from the scientific viewpoint. And this view never moves beyond thinking of death as "hermetically sealed up within the individual who died" and birth also as "life limited strictly to the individual being born." The result is that the debate concerning the handling of fertilized embryos has remained shallow, and it has become almost a foregone conclusion that the critics of this practice will lose out with enough passage of time.

Dealing with a New Barbarism

As societies modernized, they saw the buying and selling of the human body as objectionable, as demonstrated by their prohibiting slavery. In most societies the ethical opposition to prostitution also arose, because it too came to be seen as another form of buying and selling of bodies. Our present and ongoing "corporeal revolution" also involves the sale and purchase of the human body, although it is not carried out so openly or in so easily recognized a form. By disassembling and reassembling the body's parts and packaging them in unrecognizable ways, we have begun to commodify humanity itself on an unprecedented scale. Our bodies are becoming trivialized as mere resources for medicine and mere "things." Calling this a new kind of barbarism is not an overstatement.

And it is a barbarism that, as noted above, we can scarcely curtail with arguments grounded in the "dignity of life" and "theories of personhood." Therefore, if we intend to protect the principle of "dignity" at all, we need, I suggest, a new concept—what I refer to as the "dignity of *the body*," specifically the human body. Should this not be our principal concern in an age of corporeal revolution? By keeping our sights on this new concept, I suggest, we can inject a sense of reality back into our debates.

To demonstrate this point, one need only think about the uses of brain-dead patients in medicine. Although organ transplantation is probably the first thing that comes to mind, it is merely one among many potential ways of using a brain-dead patient. As early as 1974, Willard Gaylin, an American psychiatrist, in a famous essay recognized how their "usefulness" to medicine was increasingly the way in which human bodies were being viewed. In what was likely a parody, he made his point. Brain-dead patients could, after all, he conjectured, be used by medical students to practice surgical and examination techniques; to test the effectiveness of new experimental medicines; to serve as "laboratories" for treatments, if first infected with viruses and given cancer; to serve as storage containers, preserving organs for later transplantation; to be an endless source for generating new blood, bone marrow, and skin; and to be factories producing hormones and antibodies (Gaylin 1981, 524).

When Gaylin wrote in 1974, the technology for "preserving" the bodies of brain-dead patients for long periods of time had not yet been developed. But in the 1980s, "preserving" the bodies of the brain-dead for approximately one month by the hormones ADH and epinephrine became possible. Then, in 1998, UCLA neurologist D. Alan Shewmon published a study showing that 175 of approximately 10,000 brain-dead patients, even without administered hormones, maintained circulatory functioning for over a week. The most lengthy case, at the time of the study's writing, had reached 14.5 years (Shewmon 1998, 1540).[6] What Gaylin envisioned back in 1974 is today coming within the realm of possibility.

Certainly other ways of using the brain-dead body will be found. Given that it has already been possible for brain-dead women to give birth, already fertilized ova could be implanted in the uteruses of brain-dead women, thus "solving" many of the problems that, till now, have dogged surrogate motherhood.[7] Or again, since the pace of human embryonic stem-cell research is hindered, even where it is legal, by the difficulty of obtaining unfertilized and fertilized eggs, this "resource" problem could be solved by obtaining unfertilized ova from brain-dead women. The brain-dead thus become an inexhaustible lode to be mined for medicine and pharmaceuticals. In Japan, the main significance of the much-rumored emendation of the "Organ Transplantation Law" will not so much be that children will be permitted to qualify as donors but, rather, that through such changes a wider use of a greater diversity of human body parts will become available.

This cannot be prevented by invoking the "dignity of life" or theories of personhood, because the "brain-dead" are classified as "dead," and "dead bodies" are seen as lacking "personhood." Thus, I suggest that making the concept of "dignity of the human body" central to the debate has become absolutely critical. Even when we have provisionally relied on the "right to self-determination" to resolve this problem, this principle, when taken to be all we need, ends up doing nothing but giving society's "green light" to such practices. In addition, as examined in detail below, the majority of eugenic policies, such as those of the Nazi era, embraced concepts equivalent to the current one of "right to self-determination."[8]

A focus on the "dignity of the body" is one of the few means remaining by which we might control this "new cannibalism." Put differently, our uneasiness, even disgust, vis-à-vis such usage made of the dead probably arises from an instinctual sense we have that the human body must be treated with dignity.

The way we, while touting the body's marvelous potential, are in fact treating it as a mere *thing* to be used is eerily reminiscent of the way special research groups, such as Unit 731 of the Japanese Imperial Army, made the living bodies of as many as three thousand Chinese, Russians, and Koreans (by a low estimate) into raw materiel—dubbing them "logs"—for medical experiments during the Japan-China War, beginning in 1937, World War II. In development of biological and chemical weapons such "logs" were used in experiments. These "logs" were infected with diseases such as anthrax, cholera, and plague, used to test vaccines for dysentery and to try out a hot-water therapy for frostbite, and employed to gauge human physical tolerances by exposure to high and low pressure. In 1989, human bones showing evidence of surgery (including on the brain) on several dozen body parts were unearthed from the grounds of the former Imperial Army Medical School's Department of Hygiene in the Toyama section of Tokyo's Shinjuku ward.[9]

The Nazis sent an estimated 5.5 million people—mostly Jews—to the gas chambers, after which their remains were made into commodities such as textiles (from hair), objets d'art (from skin), and phosphate fertilizer (from ashes).[10] Although we are horrified by these barbarous acts committed by the Japanese Army and the Nazis, we are presently attempting to transform the human body into a resource, into various commodities, and into things marketable in the same fashion. Of course we have our "justifications," but so too did the former Japanese Imperial Army and the Nazis. Our duty today is to scrutinize all such "justifications" with the "dignity of the body" in mind. Refining the meaning and value of this term will be our challenge in the years to come.

"Resonating Death" and the "Right to Self-Determination"

The Theory of the Right to Determine One's Own Death

Here I examine more closely the "right to self-determination." One can easily imagine someone being critical of transforming the human body into a resource and so forth, but still wanting to leave concrete decisions about these things up to each individual. Among most bioethicists in both Japan and the English-speaking world, in fact, the principle of the "right to self-determination" has primacy. This, however, merely institutionalized many deeper problems, something that received scant scrutiny around the globe.[11]

Although the right to self-determination seems convincing, universal, and absolute at first sight, the fallacy within it becomes clear when applied to the case of human cloning. Were such a right universal and absolute, persons opposed to human cloning would have no case, since respecting an individual's choice would be obligatory. Yet the majority opposes such cloning and Japanese law has made it illegal. Therefore, the right to self-determination is not, in fact, all-determinative in judging the propriety of all cutting-edge medicine.

And does this principle not need to be monitored especially when it is invoked by the medical establishment? Given the stark contrast between the condemnation of Nazi-era medicine at the Nuremburg Trials (1946–47) and the deliberate *non*-prosecution of the Japanese Imperial Army's Unit 731 at the Tokyo War Crimes Trial (1946–48), some have come to view Japan's postwar medical establishment as a holdover of a so-called Unit 731 mentality.[12] In other words, some blame the strong paternalism, bureaucracy, and hierarchical organization of Japan's medical establishment for numerous tragedies—such as the iatrogenic AIDS infections. In such a context, within which each individual must protect him- or herself, self-determination has tended to be taken as the rule. However, even if the right to self-determination might protect competent individuals, this principle alone is unlikely to be able to reform the old "731 mentality." This is an example of what I mean when I say that the right to self-determination cannot resolve any systemic problems.

To make this point more sharp I wish to analyze the theory of the "right to die." When speaking of a life we tend to refer to "so-and-so's life" and to death as "so-and-so's death." We have already affixed a possessive modifier as if a life or a death *belongs to* some individual. Everyday speech reinforces this: "*her* life was saved," "*his* life is in your hands," and "he decided to take *his own* life." Examples could easily be multiplied. Even major thinkers such as Philippe Ariès, Ivan Illich, and Michel Foucault, though critical of modern medicine, slip into the use of such terms.[13]

In these terms, however, lies the mechanism by which we become able to conceive of a "right to die." That we use them with no compunction suggests how deeply this conceptualization of death has become ingrained in our minds. Even persons unconvinced of a "right to die" end up fighting the battle on their opponent's conceptual turf, merely by using such phrases.

A phrase such as "my death" has, at least for our analysis here, two important significations. The first is that "my death is my own affair" and the second is that "my death pertains to an internal process within my body." The two are conceptually connected, and the argument for a "right to die" follows the fundamental logic assumed here.

If we think back to how we drew the figures of people in our childhood, we notice that most of us began by demarcating the outline of the body in black crayon, paint, or pencil. Then, within that outline, we colored in the clothing and painted in the face, arms, and legs. This shows that we think of ourselves as that which is inscribed within the body's boundaries. However, has not everyone experienced some sense of stress when interacting with others when they come too close? When alone, we retain our "normal self"-composure, but when another oversteps the usually acceptable distance, that self is affected. In other words, although we believe that the self ends with the body's limits, in reality we are *made up of* a self that extends into our surrounding space. Furthermore, depending on who the other person is and that person's relationship to us, we expand and contract. If that "other" has an aggressive nature, the mere sight of him or her is enough to trigger stress, whereas if he or she is a loved one, personal space virtually disappears. We have an ever expanding and contracting existence, depending on the "other."

In spite of this we go on believing—without question—in a self that is bounded by the body's outer limits. And because I misconceive death as happening "within my body," it becomes something like a possession of mine. And because I own it, I imagine I am free to dispose of it as I wish. This is how we get today's notion of a "right to determine one's own death" or a "right to die."

Going from "Reverberating Death" to "Sealed up Death"

Many will dismiss my criticism of the idea that one's death pertains to one's own self and is something like a possession. Because this idea is so common today, they assume it is a given. But, in fact, it is nothing more than an idea that became pronounced in Western Europe since around the mid-eighteenth century. What is called the "right to die" could have sprung only from the particular way we grasp death in the modern age.[14]

People living in Western Europe during the Middle Ages appear to have had a strong awareness about the approach of death,[15] and in that epoch those who were going to die—knowing that there was nothing anyone could do to help them any longer—would call their relatives and friends to their deathbeds. There, conversing with each other and making amends, the dying would provide the last will. If a priest was present, last rites would begin; if not, the dying and those attending would pray together. When the last breath had been breathed, the funeral ceremony would begin. Only after being buried long enough for the body's form to disintegrate entirely was it thought that one had been fully visited by death (see Ariès 1975, chap. 4).

This conception of death is completely different from the way we typically think of death today. Then, unlike now, death was not the instant the heart stopped beating or the brain ceased to function. Death was not a point in time. Interment after family and friends had gathered, the continuous chain of events over time until the body's last remnant had finally disintegrated—this entire process was death. But this process was not merely the series of changes in the physiological condition of the dying. Death was not a phenomenon that occurred only in and to the individual dying. Conversing with those who have rushed to be there, praying together, and reaffirming with each other the importance of sharing that time together in those ways in particular—the integral passing of time that was shared *between* the person who was dying and those who were attending him, the deceased and those who would soon be bereaved—*that* was death in the Middle Ages. It interwove many people. As has been suggested above, death during that era could be analogized to a sound that reverberates outward and resonates within many others.

Things changed in the eighteenth century, and our view of death as an objectifiable phenomenon derives from that change. It was triggered specifically by the widespread incidence of premature burial. Being thrown into a state that mimicked death was a common occurrence in Western Europe then. Some, still alive, managed to escape the buried condition, but word of such incidents swept through Western Europe in the mid-eighteenth century and became a major issue. These incidents were first chronicled by J. B. Winslow in his 1746 work *The Uncertainty of the Signs of Death*. Winslow's book alone introduced some fifty horrifying cases of premature burial, but my own research turned up nearly two hundred similar *medical* texts on the topic, primarily from Northwestern Europe. Thus, in order to draw a *distinct* line between life and death, people in the field of medicine began researching the various symptoms of death and developing methods to test them. The tests for life or death were multiple: piercing the heart and veins with a needle to which might be attached a small flag that would flutter in the presence of a pulse; checking for discoloration when a needle inserted into muscle tissue had been removed; checking for reaction to ammonia solution injected under skin; testing for a response in the pupils to light or atropine drops; and scalding a person to check if blistering would occur.[16]

Mortuaries were also created in Germany during the latter half of the eighteenth century. The "dead" were kept in open coffins for two or three days and periodically checked by physicians and family members (see Stevenson 1975, 493, and Marshall 1966, 18–19). Another way to prevent premature burial was the invention, in England, of what was known as "Bateson's belfry," a bell in the night watchman's quarters that was attached by a very long string tied to the finger of the deceased in his coffin. If the "deceased" moved even slightly, the bell would ring loudly, and the coffin or crypt could be opened.

One might wonder how such developments relate to how we today comprehend death; we need to recognize that just by becoming engrossed in observing the biological signs that may be death's symptoms, we can completely forget the societal dimension—that is, the multiple ways the death reverberates outward into others. Our tendency to think what we first perceive with our eyes is somehow an objective phenomenon that is completely independent of us leads us to treat death as an instantaneous biological phenomenon that happens only to the individual "out there." In other words, equating such things as the absence of blistering, fully open pupils of the eye, or the lack of a heartbeat with death, we have trapped or sealed death within that individual.[17]

This is how it became possible to regard death as something like an individual's personal possession. This is what I call conceptualizing it as "sealed-in death." It is the way we think of it today. We are so inured to it that it has lost its strangeness and now functions as the logical basis for the modern "right to die."

Theoretical Weakness in the "Right to Die"

Whatever the issue today—brain death, euthanasia, death-with-dignity, and end-of-life care—the discussion quickly becomes medicalized. That is, we tend to treat these only within the framework of "sealed-in death." What we wind up debating is little more than a standard by which death is measured, such as death of the brain or heart. Actual death as something that resonates gets reduced to the single entity that has deceased, death "sealed in." However, upon reflection, we realize that during a person's final moments, friends, acquaintances, and a caretaking hospital or nursing staff are present. Even in this modern day, death includes such interpersonal relationships. In reality, each time we perform funerary or memorial rites, are we not reliving that "resonating death" resulting from our relationship(s) with the deceased? Simply put, death in our actual lives—in medieval Western Europe as well as today—is not restricted to an individual but exists in and through the interpersonal bonds between people.

According to the laws of modern civil society, we can freely handle only those things over which we have definite rights of possession.[18] For example, I am fully free to wear a watch that I own on my left or right arm or not at all. However, appropriating another person's property or disposing of another's property is against the law. In the same way, if death *belongs* to be a specific individual and ownership can be determined, then that person should have the right of disposition. His death is his. He can do with it as he pleases.

If, however, death is a reverberating something and occurs along and within a set of human relationships, it is not a private possession. This being the case, any notion of "self-determination of death" is a kind of illusion. No single individual has the *right* to die.

Practical and Historical Problems with the "Right to Self-Determination"

Problems in the "Right to Die"

Here I examine euthanasia—the earliest form of bio-manipulation and an issue that recently resurfaced on the world stage. Euthanasia is often separated into three categories: "active euthanasia," "passive euthanasia," and "doctor-assisted suicide." However, in each type the common feature is that death is prioritized over a continuation of treatment. They share a common logic: the choice for a dignified, peaceful death over an undignified, painful life. We can take issue with this supposition in a couple of ways.

The first issue is its distortion of language (see Tsuruta 1996). The actual opposite of an "undignified painful life" is not a "dignified and peaceful death" but, rather, a "dignified and peaceful life." So, if the problem is one of "undignified and painful life," what needs pursuing are ways of bringing about a "dignified and peaceful life." We overlook this because our thinking about this matter has gotten so twisted that we do not even notice that the presented alternative is a false one. Language about a "right" to choose euthanasia masks this distortion.[19]

A second issue has to do with background information about persons seeking euthanasia and the hiding from them of possibilities for alleviation of suffering in alternative ways. Those who want euthanasia are suffering either acute physical pain or mental anguish. For those in the former group—such as those in advanced-stage cancer—more emphasis could be given to easing the intolerable pain. According to the World Health Organization palliative care through, for instance, morphine, can do much to alleviate pain of late-stage cancer. This is not done in Japan because our technical infrastructure to administer such amounts of morphine is inadequate. Rather than fix that infrastructure, the fear of abuse leads to inadequate use of the palliative. And, as a result, people think that euthanasia may be their only way of release from such pain. My point is that, although there are problems in this area, we should not stop seeking ways to improve palliative care. Euthanasia should not be thought of as the only recourse for such pain.

Others suffer from mental anguish. Representative of what they will say, then, is: "I can't bear the thought of receiving futile life-prolonging treatment just to be kept alive by a machine." This argument only *appears* to be persuasive. Lots of means, in fact, are used to keep us alive—pacemakers, flu shots, appendectomies, and organ transplants, for instance. Why are certain procedures singled out as applied *just* to keep a person alive? What is meant by "just" in such cases?

Some might say that euthanasia should be allowable when there is no hope of recovery. Yet it is, in fact, impossible to predict recovery or its impossibility. We should not be predisposed toward the recourse of euthanasia when there is no certainty in this. Even cases diagnosed as "persistent vegetative states" have, although very rarely, shown recovery.

In Japanese we often use the phrase *ishiki fumei*—which literally means "lack of clarity whether or not consciousness exists"—as if taken to mean that a lack of consciousness has been proven. But, in fact, all we have determined is that there has been no response to external stimuli. We equate unresponsiveness with unconsciousness when the patient might in fact be conscious but simply unable to respond. Actually, today studies in the field of brain resuscitation suggest that persons in a "vegetative" state, although unable to respond to stimuli, may merely have their capacity for *communication* blocked. Some have learned how to communicate by trained eye movements. Some of this research has been done in Japan (see Horie 1997). Furthermore, electroencephalogram (EEG) records electrical activity only on the scalp; it does not directly measure activity of the brain itself. In some cases deep brain-wave activity exists but cannot be detected because the waves did not reach the scalp.[20]

I have shown the need for much more study in this area—for persons suffering both physically and mentally. Premature and unjustified recourse to and talk about "self-determination" and euthanasia short-circuits those efforts.

A Euthanasia Case in the Netherlands

When an NHK television camera crew first visited the home of Karl Coolemans in March 1994, he was seventy-four years old.[21] He had been experiencing severe abdominal pain since the end of 1993 and entered the hospital in January 1994. He was diagnosed with late-stage colon cancer that had metastasized to his liver and was told that he had three months to live. Surgery was no longer an option, and he refused chemotherapy because of its strong side effects, instead resolving to battle the pain and "when it becomes too much to bear, to elect for euthanasia" (NHK jintai purojekuto 1996, 28). He desired to be allowed to meet a "peaceful death" in the house where he had lived for most of his life. He only wanted to live until July nineteenth, the date of his seventy-fifth birthday, although his doctor thought that might be impossible.

Coolemans had thought about euthanasia even earlier. Ten years before, after a discussion with his wife, they decided to draw up a document declaring their intention to elect euthanasia should one of them become ill or injured beyond the reach of medicine. Accordingly, his wife agreed with his current decision, and his two daughters, who were working in a hospital, also agreed, saying: "I think Dad's is a respectable decision. Every day, we see people suffering from the side effects of chemotherapy. That's why we support our father's decision" (NHK jintai purojekuto 1996, 31).

In the Netherlands, euthanasia is carried out by doctors in a patient's home rather than in a hospital. When Coolemans informed his physician, Dr. Anton R. de Hoog, of his decision, the latter scolded him for drinking alcohol instead of taking his pain relievers. Even then, however, the doctor thought that euthanasia might be the only recourse.

In early December, the NHK crew revisited Coolemans's home, nine months after their first visit. To their surprise, not only was Coolemans still alive, but he had overcome his dislike of medicine and was taking his morphine. He had changed his mind about euthanasia due to something that had happened at his seventy-fifth birthday party in July. On that occasion, Coolemans, taking drink after drink, had been scolded by his ten-year-old granddaughter. She poured his drink down the drain and then hurled the liquor bottle out the window. Recollecting that incident for the Japanese TV crew, Coolemans said, "I couldn't believe it. She actually seemed to care about my health. . . . It was then that I realized how terrible it was of me always to be talking about euthanasia" (NHK jintai purojekuto 1996, 97). After this incident, Coolemans survived even a second winter, although originally told he had only three months to live. He died naturally in his home on May 29, 1995.

From this case alone we can pinpoint various problems with euthanasia that come to light:

1. Coolemans, refusing chemotherapy, drank alcohol daily in lieu of painkillers. Thus, it is possible that if he had not changed his mind, the euthanasia would have been carried out even though the conditions for it had not been satisfied.
2. Although the physician's three-month prognosis was no more than a guess, it carried special weight by virtue of being a *doctor's* judgment and, thus, affected the situation.

3. Although this prognosis became a basis for Coolemans's decision to elect euthanasia, the extent to which the physician realized his prognosis could have such an influence is unclear.
4. In reality, Coolemans outlived his three-month prognosis by over a year, and if he had been euthanized, he would never have had the important interaction with his granddaughter.
5. Because Coolemans's decision was predicated on the doctor's prognosis, it cannot really be considered "self-determined" in any strict sense. (Moreover, since euthanasia is performed by a doctor, it violates the very spirit of autonomy upon which the concept of euthanasia is supposedly based.)
6. Assuming that the goal of medicine is to save the lives of patients, whether or not euthanasia falls under the category of medicine is doubtful.[22]

Far more problematic than any of the above, however, is how the so-called right to self-determination operates in a case of euthanasia. The camera crew noted that the family—as especially in the case of the granddaughter—was much involved in what went on. In this we see how, when the concepts are limited to the notion of a "right to self-determination," the family and its actual role tend to become a mere abstraction. This is an extremely important issue.

As noted, Coolemans's wife and daughters went along with his decision to be euthanized. However, the wife's suffering was obvious as she spent day after day living with her husband as he waited to be euthanized. "Around this time of year, I wash his shirts and wool sweaters, fold them neatly, and put them away. But this year I just couldn't bring myself to do it when I thought about the fact that my husband would never wear them again" (NHK jintai purojekuto 1996, 41). In other words, instead of trying to bring maximum life out of his remaining days, they had all been occupied with the running out of the clock prior to his euthanization. This caused her to be overcome with despair. And that is because death reverberates.

Only the ten-year-old granddaughter, however, could express her true feelings through direct action. In contrast to the adults whose minds had been saturated with the notion of a "right to self-determination," the young granddaughter—precisely because she had not yet been inculcated with that idea—was able to act freely. This is the all-important point to be derived from this case.

Ironically, the "right to self-determination," which is supposed to set people free, binds them instead. Without question, the reason for this is that death is not something that happens only to an isolated individual. Because it affects not only the dying but also their caregivers and not only the dead but also their bereaved, death is not something that can be decided by an autonomous individual. The fundamental problem with autonomy lies in the way in which, because our view is distorted, those to whom and into whom the dying is actually reverberating feel compelled to act as if this were not so.

To go even further, a crucial problem lies in elevating self-determination from a simple action to the status of a *right*—as in the "right to die." When self-determination becomes a right, it is invested with power—a power to exclude intervention by any other. The force of this is what quashed the true feelings of Mrs. Coolemans, resulting in a loss of her freedom and causing her unhappiness. On the other hand, this power did not extend to the granddaughter, who was uninhibited by the notion of self-determination. Surely the right to self-determination and the concept of "rights" in general have led to major improvements—in combating feudal authority and inequities in the workplace and in the medical clinic, and countering sexual discrimination. In these cases, however, the exercise of "rights" was to combat an existing power that was already engaged in the exclusion of persons vitally involved. However, we need to question whether "rights" ought to be exerted in cases where—as in the Coolemans family—subtle interpersonal relationships are involved. This was a conspicuous case of the exercise of a "right" having such power over the situation that others were pushed aside.[23]

Past Consequences of the "Right to Die"

The matter of a "right to self-determination" has come up before—and in a context especially relevant to our considerations here. Its deeply problematical nature debuted on a national scale during the era of Nazi control in Germany. Although put forward even earlier in Germany, this *right* became the leverage for eugenics and became the so-called right to die. I here examine some specifics of Nazi eugenics policy and see how the "right to die" functioned within that framework (see Ichinokawa 1996).

Eugenic policy is the application of Darwinian evolutionary theory, theories of genetics, and statistics to human society, with the intent of improving the human gene pool by eliminating "inferior genes." Even prior to the mass murder of 5.5 million Jews and others in the Holocaust, the Nazis had euthanized several hundred thousand "undesirables" through policies targeting those with genetic diseases, intellectual disabilities, and mental illnesses.

After their rise to power in January 1933, the Nazis actively implemented such a policy. The documents of the time show four specific ways of carrying it out. The first was forced sterilization, by which genetic "undesirables" deemed likely to give birth to more "undesirables" were prevented from having children. The second was an abortion policy, by which genetic "undesirables" who were exempt from sterilization were forced to have abortions if they had become pregnant. The third disallowed marriage to genetic "undesirables." The fourth was euthanasia, the most expedient method to eradicate genetic "undesirables" who had managed to get born in spite of the first three strategies—or persons already alive before their implementation.

It is of utmost importance to note that such policies were not simply enacted by authoritarian dictum but came into being *legally* via parliamentary deliberation and sanction. It was comparable to the way in which Japan commenced the hostilities in the Pacific War—not by unilateral acts on the part of the military but, rather, by working within the bounds of the imperial constitution. An "Outline for Implementing Imperial Policies" was passed by the Imperial Court on November 5, 1941, and on December first the Imperial Court decided to commence hostilities against the United States, Great Britain, and the Netherlands. Soon after that Pearl Harbor and Malaysia were attacked (see, e.g., Inoue 1966, 201–203).

In the same way the Nazis remained technically *legal* in implementing their eugenics policy. In July 1933 they passed the "Law to Prevent Having Descendants with Hereditary Disease" and with it legalization of forced sterilization. In June 1935, they amended this law to also recognize induced abortion. In October of the same year, the German parliament enacted the "Law Protecting the Genetic Health of the German People," which legalized marriage control. Then, in August 1939, the "Euthanasia Bill" was drawn up in the fourth group of the Criminal Law Commission of the Reichsjustizminister. In this way, step by step, the eugenics policies were implemented, always within the letter of the law (see Roth and Aly 1983; and Ganssmüller 1987, 163–64).

What I want to draw attention to is the following: With the exception of the marriage law, each of these two laws and the bill was articulated in such a way that their fit with the principle of self-determination was presented. The gist of this came out as follows: "Persons with genetic diseases have every right to have an abortion. And if the person herself does not have the capacity to exercise that right, a legal surrogate or the head of a medical facility may do so in that person's stead." The most relevant portions of the Eugenics Bill were the following:

Article 1. Persons with untreatable diseases who are a heavy burden on themselves or others, or those with unquestionably terminal illnesses may, on the patient's explicit request and with the consent of an authorized physician, be assisted into death by a physician.

Article 2. Persons needing permanent institutionalization due to untreatable mental disease and persons with diseases making them incapable of providing for their own lives, may be terminated by medical decision—provided it is done without awareness on the part of the subject and painlessly. (Roth and Aly 1983, 55; Ganssmüller 1987, 163–64)

These provisions very clearly show that the state and the medical establishment may decide to euthanize persons who are incapable of exercising their own "right to die." These comprise the *very first* provisions of the bill. There even the Nazis, who are known for the savagery of their deeds, tried to clear the way for their euthanasia policy legally and by connecting it to a "right to die."[24] Hitler's invasion of Poland and the initiation of World War II interrupted debate and ratification of these bills, and therefore the Nazis carried out euthanasia extralegally. But the significant feature in the above is that the initial intent was to do all this legally and to link even forced euthanasia to the concept and rhetoric of "self-determination" in dying.

I stress the employment of language about "rights" and "self-determination" in all of these matters. This appears to been a subtle means of inducing their public acceptance. Bringing up this history and seeing parallels between it and our current debates does not mean we will simply repeat the history of the Nazis. However, the *logic* bears too much resemblance to ignore. The entire eugenics policy of the Nazis and how it was rationalized are not things we may forget.

The Dangers of Criticizing the "Right to Die"

In the above I have critically analyzed the "right to die" in terms of theory, practice, and history. Such a "right to die," I hold, is predicated on a narrow and inadequate understanding of death—that which I have called "sealed-in death." By accepting it, however, we blind ourselves to the fact that we actually live and die in a way such that our lives and our death reverberate outward into others. And the "right to die" rhetoric severs the connections between people, uproots the possibility of expanding such ties, and lures us gently toward death. This is why I hold that we should not laud a term such as the "right to die." Modernity employs a number of dualisms, ones from which we cannot easily extricate ourselves: spirit and flesh, form and substance, subject and object, idealism and materialism, humanism and scientific positivism, the whole and its parts, national and individual, government and citizens, inside and outside. But the concept of "self-determinism" is also bound up in dualistic thought, something I will explain.

Undoubtedly in the past authority figures lorded it over others. Physicians were paternalistic. Males made autocratic decisions about births and abortions. It is, then, no wonder that patients vis-à-vis their doctors and women vis-à-vis their male partners have emphatically demanded the "right to self-determination."

But this would be merely to transfer all the decision authority from one side of a dual structure to the other. In other words, the right to decision—whether it be about therapy or about childbirth, for example—will be based firmly on the assumption that one person and *only one* makes the decision. Because patients now have complete discretion in medical decisions and women in deciding about birth, we get a whole new set of problems. We shift the power from one side to the other but the basic *dualistic pattern* remains.

Asserting the "right to die" does not get us out of such a dualistic structure. Certainly during World War II death was forced on people by their authorities. Many Japanese were compelled to die; they had no choice. So too the Nazi regime made death, including death by euthanasia, something forced upon individuals. But is our problem not one of swinging to the opposite extreme? Instead of being state enforced, death becomes the private choice of the self-enclosed individual—absurdly so.

Death precludes all other possibilities, and means the separation from our loved ones once and for all. Having a "right to die" is nothing more than having a choice between choosing such a death oneself, or having it chosen for you. It is this dualistic set of options that requires our criticism and opposition.

In daily life, is there anything about which we make a decision purely on our own and not affecting others? Countless people and things are interwoven in a world of relationships, and when something comes about through mutual connection with others, just because that result comes close to our own intention, we tend to attribute it to self-determination. But even in selecting a book to read, we have already heard or read opinions about that book, and these influence us.

We probably need to look more critically at what we mean by our human rights—that is, in spite of what the idea of "rights" has contributed to modern life, we need to preserve the *ideals* to which human rights aspire. The view of man on which human rights are premised takes him as something that exists independently, somehow apart from his relationships. It abstracts the individual from all others. Accordingly, rights become *my* freedoms and pertain to *me*, whereas *your* freedoms and rights pertain to *you*. Although this helps when individuals are threatened by powerful, outside authorities, this conception of rights has the potential to alienate others. When, as in the case of the Coolemans family, "rights" becomes the individual's shield, others, even those close to us, become unable to express opinions freely. We need a capacity to recognize certain structural flaws in our concept of rights. And, as in the case of the so-called right to die, the practical problems have become downright grotesque.

There is an entire family of issues related to the "corporeal revolution," and we need to realize that we dare not be satisfied with using "self-determination" as a solution for them all. The debates over brain death and euthanasia each have their particular issues, and therefore we must examine each on its own terms. But we need to look macroscopically as well as the microscopically.

Conclusion: Costs of the "Corporeal Revolution"

Mankind has experienced many fundamental revolutions in its long history (see Itō 1975). We can easily name the agricultural revolution, the development of the great city-states, the development of mathematics and calendars, the philosophical revolution that came via the great rational systems of the ancient Greeks, Indian, and Chinese thinkers, the Scientific Revolution, the Industrial Revolution, and so forth. Each has radically altered peoples' lives and consciousness. And many have brought increased prosperity and happiness.

However, the closer to the present day that each stage of revolution brings us, the more we discover in it elements of misfortune. Our increasing alienation from one other, various geopolitical tensions, and the environmental destruction due to science and technology are but a few examples. And, although the present "corporeal revolution" currently under way may very well bring us many great "life"-related benefits, its flip side has begun to show us its negatives. We have suggested here the need to get serious about recognizing the "dignity of the body." And beyond that we must survey the "corporeal revolution" from the widest possible perspective. Notions of simple or automatic "progress" will not suffice. While reflecting on our past, we must fulfill our obligations to our descendants.

On December 6, 2002, the Japanese Strategic Council on Biotechnology formulated its "Strategic Outline for Biotechnology."[25] The introduction boldly declared: "We have the utmost confidence that biotechnology will change the world. What will be Japan's contribution? Our strategy is contained herein." The outline then went on to predict the future scale of the biotech market, which it projects to reach an astounding 230 trillion yen globally by 2010. Japan also raised its own target levels for 2010 from the current goal of 1.3 trillion yen to 25 trillion yen.

It is probably quite unnecessary to note, however, that the capital we will use for producing such enormous wealth will be none other than "our lives, our deaths, and our bodies."

Notes

For the latest trends in Japan on the research use of the human body, see Shimazono 2003.

1. Human embryonic stem cell lines were established in November 1998. Ninety percent of the human genome project was completed in June 2000. An example of the resulting medical application is the "Project on the Implementation of Personalized Medicine," an Institute of Medical Science at the University of Tokyo proposal that was formally approved by the Bioethics and Bio-safety Commission of the Ministry of Education, Culture, Sports, Science, and Technology. This institute was granted research funds of twenty trillion yen over five years. Using the genes of three hundred thousand patients, including those with cancer, diabetes, and heart disease, these studies are intended to tailor medicine and treatment options to individual patients by searching for relationships between individual genetic variations (single nucleotide polymorphisms) and the effects and side effects of chronic diseases and medications.

2. Uemura 2003 recapitulates the arguments against cloning humans.

3. On existing commercial uses of the human body, see Kimbrell 1993 and Andrews and Nelkin 2001. On the structure of the debates in brain death, organ transplantation, assisted reproductive technologies, and cloning technologies, see Hayashi 2002.

4. This refers to the ridge that appears on the surface of an embryo when it divides into the ectoderm, mesoderm, and endoderm. By being differentiated from the ectoderm the nervous system develops.

5. Translator's note: By having a nonpejorative passive form of the verb—literally, to "be died on by X, who died," Japanese as a language facilitates awareness of these two as a natural pair.

6. Since being diagnosed as brain dead at the age of four, this person continued to live in such a condition for twenty-one years, dying in January 2004. He had reached the height and weight of an adult and showed secondary signs characteristic of maturation.

7. The concern that I raise is not idle speculation. At the forty-sixth annual meeting of the Japanese Society for the Study of Infertility held on November 8, 2001, Professor Emeritus Kazuo Takeuchi of Kyōrin University, a leading figure in Japanese medicine, gave a special lecture called "Considering Birth by Brain-Dead Patients," in which he spoke publicly in favor of using brain-dead patients as surrogate mothers.

8. For more information, see Ichinokawa 2000 and Roth and Aly 1983.

9. See Tsuneishi 1981 and in the present volume, as well as Kondō 2003 and Omata 2003.

10. Such depictions appear in Alain Resnais's film *Nuit et brouillard* (1955) (English title: "Night and Fog").

11. For criticism of the bioethics field, particularly its emphasis on an individualistic right to self-determination, see Fox 1989 and Hardwig 1997. My position is closest to that of Fox. See Komatsu 2000, where I raise these issues.

12. See Komata's analysis in Komatsu and Omata 2002.

13. The concluding sections of their works state the similar sentiment: "I will not let medicine take away *my death.*" Ariès 1975, Illich 1976, Foucault and Watanabe 1978.

14. See Komatsu 1996. Katō 2001 and Tateiwa 1997 follow different lines of argument but are likewise critical of personal ownership of the body.

15. There are many accounts in fables and folklore that begin with phrases such as "I thought I was done for this time, but . . . " For examples, see de la Fontaine 1668, chap. 5, sect. 9, and Bédier 1900, chap. 19.

16. On the symptoms of death from the seventeenth to the nineteenth centuries, see Tebb and Vollum 1896, chap. 13.

17. This view results from an epistemology that understands the subject and object of recognition as existing independently of one another. This would be like continuing to adhere to Newtonian physics despite the advent of the theory of relativity and quantum mechanics in physics. See Hiromatsu 1977.

18. This understanding can be traced back to John Locke's *Two Treatises of Government,* 1690, Book 2, chap. 5.

19. In Japanese words such as *anrakushi* (calm and peaceful death) and *songenshi* (death with dignity) are common, but ones such as *anrakusei* (calm and peaceful life) and *songensei* (life with dignity) do not even exist.

20. Shūji Karasawa and others at the Funabashi Municipal Medical Center studied this phenomenon and developed a machine that could measure deep brain activity. During the craniotomies of seven patients experiencing subarachnoid hemorrhaging, they measured and compared scalp EEGs with deep brain EEGs, confirming that there are cases in which brain activity exists even when scalp EEGs test negative (Karasawa et al. 1996).

21. Karl Coolemans was the subject of the NHK television special "Euthanasia: Those at the Moment of Truth, a Report from the Netherlands" (NHK BS1, aired March 10, 1995) and a more detailed book, *Anrakushi—Sei to shi o mitsumeru* (1996), edited by NHK jintai purojekuto.

22. In a broadcast of "Global Court: Questioning Bio-Manipulation, Part One" (NHK BS1, aired December 12, 1998), I discussed the case of Karl Coolemans with Dr. de Hoog. However, the thrust of my argument, as described later, was not aired.

23. The feminism that takes decision making about birth as a woman's right, while attempting to oppose prenatal screening based on the same "right to self-determination," leads to contradiction. This contradiction arises from the expulsive power of this right being used to pull in many different directions.

24. Concerning the First and Second Articles of this bill, see Roth and Aly 1983, especially 55, and Ganssmüller 1987, 163–64. For the full texts of other laws related to eugenics policies, see *Reichsgesetzblatt* 1933, 529–31, and *Reichsgesetzblatt* 1935, 773–74. Although this history may be common knowledge in Germany, it remains largely unknown to the rest of the world. The guidelines proposed at the International Congress on Human Genetics held in Brazil in August 1996 are emblematic of this state of ignorance. See Boulyjenkow et al. 1995. This document, created to advance and promote procedures such as prenatal diagnosis, made the following pronouncement: "The spirit of genetics today is about assisting concerned parties in making the best choices to achieve their reproductive goals. This is the decisive difference between the present-day genetics and the eugenics of the past" (p. 3). It is stated here that the watershed between "eugenics" and "genetics" consists of whether or not the right to self-determination has been exercised. This statement plainly reveals the ignorance of the realities of the Nazi eugenic policy.

25. The full text is available at www.kantei.go.jp/jp/singi/bt/kettei/021206/taikou.html.

References

Andrews, Lori, and Dorothy Nelkin. 2001. *Body Bazaar.* New York: Crown Publishers.

Ariès, Philippe. 1983. *Essai sur l'histoire de la mort en occident: Du Moyen Âge à nos jours.* Paris: Éditions Seuil.

———. 1977. *L'homme devant la mort.* Paris: Éditions Seuil.

Bédier, Joseph, ed. 1900. *Roman de Tristan et Iseut.* Paris: H. Piazza.

Boulyjenkow, V., et al. 1995. *Guidelines on Ethical Issues in Medical Genetics and the Provision of Genetic Services.* Geneva: World Health Organization.

Fontaine, Jean de la. 1668. *Fables choisies mises en vers.* Paris: Claude Barbin.

Foucault, Michel, and Moriaki Watanabe. 1978. *Tetsugaku no butai.* Tokyo: Asahi shimbun shuppansha.

Fox, Renée. 1989. *The Sociology of Medicine: A Participant Observer's View.* Englewood Cliffs, N.J.: Prentice Hall.

Gaylin, Willard. 1981. Harvesting the Dead. In *Bioethics,* rev. ed., ed. Thomas A. Shannon, 517–27. New York: Paulist Press.

Ganssmüller, Christian. 1987. *Die Erbgesundheitspolitik des Dritten Reiches: Planung, Durchführung und Durchsetzung.* Köln, Wien: Böhlau Verlag.

Hardwig, John. 1997. Is There a Duty to Die? *Hastings Center Report* 27, no. 2: 34–42.

Hayashi, Makoto. 2002. *Sōsa sareru seimei—Kagakuteki gensetsu no seijigaku.* Tokyo: NTT shuppan.

Hiromatsu, Wataru. 1977. *Kagaku no kiki to ninshikiron.* Tokyo: Kinokuniya shoten.

Hiroshige, Tetsu, Shuntarō Itō, and Yōichirō Murakami. 1975. *Shisōshi no naka no kagaku.* Tokyo: Bokutakusha.

Horie, Takeshi. 1997. Gaishōsei shokubutsu kanja to no 12 nen—shinguru kara sain e—. In *Dai rokkai ishiki shōgaisha no chiryō kenkyūkai yōkōshū.* Naha: Ishiki shōgaisha no chiryō kenkyūkai.

Ichinokawa, Yasutaka. 1996. Sei to seishoku wo meguru seiji—Aru Doitsu gendaishi. In *Seishoku gijutsu to jendā,* ed. Yumiko Ebara, 163–217. Tokyo: Keisō shobō.

———. Doitsu: Yūseigaku wa Nachizumu ka. In Yonemoto et al.

Illich, Ivan. 1976. *Limits to Medicine*. London: Marion Boyers.

Inoue, Kiyoshi. 1966. *Nihon no rekishi*. Vol. 2. Tokyo: Iwanami shinsho.

Itō, Shuntarō. 1975. Jinruishi no kyoshiteki tenbō. In Hiroshiga, et al.

Karasawa, Hideharu, et al. 1996. Nō no dairekuto monitaringu: tōhijō nōha heitanji no shinbu nōha no kentō. *Nihon shinkei kyūkyū kenkyū zasshi* (Journal of Japanese Congress of Neurological Emergencies) 10: 24–28.

Katō, Shūichi. 2001. Shintai wo shoyū shinai dorei—Shintai no jiko ketteiken e no yōgo. *Shisō* 922: 108–35.

Kayukawa, Junji. 2003. *Kurōn ningen*. Tokyo: Kōbunsha shinsho.

Kimbrell, Andrew. 1973. *The Human Body Shop: The Engineering and Marketing of Life*. New York: Harper Collins.

Komatsu, Yoshihiko. 1996. *Shi wa kyōmei suru—Nōshi, zōki ishoku no fukami e*. Tokyo: Keisō shobō.

———. 2000. "Jiko ketteiken" no michiyuki—"Shi no gimu" no tōjō—seimei rinrigaku no tensei no tame ni. *Shisō* 908–909: 124–53, 154–70.

———. 2002. Baioeshikusu no seiritsu towa nandeatta no ka—Jintai no shigenka, shōhinka, shijōka no tōkyū no tame ni. *Asoshie* 9: 34–57.

Komatsu, Yoshihiko, and Waichirō Omata. 2002. Seimei kagaku to igaku rinri. In *Tairon: Hito wa shindewa naranai*, ed. Yoshihiko Komatsu, 79–101. Tokyo: Shunjūsha, 2002.

Kondō, Shōji, ed. 2003. *731 butai: Saikinsen shiryōshū CD-ROM ban*. Tokyo: Kashiwa shobō.

Locke, John. 1690. *Two Treatises of Government*. Book 2. London: n.p.

Marshall, T. K. 1966. Premature Burial. *Medico-Legal Journal* 35: 14–24.

Naikakufu sōgō kagaku gijutsu kaigi BT senryaku kaigi. 2002. Baiotekunorojī senryaku taikō.

NHK jintai purojekuto, ed. 1996. *Anrakushi—Sei to shi o mitsumeru*. Tokyo: NHK shuppan.

Omata, Waichirō. 2003. *Kenshō jintai jikken—731 butai, Nachisu igaku*. Tokyo: Daisan bunmeisha.

Reichsgesetzblatt. 1933.

Reichsgesetzblatt. 1935.

Roth, Karl Heinz, and Götz Aly. 1983. Die Diskussion über die Legalisierung der nationalsozialistischen Anstaltsmorde in den Jahren 1938–1941. *Recht und Psychiatrie* 2: 51–64.

Shewmon, D. Alan. 1998. Chronic "Brain Death": Meta-Analysis and Conceptual Consequences. *Neurology* 51 (1998): 1538–45.

Shimazono, Susumu. 2003. Sentan seimei kagaku no rinri wo dō ronjiru ka. *Sekai* 721: 134–43.

Stevenson, L. G. 1975. Suspended Animation and the History of Anesthesia. *Bulletin of the History of Medicine* 49: 482–511.

Tateiwa, Shinya. 1997. *Shiteki shoyūron*. Tokyo: Keisō shobō.

Tebb, William, and E. Perry Vollum. 1896. *Premature Burial and How It May Be Prevented*. London: Swann Sonnenschein and Co.

Tsuneishi, Kei-ichi. 1981. *Kieta saikinsen butai—Kantōgun 731 butai*. Tokyo: Kaimeisha.

Tsuruta, Hiroyuki. 1996. Shinu kenri no kansei. *Imago* 7 (10): 202–11.

Uemura, Yoshirō. 2003. *Kurōn ningen no rinri*. Tokyo: Misuzu shobō.

Yonemoto, Shōhei, et al. 2000. *Yūseigaku to ningen shakai*. Tokyo: Kōdansha gendai shinsho.

Winslow, J. B. 1746. *The Uncertainty of the Signs of Death*. London: M. Cooper.

14 Why We Must Be Prudent in Research Using Human Embryos: Differing Views of Human Dignity

Susumu Shimazono

Justification through Comparisons with Abortion

Those who are attempting to rationalize scientific research on human embryos often bring up comparisons to abortion. The question, for example, of whether or not to approve the genetic diagnosis of a fertilized egg prior to its implantation is often discussed through that comparison. This occurred even in Japan. The Research Council in Bioethics, established by Prime Minister Junichirō Koizumi within the framework of his Commission on Science and Technology, had been charged to consider the handling and use of human embryos and began to discuss this during August 2001. Thereupon a discussion of the morality of pre-implantation genetic diagnosis became one in which comparisons with induced abortion were brought up. In "Hito hai no toriatsukai ni kansuru kihonteki kangaekata" (Basic considerations concerning the use of human embryos), a report of the interim findings submitted by this panel in December 2003, committee member and legal scholar Hajime Machino expressed an independent view in reference to the topic of abortion. He stated that "in our debate over genetic diagnosis prior to implantation, as long as we in Japan continue shelving the ethical examination of conditions related to abortion freedom here, the tendency to grant far more protection to the fertilized embryo than to the aborted fetus is a very strange outcome indeed" (Sōgō kagakugijutsu kaigi 2003, 57).

In Japan, performing an abortion was considered a criminal offense and prohibited in 1880. Abortion eventually became tolerated, however, under the Eugenic Protection Act, in 1948 (Fujime 1997). According to the Eugenic Protection Act, "eugenic surgery" was approved, and medical interventions to "prevent the birth of defective offspring" were permitted. In 1996 the Eugenic Protection Act was revised and became the Maternal Protection Act. It stipulated that "in cases where there is fear of serious damage to the health of the mother through the continuation of pregnancy to full-term, or possible physical or economic constraints," just as in cases where rape has occurred, abortion is permitted. The Maternal Protection Act of 1996, however, did not recognize "defective offspring" as a reason for abortion. Therefore, according to current law, the abortion of a fetus for the reason that it carries an inherited illness is not legal.

On the other hand, when the possibility of giving birth to a disabled child is known and a physician has *not* suggested the possibility of abortion to its parents, there have been judicial precedents that recognized physician accountability and allowed compensation to the parents. In actuality, therefore, abortions of fetuses with genetic defects are carried out frequently and are tolerated. According to Machino, this is a regulation that in actual practice operates in opposition to the provisions of the Maternal Protection Act. He writes:

> This sort of interpretation and application of the law is, according to one way of thinking, unreasonable, and both abortion and prenatal diagnoses ought to be disallowed. If this viewpoint is followed, pre-implantation diagnoses, and of course the doing of any prenatal screening not in accord with current law ought not to be recognized; and "wrongful births" will not be contrary to the civil code, but abortions of fetuses based on their gender will have to be acts that are prosecuted and punished as acts of illegal abortion. . . . However, to not allow abortion based on the fetus' gender could be seen as an infringement of a woman's right to choose whether or not she will give birth. And would this not be an injustice? If the Maternal Protection Act does not uphold this right, it is in violation and nullification of Article 13 of the Constitution (the right to the pursuit of happiness including the right to privacy). If we wish to avoid making laws that do not violate and nullify our constitution, we will have to apply the Maternal Protection Act in accord with the Constitution, using "constitutionally strict interpretation." . . . And if we do this, we ought to see the need to allow abortions for avoiding disabled children and, along with that, pre-implantation diagnoses and screening. (Sōgō kagakugijutsu kaigi 2003, 57)

Gynecologists also strongly insist on the point that, if abortion is permitted, pre-implantation testing should not be disallowed. Parents who must make the decision whether or not to abort a fetus with severe genetic defects are faced with a tremendous hardship. In addition to the physical pain of a disability, the deepening emotional bond to an unborn fetus can cause psychological distress as well. Since many physicians are loath to remove a fetus, parents often must go around searching for a physician who will help them. After all, an act tabooed because it terminates the life of a fetus is one, in the final analysis, for which the physician must bear the responsibility. In view of this, what could possibly be wrong with pre-implantation diagnoses, since what is removed is something at a much earlier stage of development (a just-fertilized ovum), which is a much lighter burden? People who worry that the standpoint adopted by Japan's disabled persons—namely that such diagnoses are inclined prejudicially against the disabled—will hold that Japan ought to take a prudentialist position on pre-implantation diagnosis. But this viewpoint tends to get drowned out by the voices actively promoting such procedures.

The logic of comparing abortion and the manipulation of embryos is also brought into play on the question of whether it is right or wrong to make use of embryos for research. Ova artificially inseminated result in so-called sur-

plus embryos that are not returned to the uterus. These can be used for research on embryonic stem cells. Newly cloned embryos having exactly the same
genetic makeup as a given patient can be produced, and from these it is envisioned that replacement organs might be made. Some insist that the question
of whether the use of such materials in this process (also known as "therapeutic cloning") is ethical is a discussion in which comparison with the morality
of abortion is appropriate. I earlier quoted Machino, who writes, "to grant far
more protection to the fertilized embryo than to the aborted fetus is a very
strange outcome indeed." Such criticism is directed not just at any restriction
of pre-implantation diagnoses but, more clandestinely, at any attempt to restrict
the use of embryos for research. It is good to recognize that this is a way of
turning any prudentialist concern into a laughingstock. This way of thinking is
presumed to be keeping human dignity in view by not destroying human life,
but in fact it is a point of view in which there is a very weak awareness of the
problems arising from the use and instrumentalizing of life, that is, of turning
life into a mere resource material.

Human Dignity and Religious Culture

In discussing bioethical questions concerning the beginning of human
life, we note that, since 1960, in both Europe and America the debate surrounding the morality of abortion has been carried on with battle-like intensity. The
points made during this debate have determined the general scheme of public understandings of the issue. In short, the focus of that debate centers on
whether or not embryos and fetuses are human life forms (life as individuated
human beings) worthy of the highest level of respect. The Catholic Church and
other denominations within Christianity that emphasize "sanctity of life" are
resolute in maintaining that life begins at conception and that the destruction
of anything from that point on is a sin and the equivalent of murder. The viewpoint that takes shape in opposition to this lays the emphasis upon a woman's
right to choose. They do not believe that at some weeks or even some months
after conception the embryo or fetus already has independent existence and
personhood. To them, consequently, abortion is above all a matter involving the
body of a woman, and it is the woman and the woman alone who has the right
to make the choice (Ogino 2001).

In Europe and America, discussions of the embryo and fetus are dealt with
in this way, and the ethical question of "when exactly life begins" has come to be
thought of as having a decisive importance and significance. UNESCO, which
takes a leading role in Western cultures, performed studies whose results on the
question of the beginning of life could be laid out within the following range.
Life begins: at the moment of conception (the Catholic Church and others);
fourteen days after conception (a criterion for using and doing research on embryos in England); at such time as the embryo becomes attached to the wall of
the uterus (authorities within the Jewish faith); forty days after conception
(authorities within Islam); at the stage at which there can be consciousness

(those within the Anglophone world whose position emphasizes "personhood") (Nudeshima 2001).

The multitude of perspectives on even the issue of when life actually begins demonstrates the limits of effective debate on this matter. In Japan, the debate over this issue has not been very lively, and, in fact, the issue is not seen as having any crucial significance (LaFleur 1992; Hardacre 1997; Tateiwa 2000). One reason for this is that among those supporting abortion rights in Japan there is also concern for the things being emphasized by the community of persons with disabilities—and this plays a significant role (Morioka 2001; Tateiwa 2000). Theories that would justify the elimination of those with disabilities can be thought of as having already damaged human dignity. And this way of looking at things subsequently comes to be recognized by those who take a prudentialist stand on prenatal testing and pre-implantation diagnoses.

In Japan, certainly, there are no large religious organizations like the Catholic Church that have developed powerful oppositional movements. There is instead a multiplicity of religions—not only Shinto and Buddhism, but also denominations within both of these. Also there are new religious organizations, which often have power and influence to vie with that of Shinto and Buddhism. It simply cannot be that among all of these, one will not find groups strongly opposed to any intervention into an embryo by therapeutic technology (Deguchi 2000; Taniguchi 2001). Nevertheless, this has not yet led to a large outcry within society. If it can be assumed that the attitudes of different religious bodies on these questions will reflect national and regional differences, can we not expect such differences to show up in approaches to the question of "the beginning of life"?

Can we then assume that the people of Japan will wholeheartedly accept medical interventions on human life forms? On the matter of brain death and organ transplantation, Japan is the nation in which more emphasis is placed on being cautious and prudent than in any other nation in the world. The result of this is that the new legal definition of death—namely, that brain death equals death—is not acceptable to the people of Japan. A lot of doubt is expressed about allowing the medical community to have the authority to decide what constitutes death, and about equating brain death with death (Morioka 2001; Komatsu 1996). Although, at the end of a protracted debate, the "Law Allowing Transplantation" was enacted in 1997, among the Japanese people the definition of brain death as constituting true death is still not accepted. As a result, organ transplantation based on brain death occurs only very infrequently in Japan.

One source of the Japanese public's suspicion of the notion of brain death is a sense that in Japan paternalistic physicians readily violate, through their medical interventions, the bodies of patients. Very soon after the world's first cadaveric heart transplantation had been performed in 1968, Jurō Wada, a professor at Sapporo Medical College, took the heart out of a twenty-one-year-old youth who had drowned while swimming and implanted it into the body of another youth, who was being treated for a malfunctioning heart valve; the recipient died eighty-three days later. A case brought against Dr. Wada as a result was eventually dismissed for lack of evidence, but many of Japan's citizens continued to doubt that Dr. Wada was guiltless in this affair.

Among Japanese, the sense that Japanese doctors will not hesitate to do medical violence against patients gathered intensity following revelations during the 1980s of details of the atrocities committed by Japan's medical Unit 731 during World War II. Unit 731, a corps of slightly fewer than three thousand active in the vicinity of Harbin between 1936 and 1945, was charged with the task of developing bacteriological weapons. The unit was directed by Army Lieutenant General Shirō Ishii, a military medic who had studied at the medical school of Kyoto University. It is estimated that, for the purpose of producing bacteriological weapons, this unit was responsible, through its experiments, for the deaths of between two and three thousand Chinese, Koreans, Mongolians, and Russians. These facts were first made widely known to the people of Japan by the publication in 1981 of *Kieta saikinsen butai* by Kei-ichi Tsuneishi and also by the three volumes of *Akuma no hōshoku* by Seiichi Morimura published between 1981 and 1983. Moreover, quite a few of the very physicians who had taken part in these wartime experiments rose, in the postwar period, to high positions in Japanese research of that time. Knowledge that its research regimen had put these medical men at the pinnacle of the research science structure, and that there had been a nonchalant commission of crimes—involving the use by physicians of the bodies of living patients for clinical research—led in Japan to an intensified distrust of physicians and of the medical research that had accepted such things as somehow normal. This had, indeed, been *dark* medicine.

In the 1980s, also, the debate in Japan about the propriety of performing transplants using organs from "brain dead" persons became especially heated. This period was also one during which there was a deepening awareness that physicians' therapies were virtually powerless to provide "care" for persons in the process of dying. Yet suddenly the establishment of facilities for therapy proliferated, there was an impressive increase in committing patients to medical therapies for help, and the average life expectancy of the Japanese was dramatically extended. This notwithstanding, the public's dissatisfaction with, and distrust of, medical therapies showed a marked increase. Many of Japan's citizens continued to have a sense that medicine was "going too far." Discontent with Western-style medicine, which is devoted to focusing on the body as divisible into multiple parts and to the function of each separate part, gave increasing support to the need to look again to holistic and alternative therapies that are based on Japan's own East Asian traditions. Within a context such as this, there arose questions about transplants performed on the basis of the criterion of brain death—and for quickly abandoning all attempts to give therapy to still-living persons in that state. This implied falling into practices that give even more power to the physician in his or her dealings with patients.

Another source of skepticism in the debate over brain death was the question whether the brain's faculties and awareness form the core of an individual's existence, or whether the body should be included. That the Japanese do not feel comfortable with making a clear division between mind and body, and with taking the former to be the locus of a person's life, is a circumstance that powerfully influences this debate. Japan has a religious culture that embraces the animistic way of seeing life and even mind in things and in bodies, and this belief is cited by those who resist the notion of brain death (Umehara 1992b). This is an instance of religious culture being used by those who would be prudentialist vis-à-vis "medical intervention in persons moving towards death," but it can also be recognized in the debate about "medical intervention in persons on the way to being born." In both cases there is a strong possibility that the religious culture with which one aligns will have an impact on the approach one takes in the debate.

In new reproductive technologies, new therapies for reviving life, new forms of genetic therapy, and the like, the potential for therapies and manipulations to intervene with "life on the way to being born" has become markedly high. In the cultures of East Asia, where high value has always been placed on the continuity of life from ancestors to their descendants, the thinking is that, precisely because so much emphasis is placed upon having male heirs, there will be a ready acceptance of getting these not only by normal childbirth but also by in vitro fertilization and even by surrogate motherhood. It is assumed that the acceptance of reproductive technologies will carry over into an acceptance of regenerative ones and of gene therapies. Not a few analysts hypothesize that, due to the influence of Confucian culture, there is a high possibility that positive attitudes will be taken vis-à-vis "therapeutic intervention on life forms on the way to being born." In Japan, however, with regard to "life forms on the way to being born," a more prudentialist attitude has penetrated the society to some extent. Therefore, although abortion in Japan is, by comparison, rather widely accepted, various kinds of technological alteration of sex organs, regenerative therapies, and genetic therapies are not necessarily receiving acceptance.

On this point, Yōichirō Murakami, who is both a researcher in the history of science and a Catholic, states that it is not consistent to oppose the sort of regenerative medicine that would require stem cell research while accepting induced abortion (Murakami 2002). What follows is based on notes taken during a public lecture by Murakami and, therefore, must be seen as something to which the speaker has not had occasion to give the same kind of scrupulous attention as he would have given something more formally academic. But it does provide a way of getting to know his thinking on these matters.

> This is my own opinion, but it seems to me that, in the case of surplus embryos that meet the fate of being thrown away, there also has been the beginning of life in them. I personally go along with that point of view. But within Japanese society there is something even more horrendous going on. Take a look yourselves at the comparison. Within one year approximately 400,000, some years even more than a million, fetuses are killed. And the question to be asked is what is the fate of those fetuses or, more precisely, what is *done with* the fetuses that are taken from the wombs of their mothers? It depends somewhat on the length of the pregnancy. If it has lasted only a few weeks, the fetus is merely flushed down the drain. Although everyone knows that pharmaceutical and cosmetic companies often get these fe-

tuses and use them in the making of medicines and cosmetics, no one takes this up as a problem to be considered with any seriousness, and there is no law formed to regulate such a practice. The professional society of gynecologists writes about handling these matters with reference to the laws concerning postmortem dissections, but this is almost meaningless. If one were to compare the fate of these destroyed fetuses with the approximately 200 surplus embryos that are discarded each year, and then go on to censure only one side, the latter, it becomes abundantly clear that the reasoning here is faulty. This is the basis for the position I am taking on this matter. (Murakami 2002, 3–4)

Comparatively, Japanese society has traditionally dealt with the human fetus quite loosely. In 1549 when Francis Xavier's group came to Japan, they were surprised at the high ethical standards and morality of the Japanese, which they wrote about in a report to Rome. However, in this Japanese society where high morals were maintained, the one thing that the foreigners just could not stand was the fact that infanticide and abortion were common occurrences. It is within this mindset that Luis d'Almeida is said to have built Japan's first Western style hospital in Northern Kyushu. However, this was in fact not a hospital but rather a place for another type of "child dumping." He asked people who were planning to throw away their child to leave the baby in a box he had placed in front of the church, saying that he would raise it himself. (Murakami 2002, 6)

This remark resonates with the Christian critical stance regarding Japanese religious culture and ethical consciousness based on the idea of dignity of human being as individual. Concerning the treatment of aborted fetuses, it is necessary that we reexamine whether or not everyone really knew about these practices and tolerated them, or merely whether there simply had never been much discussion concerning them. In either case, Murakami presumes a Christian stance of "sanctity of life" and is critical of Japanese culture. Therefore, he presents strong points of contention.

However, his criticism is based on the concept of respect for each human as an individual, and I do not think we can say that this is a criticism arising from bases intrinsic to Japanese religious culture. In Japan there is little support for that line of thought, that is, the idea that respect for the human as an individual is the absolute basis for the ethics of life and death. I think this is because when the Japanese think about respect for humanity, they think about this not only on the level of "individual human life," but also as "life within the community," or "life as a shared body." In other words, Japanese think of life also on the level of "one among many existing together." I wish to use this as a key to continue the discussion, but first I will offer a historical perspective on the subject of infanticide and abortion in Japan.

From Coexistent Life to Life as an Individual— A Change in the Nineteenth Century

In Japan it was during the late Edo period (1600–1868) that interest in dignity for fetal life heightened. During this period, as anti-infanticide and anti-abortion sentiment increased, there was also a drastic change in thinking about conception and childbirth (Chiba and Ōtsu 1983; Shinmura 1996; Sawayama 1998). The Meiji Restoration in 1868 gave rise to even more change, but there appear to be two ways of viewing this change: as continuous with the late Edo period, or as a new development in thought. In this discussion I will use the nineteenth century as the time frame and explore the changes in attitudes about the lives of fetuses and infants during that period. Further, I will consider how these changes are related to Japanese religious culture.

Evidence suggests that in the earlier part of this period, abortion and infanticide remained widespread. Though we can only speculate as to the incentives for such behavior, it appears that there was fear of future financial burdens caused by having too many children. Another probable explanation is that people would abort or kill babies for health reasons of the mother, or because it might be an obstacle to her work capacity. Particularly under the imminent danger of famine, when population growth could potentially threaten the life of the family and community, the desire to prevent excess numbers became prevalent. This way of thinking connects to the idea that preservation of the group is most valuable, even at the expense of sacrificing the lives of certain individuals. On the other hand, during this same period, many put increased effort into the care of individual children, and limiting the number of children was a result of a desire to raise each child properly. In the background of such self-controlled birthrate restrictions was the fact that the independent farming households, having a limited amount of land, constructed "budgets" of children for themselves, resulting in a prosperous agricultural management system. It is within this environment that recognition of the value of a child's life grew.

This is not to say, however, that there was no consciousness of sin vis-à-vis those lives that were sacrificed. According to Emiko Namihira, a cultural anthropologist who has accumulated surveys about individual Japanese communities, the Japanese during this period viewed abortion and infanticide as sending the "little spirits" back to a place that can be characterized as a "life pool" or reservoir, asking for them to be reborn later (Namihira 1996).

> [I]n the background of beliefs about children's reincarnation is the idea that people are who they are by virtue of their families or where they live rather than by their individuality. People are constantly re-cycling through birth and death— each life comes from a large place somewhat like a reservoir and is allotted a given amount of time in this world. When one dies, his/her life returns to the reservoir. This reservoir metaphor leads to a conceptualization that does not emphasize the individual life. It happened frequently that the name of a child who died soon after birth would be given to another child born before much time had elapsed. Furthermore, there are many regions of the country where funerals were not performed and posthumous Buddhist names were not given to those who died as children. If we align our thinking with those people who accepted this immediate re-cycling of names "so that it (the young child's life) could be re-born immediately," we see that the tendency to think of life as an individual unit was still slight during their time. However, the concept of life *today* is definitely headed towards individualism. The life of a child who dies young is different than the life of the next

child born. We do not draw a connection between the life of the aborted fetus and that of the child who is born next. In the background of today's memorial service for *mizuko* (fetuses and children that died in infancy), do we not see a "tendency toward individuation of lives"? Likewise, if we look at the fact that beliefs pertaining to children who either die as babies or in the womb flourish more among urbanites than among the rural people, we see that the traditional ceremony for dead babies has not so much changed in modern times, as it has had added to it a new belief (Namihira 1996, 44–45)

Folk sayings such as "a child until seven belongs to the gods" expressed a way of thinking in which praying for a child's rebirth without holding any of the normal funeral ceremonies was justified. The Japanese during the nineteenth century believed that the individual person preserves the soul of the group and exists in connection with the other world. When she or he is born into this world, her or his individual life becomes precious, yet naturally the collective life from the other world is also still valued. This tied into the idea that children are an endowment to us by the gods.

Prior to the Meiji Restoration (1868), there were public declarations that children already born had to be valued, and admonitions warning against abortion and infanticide were widespread. Those insisting on this were people with political or religious power. In the beginning of the nineteenth century the government and powerful clans cautioned against abortion and infanticide, and in order to prevent such behavior some regions forced people to report pregnancies. This anti-abortion, anti-infanticide stance was due to the fact that if the birth rate of a region was low, the population also remained low, and the government's and clans' economic success hinged on population growth. Abortion and infanticide were therefore directly connected to economic issues. Teachings that preached the value of individual lives were closely tied to policies that presupposed population growth. The prohibition of abortion was adopted after the Meiji Restoration and was molded into governmental policy by the Meiji leaders, who had their eyes set on increasing national power. During the same period, the True Pure Land Buddhist sect preached against taking lives and cautioned against abortion and infanticide. This sect stood out as a religious group with a religious incentive for preaching the value of each individual life. Although True Pure Land Buddhists emphasized the salvation of each individual person, they were also motivated by a passionate desire to collaborate with the government. They regarded killing the weak as an indisputable violation of the commandments of the Buddhist canon. They preached that because humans are hopeless sinners we should rely all the more on Amida Buddha's grace. During this period they are said to have been strong condemners of taking lives (Arimoto 1995). Masao Arimoto writes:

In research on the history of modern society, or more specifically the history of modern religions, we do not know of any concrete records of discussions among True Pure Land lay people regarding the precept against killing. Primarily what we have are the founder, Shinran's, doctrines—particularly his "teaching that even hunters are acceptable" and that, as a principle of the True Pure Land, "eating meat and having a spouse" did not estrange persons from the faith—so much so that at that time they did not realize that this was a virtual inversion of traditional [Buddhist] understandings. . . . Nevertheless actual history forces us to recognize discrepancies between theory and practice, and we observe that there are differences between regions of Japan where the True Pure Land faith was strong and regions where it was weak. For instance, although interdictions of abortion and infanticide often showed up in places where there were very few True Pure Land temples and the authorities worried about a declining population, in areas where there was a fervent adherence to the True Pure Land sect we note that the population was growing and nothing like interdiction on abortion and infanticide seems to have appeared. There probably was not a decided difference in the daily living conditions of both groups.

In other words, whether or not people would take recourse to abortion and infanticide, whether or not they would risk their own future existence, and whether or not there would be prohibitions on abortion and infanticide—all these were matters where a division into two substantially different approaches seems to have depended very much on matters of faith and ethos. The result was thoroughly paradoxical. The group that agonized over their future and took recourse to abortion and infanticide experienced a narrowing of its livelihood base, one that brought about the ruination of agricultural hamlets. The latter group, in contrast, realized an increase in the base of its livelihood so much that "family productivity strongly contributed to local prosperity." . . . The development of Hokkaidō went forward during the third decade of the Meiji period [1887–96], with people from the latter group putting their energies into that development. And the treaty between Japan and the government of Hawaii allowing immigration [beginning in 1885], stipulated "permission to immigrate granted to working families from four Japanese prefectures"—namely Hiroshima, Yamaguchi, Kumamoto, and Fukuoka, where the faith was strong. And soon they were arriving on the North American continent. . . . This meant the emigration of high-quality workers and merchants away from their home base in Japan and especially from the areas where there were fervent followers of the True Pure Land sect. This emigration not only took care of the problem of population growth otherwise handled only by restricting births but also demonstrated that population growth could occur easily among persons invited to emigrate from areas of strong True Pure Land faith and an ethos of prohibiting abortion and infanticide. When all of this fit into an ethos that made honesty, industriousness, thrift, endurance, and the like into virtues, there was a natural burst of social and economic energy, and the economic activity that resulted was impressive both in quality and quantity. (Arimoto 1995, 243–44)

In regions of Japan where True Pure Land Buddhism was thriving, the population was large, the inhabitants worked hard, there was much emigration, and there were many people who had what it took to accommodate to modern conditions. There were a great many True Pure Land followers who in the process of modernization moved to new territories. Among the colonizers of Hokkaido and Manchuria and emigrants to places such as the United States and Brazil, many came from areas of strong True Pure Land belief. Then, in the modernization process, when the recognition of dignity for each individual human life increased, it was not merely that an individual's standard of living went up, but also that stronger ethical value was given for an individual's life. It is important not to forget that in some cases the recognition of the value of each human life was closely tied to an expansion of the power of that group we call the "nation." And the expansion of the nation's power was a cause of the development of imperialism and the creation of environmental problems.

With modernization a religious culture developed that moved in the direction of placing emphasis upon the dignity of individual lives; this certainly implied a refinement of ethical sensitivities. Movement in the direction of a sharpened ethical sensitivity is no doubt part of why religious culture today is directed toward valuing each individual life. Modern Japanese people too have a heightened consciousness of human rights and, much more than in the past, have become keenly aware of the preciousness of each human life. There is absolutely no need to reverse this trend and make a case for a return to the earlier way of thinking and acting. However, I cannot deny that the respect for human lives as "existing with other lives," as "life as a shared entity," and of "life in a group" has moved in the direction of becoming lost. There have been more than a few instances in which respect for the value of the individual overrode the effective strength of the group. One result is pressure on, and collapse of, any sense of life shared as a group. There is a necessity now for us not only to place value on the individual life but to renew attention to how this relates to the value that should be recognized in "existing with other lives," in "life as a shared entity," and in "life in a group." Likewise, it is necessary to make clear the role to be taken by religious culture in carrying out this task.

That again is related to the work of illustrating how deeply sexual reproduction in modern and contemporary times is connected to incentives for the continuation and also the development of the family, the nation, and the group. Bioethical problematics that start out with questions centered on "the beginnings of life," while necessarily giving consideration to the dignity and rights of an individual life, ought also to bring about an understanding of why it is important to reflect deeply on the value and morality of holding that life is also "life as a shared entity."

Why Should We Refrain from Making Use of Human Embryo Research?

Up to this point, I have attempted to provide a brief historical outline of birth control and reproductive principles in contemporary Japan. I have reflected upon a broad range of judgments toward human dignity and regard for human life. My main goal has been to point out the necessity of thinking critically about varying forms of human dignity, as well as the different ways we place value on human life. Now, while keeping in mind these past inquiries, I would like to tackle the bioethical problems surrounding current research being conducted on human embryos, and to see what sort of implications we can extract from it.

If we were to take the stance that embryos hold the same status as children who have already been born, then the destruction of an embryo, or an abortion, would be equivalent to murder. Matters related to this have been dealt with exhaustively in the West over the past half-century, with the debate becoming particularly intense in the 1970s and '80s (Ogino 2001). In the context of this dispute, the central question was at what point, from the time of fertilization to the time of birth, individuated human life begins. An individual's life cannot simply be destroyed or used (for research purposes), but if there are thought to be embryonic stages that exist prior to the creation of human life, then destruction could be permitted during these stages. The opposite argument is that individuated life begins at the instant of conception, and that the use of the embryo at any stage therefore cannot be permitted. This is the standpoint adhered to by members of the Catholic Church.

To many people, the embryo does not have exactly the same life status as that of an individual (who has already been born), and as such it does not have exactly the same rights. Thus the opinion of these people is that any sort of destruction or research must be carried out with prudence. They argue that even if there are embryonic stages when the embryo does not appear to be an individuated human being, since the embryo would inevitably become a person, its very existence corresponds nearly to being a full-fledged human being. In the interim report of the Japanese Bioethical Research Committee, the embryo was said to be "the bud of human life," which presents a way of thinking about embryos that is in line with the aforementioned assertions.

These are important themes, of course, but this type of argument can cover only a limited aspect of the actual ethical issue. The bioethical position of the embryo has been abstractly discussed, but from this point on, I would like to focus instead on the *use* of embryo research, a topic that has not yet been discussed in depth. A careful investigation of the contents of the research being carried out on embryos that may violate or threaten human dignity is imperative.

It is not sufficient simply to discuss the advantages that are brought about by human embryo research. The people arguing *for* the utilization of embryos for research purposes emphasize the good things (benefits, welfare, and usefulness) that can come from such research. The main objective of utilizing embryo research in this case is to help alleviate the many serious problems faced by people who are suffering from illness or who are under distress. An important point is that the interests of those suffering from grave illnesses should always be considered.

That said, in actual practice, the field of regenerative medicine has not yet realized these objectives. People who are suffering should be kept in mind above all else when considering the above-mentioned objectives, but this is not usually the case, as economic gains often are being sought concurrently. For example, the provision of "spare parts" for people seeking longevity or enhancing physical appearance and abilities has come to be included within the range of objectives of regenerative medicine. The question becomes whether or not it is acceptable to destroy embryos in research geared toward this kind of medical practice. This would be essentially making implements and/or resources out of human lives, so should the answer not be a resounding "no"? Supposing that we say "no" to the use of embryos for this kind of research, then for what kind of medicine and research *can* we approve of the destruction of life as the sacrifice to be paid for advancement? This is the main question concerning the objectives of using research done on human embryos.

Next, there is the question of whether or not results that could benefit human welfare in various ways can arise from research that is conducted on human embryos. Despite the need to provide relief to individual patients who are suffering, such research is not always linked to the promotion of the welfare of society. The grieving parents of children who have died might see the prospect of human cloning as wonderful news if they were able to use their deceased child's genes to create an exact clone. A valuing of that which is appropriate to humans and to a community of orderly cohabitation, along with a realization of the unfavorable situations that would be thrust upon people, has prevented such procedures from being carried out up to this point. Such research could violate human dignity, and the results arising from such research could ultimately go against human welfare.

Among the themes central to the examination of the rights and wrongs of human embryo research is the aforementioned possibility of making useful things or resources out of human lives. A thorough reflection on what kind of benefits will result from human embryo research is imperative. If we look at the long-term growth of human embryo research and regenerative medicine, we can see the profound impact that it could potentially have upon our lives. Whether we experience these impacts in our own lifetimes or not, they are likely to occur at some point in the future. With respect to growing technology, the way that people live their lives (their values and life routines) is fundamentally changing such that a new kind of power is now at their disposal. Since the technological innovations being pursued at present will have the most profound effect on future generations, it is our responsibility *now* to thoroughly examine what these effects will be (Yonasu 2000 [trans. of Jonas 1979]). Our responsibility to question the rapid growth of modern medicine for the sake of future generations is becoming increasingly urgent. An ethics that takes responsibility seriously is one that thoroughly assesses what kind of results present actions will have in the future, and is an ethics that requires the taking of a prudentialist position. It is natural for us to place emphasis on our own lives, instead of considering the lives of those who came before us or those who will come in the future. Should not an ethics of responsibility emphasize the dignity of shared life? Of all the things that can result from manipulating or using embryos for research, perhaps the most important to understand is how it poses a threat to our shared humanity, and how in many cases it will bring along things that run contrary to humankind in the future. I will list a few of these:

- The current system of scientific research is such that scientists cannot maintain the attitude that the embryos produced through in vitro fertilization or cloning will be treated as existences that would grow into full individual human beings. We have not yet formulated a research ethics that gives serious consideration to the necessary conditions for treating early forms of human life. Thus, while there might be the possibility to sacrifice the "bud of human life" for deriving stem cells from in vitro fertilization and cloning, and for using them to save patients suffering from serious diseases, there is also a fairly large possibility that the use of this research will cross the line and use them for various benefits that do not merit the sacrifice of the "bud of human life."

  There must be a thorough investigation into the rules that govern laboratory research when experiments utilize types of existence close to human lives. There has not been such an attempt. We have strict ethical rules for making research on full human beings, but we also need ethical rules for the research that involves the use of human embryos. If these are not made more clear, then the possibility is high that the "bud of human life," or even the forms of life that result from it, will be treated on the same level as inanimate objects, plants, or animals—that is, in the way things have been treated in laboratories up until now. In order for the use of research derived from human embryos to be handled appropriately, a completely new set of experiment and research rules must be created.

- Even if the use were limited to the very initial stages of the embryo (for example, the stage up to fourteen days following conception, when the "primitive streak," which later develops into the fetus's central nervous system, appears), the fact still remains that the stem cells that exist in the embryo hold the potential for creating more highly developed forms of life. A large element of stem-cell research has become the production of body tissue and subsequently various human body parts. That is to say, research now tinkers with the human body being cultivated outside of itself. Many laboratories have been established that work with human body tissue. The possibility of threatening human dignity is very high when, in this way, human body parts are cut off from the individual and used as raw materials. Even if not as extreme, "human tissue experimentation" ought to be more widely considered as on par with "human experimentation."

  There needs to be a vocabulary that expresses the dignity of the human body. This sort of mutual understanding was brought to light by the "Three Laws of Bioethics," established in France in 1994 (Sōgō kenkyū kaihatsu kikō [General Research and Development Forum] and Kawai 2001, 192). While stem cells have the potential for becoming nearly all parts of the human body, they also have even greater possibilities, and it is thus necessary to exercise extreme prudence when considering issues that concern the dignity of the human (which is latent in these cells). Although we can say the above about research involving stem cells from surplus embryos, if we then move on to how to make use of cloned embryos, the extent of such research gets even broader, and the importance of the ethical problem becomes all the greater.

- When manipulating human embryos, and in fusing together stem cells with other forms of life, there is a distinct possibility of creating existence or tissue that will have a nature that is partially human. If embryo and stem-cell research progresses, it will become easy to produce chimeras (organs/organisms made up of two or more different genetic components) and hybrids. If reproductive cells created from stem cells are used, the resultant chimeras and hybrids cross the line into a whole new category of life form. How great would be the profits and benefits that would result from such a process!

However, the possibility then arises for a blurring of the distinction between human and nonhuman. For example, in the field of regenerative medicine, it has been speculated that human organs could be created inside the body of an animal, which would be creating none other than a human-animal chimera. This tinkering with the nature of humans and the implanting of human body parts into other animals could fundamentally jolt our concept of the uniformity of our species, and our concept of the human race having a uniform body.

- When creating human embryos artificially, technicians need to gather ova from women. There then arises the high possibility of utilizing women's bodies like instruments and material resources. If we can create cloned embryos, establish embryonic stem cells from them, and cultivate stem cells with one's own genes, there may be a considerable possibility of producing various therapeutic effects. At least at the present stage of technology, however, we must first get many ova to create cloned embryos, and then we again need many cloned embryos to establish embryonic stem cells.

  Where do we get these ova? Women from whom ova are taken have to endure a severe bodily burden. There have been reports that patients have died from the side effects of induced ovulation. We cannot investigate the long-term side effects of sterility therapy at this stage. And there is the question of motivation— there must be something that leads women to undergo this type of potentially dangerous treatment. It is possible that women offering ova expect monetary compensations; there is also the possibility that women close to patients would be coerced to offer them. If medical treatments use ova as if they were instruments or resources, women in weak positions could be forced to bear burdens and risks. This is because, at bottom, medical use of embryos presupposes the use of human life in its early phase or the use of body parts such as ova—the great sources of future human life—as mere instruments and resources.

- If human embryo research continues, we will soon see eternal youth and longevity, people living to a super-old age, women giving birth at older ages, and the individual's expectations and capacities becoming ever higher. As a wealth of medical services continues to mold and remold the human body, passage beyond the human limits that up to now people have not been able to escape will become a possibility. This ought to be called "medical therapies gone wild," and if the principle of accommodating every desire of individual clients continues, then it will unavoidably lead to medicine going too far. The possibility of this happening is particularly acute in the field of regenerative medicine (Shimazono 2002). And yet, could the further development of these "excesses" in the medical field possibly contribute to the welfare of humanity (Fukuyama 2002)? In addition, can it really be the case that the use of such embryos fits the view of the embryo having the same status as the "bud of human life"?

  Furthermore, with this field of therapy developing to excess, there arises great potential for growing disparities between those who have a share in the benefits of the research and those who do not (Silver 1997). People from wealthy nations and the most affluent people from less wealthy nations will receive these medical services, while poorer nations and people will not, and the disparities between these groups could consequently become magnified. If this happens, a questioning of the foundation of social justice would become stronger, as the wealthy and the poor might not even feel that they are part of the same human race any longer. We could lose sight of the idea of equality across the human race, as we would essentially be living in a society organized by social status. Such extreme social stratification could result in a hostile spirit all across society. Instead of risking all these dangers, might it not be better to devote concentrated effort to further develop medical technology that promotes the essential health of people around the world?

The Dignity of Human Life and Religious Culture

From the above consideration of the use of human embryos for research, what can we learn about the relationship between the notion of "dignity of human life" and religious culture? In treating both the rights and wrongs of using human embryos for research and the problem of when life begins, we must move beyond limiting ourselves to a discussion of the preservation of the dignity of *individual* human life and proceed to consider the possibility of teasing out ideas with more diverse, broad, and cross-cultural implications for the dignity of human beings.

The basis for the Catholic Church's opposition to abortion is the theological notion that human life, held to be sacred, begins at the moment of conception. Although the official expression of this idea began with Pope Pius IX's 1869 pronouncement, the underlying basis lies in systems of medieval theology (Hēringu 1990 [trans. of Häring 1980]). In other words, although human life starts, biologically speaking, with the union of sperm and egg (that is, with conception), the thing that makes humans "human" does not occur through a biological process but through a deity's granting of a soul. This is called "ensoulment." The discussion of when this "ensoulment" happens had already begun, and the explanation that it occurs at the moment of conception had already been indicated, by the thirteenth century. With the advancement of biological knowledge, this argument became the Church's official theological position in the nineteenth century; however, this position was defined firmly when abortion came to be the topic of intense political debate in the 1960s and continues to the present.

However, the theoretical notion of "ensoulment" has moved beyond the Christian sphere and has greatly influenced Western ethics. The person responsible for charting the idea of "dignity of human life" in theories of modern philosophy, and for greatly influencing the ensuing discussion, is Immanuel Kant (Nakayama 2002). According to Kant, humans are endowed with reason and morality, and the fact that they have individuality is therefore especially valuable. This grants dignity to humans. Thus, humans have their own value by existing, and Kant argued that this existence must therefore not be treated merely as a means to another end. Moreover, he held that humans, because of this sanctity, enjoy a completely different ethical status than do other living creatures. According to the bioethics that has developed in the English-speaking world since the 1970s, dignity of human life is bound up in notions of personhood;

the protracted debate over when individuality develops (the theory of "personhood") and over medical intervention in the beginning of life (Engeruhāto 1988 [trans. of Engelhardt 1982]; Toūrī 1988 [trans. of Tooley 1980]) tells the story of the great influence of Kant's ideas, entwined as they are with the "dignity of human life."

This argument of Kant's is structurally comparable to the "ensoulment" position from medieval Christianity, which says that humans are granted souls by God and are therefore especially valued. In Western cultural traditions, that humans are imagined to bear God's image and therefore enjoy a special relationship with the divine has meant that humanity's existence is isolated from that of other creatures. Moreover, the idea that the exalted nature of humanity's position is related to God-granted reason and morality is deep-seated. According to this notion, humans enjoy a special status within the system of existence ordered by divine will, and the idea that human life has dignity naturally follows. The commandment that "one must not kill humans without just cause," too, is tied to just such an interpretation of "dignity of human life" and gains approval in this way.

Although the commandment that "one must not kill humans without just cause" is acknowledged in Buddhism, Shinto, and Confucianism as well as in Japanese folk culture, rhetoric explaining the foundation for this belief differs greatly from that found in the Western cultural sphere. In the background of this difference in explanation lies a difference in the embodied thought processes and feelings with respect to life and death. Broadly defined views of life and death, and culture and values that focus on "life" themselves, differ. For example, the fundamental Buddhist injunction against taking life pertains to animals as well as to humans. According to the India-derived Buddhist notion of karmic rebirth, humans may be reborn as animals, and any human might have been an animal in a past life. The idea that humans enjoy special status does not come to the fore in the prohibition against taking life.

Moreover, there are also beliefs in Shinto and Japanese folk religion that divinities may take the form of animals or that animals may act as messengers of the gods. The mythic, totemistic idea that ancestors were in fact animals has also survived. Human and animal life is seen as linked, and the special high status of humanity within the order of life is not emphasized. Instead, living in harmony both with nature and with other living beings is held to be precious. In this way, a religious culture different from Western thought exists in Japan, and when the notion of "dignity of human life" is used in Japan, it reflects a religious culture with different nuances from those evoked in the West. However, Christian believers exist in Japan as well, and there are more than a few people in the West who feel an intimacy with Japanese culture. Contemporary values and spirituality held worldwide about the dignity of individual human life reflect the influence of various religious cultures; on the other hand, these are also influenced by the modern individual-based notion of the "dignity of human life," and these beliefs are thought to be manifested in diverse forms.

There are many cases of individuals who are influenced by Japanese religious culture but who nevertheless take the idea of "human dignity" to mean that humans occupy a completely different and higher level in the order of existence than do animals, and that animals are not therefore worthy of dignity. Moreover, these things are related to how one views the relation between body and rationality (or knowledge, or consciousness). The idea that dignity stems from the existence of something that supports humanity's unique position based on physical difference is not necessarily felt. This problem, revolving as it does around debates over brain death and organ transplantation in Japan, is a deeply questioned issue there (Morioka 2000; Umehara 1992a; Umehara 1992b; Komatsu 1996). Moreover, rather than conceiving of humans as independent ethical subjects who make moral judgments, Japanese culture patterns stress knowledge and feeling in concert with others, with having a corporeal existence that responds bodily to the environment and to other people—in other words, "coexisting life."

On the other hand, Japanese culture may be weak in understanding the importance of the independence of the individual and the idea of human rights. We should recall the fact that during World War II Japanese scientists and physicians conducted violent experiments on innocent human beings and killed them. This can be explained at least partly by the fact that people in the Japanese army, in the medical professions, and in Japanese society overall were not strongly attached to the ethical idea that humans should not violate the dignity of human beings as individuals. By the 1970s and 1980s, when brain death and organ transplantation were being discussed, the concept of human rights had taken root widely among Japanese citizens. While accepting the importance of the respect for dignity of human beings as individuals, the Japanese public at the same time strongly insisted on a difference in values between Japan and West.

The value that the Japanese place on human life and the principles and regulations that prohibit violence against it are based on elements quite different from the notion that it is humans who lead a conscious and reason-based existence and therefore have a more highly valued existence than do other forms of life. When above in this chapter we referred to the Japanese consciousness of the value of life, I used the concept of "the dignity of coexisting life" in considering why we must refrain from using human embryos. This was an attempt to liberate the values and spirituality that accompany the idea of "dignity of human life" from the notion of respect for the human *as an individual*. The ideas of calling attention to "the dignity of coexisting life" and of seeing the basis of the dignity of humans in nonhuman life and nonhuman bodies are linked.

By making this point, we emphasize the characteristics of Japanese culture so that differences from the Christian cultural sphere may become clear, and, in addition, we can provide an argument for the diversity in concepts of "human dignity." However, the problems involved in using human embryos mentioned above should not be seen as misgivings that happen to be found in one, somewhat local, religious culture. Doing so would dismiss the matter far too easily. If we conceptualize the use-of-embryos problem as one that should be viewed through the perspective offered by the wider concept of "the dignity of coexisting life," it would be wrong to trivialize this as a religious viewpoint locked up within a single culture. In fact, one reason why this larger perspective has never surfaced in Europe and America may be because societies there have been totally caught up in a single-minded focus—that is, debating the point at which human life begins. The "blind spot" may very well have been the West's.

Presently, the fact that differences in value systems and spirituality on the "human dignity" question greatly influence bioethical considerations causes apprehension. Because cultures are different, great differences in judging problems arise, and the number of such problems that must be solved is considerable. If so, we are coming to a point where we must seek some understanding based on a standard shared by all of us humans. The value systems and notions of spirituality based in particular religious cultures confront one another and are diverse. Must not then bioethics be constructed on the basis of value systems and notions of spirituality that are in turn built on the commonalities of human values and spiritualities?

But what *are* these human value systems and spiritualities? They are not already in evidence; moreover, it is not necessary to conceive of them as fixed. There exists a range of individual value systems and notions of spirituality that mirror the diversity of human cultures. However, if we inquire into a particular problem, then shared tendencies can emerge. The number of possible understandings corresponds to the multitude of human beings, and we should also be able to find points of compromise within the tendencies we share. Thus, such shared inclinations can be recognized as such, and the reason for being able to achieve unanimity is based in our common human nature.

For example, regarding the intervention of life sciences in the question of when life begins, various religious and ethical ideas regarding the prohibition that "one must not kill humans without just cause" should be considered. In this, the question of why human life must be valued more highly than other life for us can be asked through philosophy, through religious studies, through comparative cultural theory, and through sociology. We can ask what sort of practices and ideas of life and death have been preserved in Christian, Buddhist, Shinto, or local animistic religious cultures. Then the various versions of "the dignity of human life" or "the precious nature of human life" based upon those religious practices and ideas may become clear. Moreover, we can also investigate the biological reason for the particular importance that humans themselves place on the existence of humans. For example, following the natural sciences' explanation of empathy, we may also be made aware of important insights regarding the bioethical problems with the use of or research on fetuses. While this incorporates a biological approach (in the sense that physiology incorporates psychology), it can also offer an explication of a value system and a notion of spirituality that contribute to the deliberations of bioethics.

The important bioethical questions concerning the beginning of life, however, are in no way limited to the problem of "reason for prohibiting the destruction of human life." As I showed above, in those cases where the use of embryos or research on them is being approved, a consideration of what sort of *result* might occur is also crucial. In our asking this question, the problem of transforming human life into tools or resources may be greatly clarified by considering the matter of "coexistent life."

However, we should recognize that this perspective cannot be seen as *the* key to solving every problem. These matters should be investigated through mobilizing the knowledge of various fields, including the natural sciences, the social sciences, and the humanities. However, once we grapple with the problem of the dignity of life, does it not become impossible to avoid engaging with issues of value and spirituality?

As I noted above, any consideration of the consequences that the life sciences are bringing forward must be related to the new proposed ethics that Hans Jonas calls the "ethics of responsibility to future human beings" (Yonasu 2000 [trans. of Jonas 1979]). The human species, with highly advanced technology at its disposal, may have become able to change fundamentally the conditions of its own existence. For those living in these times, a new perspective on the responsibility toward future humans is called for.

In any case, when we imagine the existence of future human beings, and we think of what we can do on their behalf, this calls into question the adequacy of an ethical system based on rational deduction alone. We need a broad definition of spirituality. Such a spirituality, bound to a sense of responsibility to the future, will bring forward a variety of points based within particular religious and cultural traditions. However, at the same time, certain deductions that transcend individual religious or cultural frameworks will also come out. This effort will cross the boundary between science and the humanities, requiring the united work of specialists in many disciplines, and begin to engage the world's citizens at large.

Note

A French bioethical law, "Code 94-653 Concerning Regard for Human Bodies, of July 29, 1994," is being inserted into the Civil Code with the following text: "Article 16, Point 1: Every person is endowed with the right to receive respect for his or her body. The body is inviolate. The body, its parts and its products, cannot be the subject of property claims/ property rights. (Section omitted.) Article 16, Point 3: Excluding cases of therapeutic necessity, the integrity of the human body may not be violated."

References

Arimoto, Masao. 1995. *Shinshū no shūkyō shakaishi*. Tokyo: Yoshikawa kōbunkan.
Chiba, Tokuji, and Ōtsu Tadao. 1983. *Mabiki to mizuko: kosodate no fōkuroa*. Tokyo: Nōsangyōson bunka kyōkai.

Deguchi, Itsuki. 2000. *Hito ES saibō wa yōnin dekiru ka.* Kyoto: Ōmoto honbu mioshie sendenbu.

Engeruhāto, H. Torisutoramu [Englehardt, H. Tristram]. 1988. Igaku ni okeru jinkaku no gainen. In *Baioeshikkusu no kiso: Ōbei no "Seimei rinri" ron,* ed. Katō Hisatake and Iida Kōsuke. Tokyo: Tōkai daigaku shuppankai. Translation of Engelhardt 1982.

Engelhardt, H. Tristram, Jr. 1982. Medicine and the Concept of the Person. In *Contemporary Issues in Bioethics,* ed. Tom L. Beauchamp and LeRoy Walters. Translated into Japanese as Engeruhāto 1988.

Fujime, Yuki. 1997. *Sei no rekishigaku: Kōshō seido, dataizai taisei kara baishun bōshihō yūseihogohō taisei e.* Tokyo: Fuji shuppan.

Fukuyama, Francis. 2002. *Our Postmodern Future: Consequences of the Biotechnology Revolution.* New York: Farrar, Straus, and Giroux.

Hardacre, Helen. 1997. *Marketing the Menacing Fetus in Japan.* Berkeley: University of California Press.

Häring, Bernhard. 1980. *Frei in Christus: Moraltheologie für Praxis des christlichen Lebens.* Freiburg im Breisgau: Verlag Herder. Translated into Japanese as Hēringu 1990.

———. 1981. *Free and Faithful in Christ.* Vol. 3: *Light to the World.* New York: Crossroad.

Jonas, Hans. 1979. *Das Prinzip Verantwortung: Versuch einer Ethik für die technologische Zivilisation.* Frankfurt: Insel Verlag. Translated into Japanese as Yonasu 2000.

Komatsu, Yoshihiko. 1996. *Shi wa kyōmei suru: Nōshi, zōki ishoku no fukami e.* Tokyo: Keisō shobō.

LaFleur, William R. 1992. *Liquid Life: Abortion and Buddhism in Japan.* Princeton, N.J.: Princeton University Press.

Morimura, Seiichi. 1981–83. *Akuma no hōshoku.* Tokyo: Kōbunsha.

Morioka, Masahiro. 2000. *Zōho ketteiban: Nōshi no hito.* Kyoto: Hōzōkan.

———. 2001. *Seimeigaku ni nani ga dekiru ka: Nōshi, fueminizumu, yūseishisō.* Tokyo: Keisō shobō.

Murakami, Yōichirō. 2002. "Seimei no hajimari" sono yukue. *Seimei sonchō nyūzu enburio nihon.* Fall issue, part 2.

Nakayama, Susumu. 2002. "Ningen no songen ni tsuite." In *Hito no seimei to ningen no songen,* ed. Takao Takahashi, 133–66. Fukuoka: Kyūshū daigaku shuppankai.

Namihira, Emiko. 1996. *Inochi no bunkajinruigaku.* Tokyo: Shinchōsha.

Nudeshima, Jirō. 2001. *Sentan iryō no rūru jintai riyō wa doko made yurusareru no ka.* Tokyo: Kōdansha gendai shisho.

Ogino, Miho. 2001. *Chūzetsu ronsō to amerika shakai: Shintai o meguro sensō.* Tokyo: Iwanami shoten.

Sawayama, Mikako. 1998. *Shussan to shintai no kinsei.* Tokyo: Keisō shobō.

Shimazono, Susumu. 2002. Ningen no hai o kiyō suru koto no zehi. *Sekai.*

Shinmura, Taku. 1996. *Shussan to seishokukan no rekishi.* Tokyo: Hōsei daigaku shuppankyoku.

Silver, Lee M. 1997. *Remaking Eden: How Genetic Engineering and Cloning Will Transform the American Family.* New York: Avon Books.

Sōgō kagakugijutsu kaigi, Seimeirinri senmon chōsakai (Committee on Science and Technology's Research Council on Bioethics), ed. 2003. *Hito hai no toriatsukai ni kansuru kihonteki kangaekata* (Basic Considerations Concerning the Use of Human Embryos). Tokyo.

Sōgō kenkyū kaihatsu kikō (General Research and Development Forum) and Ken Kawai, eds. 2001. *Seimei kagaku no hatten to hō: seimei rinrihō shian.* Tokyo: Yūhikaku.

Taniguchi, Masanobu. 2001. *Kami o enjiru mae ni.* Shūkyōhōjin: Seichō no ie.

Tateiwa, Shin'ya. 2000. *Yowaku aru jiyū e: jiko kettei, kaigo, seishi no gijutsu.* Tokyo: Seidosha.

Tooley, Michael. 1980. Abortion. In *Matters of Life and Death,* ed. Tom L. Regan. New York: Random House. Translated into Japanese as Toūrī 1988.

Toūrī, Maikeru [Tooley, Michael]. 1988. Eiji wa jinkaku o motsu ka. In *Baioeshikkusu no kiso: Ōbei no "seimei rinri" ron,* ed. Hisatake Katō and Kōsuke Iida. Tokyo: Tōkai daigaku shuppankai. Translation of Tooley 1980.

Tsuneishi, Kei-ichi. 1981. *Kieta saikinsen butai: Kantōgun nanasanichi butai.* Tokyo: Kaimeisha.

Umehara, Takeshi, ed. 1992a *"Nōshi" to zōki ishoku.* Tokyo: Asahi shimbunsha.

———. 1992b. *Nōshi wa shi de nai.* Kyoto: Shibunkaku shuppan.

Yonasu, Hansu [Jonas, Hans]. 2000. *Sekinin to iu genri: kagaku gijutsu bunmei no tame no rinrigaku no kokoromi.* Trans. Katō Hisatake. Tokyo: Tōshindō. Translation of Jonas 1979.

15 Eugenics, Reproductive Technologies, and the Feminist Dilemma in Japan

Miho Ogino

In the last few decades, people living in the highly industrialized world have witnessed the rapid and rampant development of reproductive technologies in the areas of fertility treatment and prenatal screening. Changes in technology can bring important changes in the way people think about reproduction, family and children, and life itself—but development in the medical field tends to proceed without waiting for sufficient discussion and agreement in society.

There have been attempts in some nations to control the development and clinical application of new reproductive technologies by enacting restrictive law, but in this era of globalization, both the news of and the desire to try newly available technologies cannot be stopped at national borders. In Japan, for instance, both surrogacy and egg or embryo donation as a means of assisted reproduction are inhibited by the professional guidelines of the Japan Association of Obstetrician-Gynecologists (new legislation regarding reproduction is now underway). However, we know that there are many Japanese couples who travel to the United States, where in some states they can find doctors and women who, in exchange for money, will help them to have "their own" babies. A Japanese woman who is a television personality recently published books describing in detail the process by which she and her husband finally got twins through a surrogate birth contract in Nevada. We also know that some of the Japanese women who succeeded in becoming pregnant with the help of the reproduction business in the United States were well past their biological age of childbearing.

It is an undeniable fact that women bear a disproportionate part of the burden of the new reproductive technologies, because it is not men but women who provide their bodies as the essential site for the production of ovum, implantation and pregnancy, childbirth, and, as in the case of selective prenatal diagnosis, abortion. It is women's bodies that undergo technological intervention, whether it is to get pregnant or to terminate pregnancy. Accordingly, evaluating the meaning of new reproductive technologies has been an inevitable and pressing problem for feminists in many countries. Do they provide women with more alternatives and thus liberate them from biological destiny? Or are these technologies another example of the manipulation and exploitation of women's bodies and reproductive capacities in a profit-oriented world?

The answers cannot be simple, because there are differences of interest and opinion among individual women. Nevertheless, one can find common ground in the attitudes of women of a given country because their attitudes toward reproductive technologies often reflect the specific historical conditions of that country and women's experiences in their respective societies. For example, in America, one cannot ignore the impact of *Roe v. Wade* and the subsequent abortion controversy if she or he wants to understand reproductive politics and culture in the United States. In the case of Japan, it is the Eugenic Protection Law and problems related to it that have heavily impacted feminist thought. Accordingly, it is necessary to examine in detail the experience of the Japanese people under this law.

Following its defeat in World War II, Japan immediately faced a serious problem—overpopulation. While the national territory was reduced by 40 percent due to the loss of overseas colonies, large numbers of Japanese returned home as demobilized soldiers or repatriated citizens. With the help of the postwar baby boom, the population expanded at an alarming rate. Amid starvation and confusion due to the near-complete devastation of the social and economic infrastructure, people resorted to illegal abortion, child abandonment, and infanticide to deal with unwanted pregnancies. The Japanese government and the occupation administration, headed by General Douglas MacArthur, quickly responded to this "state of national emergency" by passing the Eugenic Protection Law in 1948. Under this law, induced abortion was made legal either for eugenic reasons or when pregnancy was a result of rape or was a grave health hazard for the woman. In the next year, economic reasons were added as legitimate grounds for abortion. Another amendment in 1952 made the previously required investigation of each abortion application by a local screening committee unnecessary, and consent of the woman's husband and the attending obstetrician-gynecologist became the only prerequisite for the operation. The preexisting penal code that banned abortion was never repealed, but since there was no stipulation of specific economic criteria for the physician to apply in deciding whether or not the applicant was qualified for legal abortion, Japanese women were given de facto abortion on demand.

Under the new law, the number of induced abortions skyrocketed, and in concert with this the crude birthrate dropped from 34.3 per thousand in 1947 to 28.1 in 1950 and 17.2 in 1957. That is, the halving of the birthrate was realized within less than a decade. In comparison with such prompt "popularization of abortion," changes in contraception and family planning were relatively slow to occur. It was only in the mid-to-late 1950s that the Japanese government formally endorsed diffusion of contraceptive knowledge, launching the nationwide family-planning movement among the Japanese people. The government's great success in suppressing fertility and the subsequent economic reconstruction and growth in postwar Japan undoubtedly would have been impossible, or at least much retarded, without the early enactment of the Eugenic Protection Law.

Unlike women in other countries who have had to fight a long battle for their right to have safe and legal abortions, Japanese women were thus given from above the "liberty" of controlling their fertility by legal abortions. The Eugenic Protection Law, however, had another face. As is implied by its name, this law was a descendant of the National Eugenic Law that was enacted in 1940 during World War II. This former law was proposed by medical scholars and bureaucrats and was patterned after the 1933 German Law on Preventing Hereditarily Ill Progeny, the so-called sterilization law of the Nazi regime. It mandated the sterilization of people with "inferior" heredity while banning abortion except for eugenic reasons. However, unlike Germany, where three to four hundred thousand people are said to have undergone forced sterilization during the Nazi era, the number of sterilizations conducted in Japan under the National Eugenic Law during the war period was relatively small, 538 cases in total (Tsuge, Ichinokawa, and Katō 1996, 380).[1] Although the law had a clause for compulsory sterilization, its execution was suspended due to opposition from conservative Diet members who were afraid that the idea of "extinction of blood" was detrimental to the patriarchal family system of Japan.

After the war, while the new Eugenic Protection Law decriminalized abortion as described above, it inherited the eugenic character of the former law and even strengthened it by stipulating the compulsory sterilization of people with physical or mental hereditary diseases. Furthermore, in spite of the fact that Hansen's disease (leprosy) was already known to be a nonhereditary disease, patients with Hansen's disease or their spouses also became targets of eugenic sterilization and abortion. Most of the Diet members who designed this law were medical professionals, except for Shizue Katō, a feminist and birth-control activist who has frequently been called the "Japanese Margaret Sanger." They anticipated that the diffusion of birth control among the "worthy" population in the democratized postwar society was inevitable and feared that this would result in "counter-selection," or the degeneration of national quality.

Under this law, during the period 1948–96, more than eighteen thousand operations of compulsory or semi-compulsory sterilization were conducted (Matsubara 2002, 43). For instance, institutionalized patients with Hansen's disease were not allowed to marry among themselves unless they consented to sterilization; if female patients became pregnant, they were compelled to have an abortion. According to the statistics of the Ministry of Health and Welfare, the total number of sterilizations and abortions conducted in sanatoriums during the period from 1949 to 1996 is reported to be 1,400 and 3,000, respectively (*Asahi Shinbun* 2001). Furthermore, although there was no such stipulation in the law, hysterectomies of normal uteri were carried out clandestinely on female patients with physical or mental diseases in some institutions, for the sole purpose of removing their menstrual cycles and lightening the burden of caring for them. Because of such discriminatory provisions and actions, from the 1970s on, the Eugenic Protection Law came to be increasingly criticized and protested by the nascent disability rights movement. It was nearly three decades, however, until in 1996 the eugenic clauses were finally deleted.

While the Eugenic Protection Law was in existence, two major crises threatened Japanese women with losing their access to abortion on demand, one in the early 1970s and the second a decade later. With the advent of economic growth, the low birthrates among Japanese women came to be regarded as detrimental to further development of the Japanese economy. Under such circumstances, the political campaign to eliminate the economic reasons clause from the Eugenic Protection Law was organized by a religious body called Seichō no ie (Home of life) and conservative members of the Liberal Democratic Party. Seichō no ie is a new religion with an eclectic creed consisting of elements borrowed from Buddhism, Shinto, and Christianity. Since more than 99 percent of abortion cases were legalized by the economic-reasons clause, its elimination actually meant a ban on abortion on demand. The group claimed that Japan was sufficiently affluent and that it no longer needed to permit the "murder" of innocent fetuses for economic reasons.

In 1972, a revised bill was submitted to the Diet by the anti-abortion group. In addition to the deletion of the economic-reasons clause, it proposed to allow abortion if the fetus was suspected of having a serious mental or physical defect, and also to exhort Japanese women to give birth to their first children at a suitable age. While aimed at increasing fertility rates, the bill simultaneously advocated that eugenically "undesirable" children should not be born.

Two different groups immediately took action to oppose the bill. One was composed of the activists of the women's liberation movement that had been rising spontaneously and fervently in Japan from around 1970. For these advocates, the campaign to defeat the attempt to revise the Eugenic Protection Law and defend the right to abortion became an important opportunity for articulation of "women's autonomy" and "women's right to control their own bodies." A famous slogan, "It is I, a woman, who decides to bear or not to bear," was coined for their anti-revision campaign.

Another group was composed of people with disabilities, mainly those with cerebral palsy belonging to a group named *Aoi shiba no kai* (Green Grass). They felt that the new provision for "defective" fetuses would justify discrimination against people with disabilities by legitimizing eugenic selection and would thus infringe upon their fundamental right to live. They argued that social tolerance for killing a disabled fetus is synonymous with saying to those living with disability, "You are not supposed to exist in this world. You'd better die." At the same time, they questioned the fundamental validity of abortion sanctioned by the Eugenic Protection Law and criticized the claim that abortion was a woman's right to choose, saying that this was nothing but a "healthy person's egoism" and that women were taking part in sustaining discrimination against the disabled. Thus, two socially marginalized groups were placed in awkward confrontation in connection with the Eugenic Protection Law.

Women advocating reproductive freedom were both disturbed and moved by the criticism of disabled people. While they fully recognized the vital importance and necessity of legal abortion for women's lives, they realized at the same time that their claim of right to abortion under the present state of the law could easily be exploited and used in such a way as to eliminate the rights of the disabled. The following words of Mitsu Tanaka, one of the most famous figures of the Japanese women's liberation movement, reflect the peculiar dilemma with which Japanese feminists were confronted:

> Women's liberationists in Europe and America claim the freedom of and right to abortion because they primarily seek liberation from religious moral systems such as that of Catholicism. In Japan, however, induced abortion has been legalized since 1948, though not in a quite satisfactory manner. We Japanese women have not been forbidden abortion by religious morals but have resorted to abortions because we think we should not give birth, and in doing so have contributed to increasing the benefit to corporations. We cannot and dare not say so readily that abortion is our right. . . . If we do not perceive our pain in conducting forced infanticide and keep resorting to abortions for the reason that there is no way to escape from such a society, we will inevitably be caught up in the stink of this efficiency-oriented, dog-eat-dog world that attaches higher value to production of automobiles than to children's lives. (Tanaka 1973, 3–4)

Despite their strained relationship, the two groups, women and people with disabilities, formed a tentative joint struggle for the common purpose of defeating the revision forces, and they succeeded in 1974. However, the problem of "eugenic thought internalized by women themselves" pointed out by the disability activists was left as an unresolved issue for the women's movement.

In the early 1980s, Seichō no ie and its political agents resumed their campaign for the revision of the Eugenic Protection Law. This time, they carefully avoided mention of "fetal disability" and focused exclusively on the economic-reasons clause, asserting that abortion on demand is counter to "sanctity of life." It was rumored that there was close contact between Seichō no ie and the Moral Majority and the pro-life movement in the United States.

This time, not only women's liberation activists but also women belonging to more traditional organizations and even some female politicians of the Liberal Democratic Party, the ruling conservative party that submitted the revision bill, rose to offer wide opposition to the proposed revision. Due to the concerted efforts of the anti-revisionists, the second attempt at revision failed, and Seichō no ie eventually decided to withdraw from political activities.

During the 1994 Cairo International Conference on Population and Development, the problematic character of the Eugenic Protection Law was brought to international attention by Yūho Asaka, a Japanese woman activist with a disability. She reported that in Japan the law, or rather the eugenic idea embodied in it, had been used by doctors to prevent disabled women from having children, sometimes conducting unnecessary hysterectomies. Partly as a result of the international stir caused by Asaka's report and partly due to the pressure from the disability rights movement, the Eugenic Protection Law was suddenly revised in 1996, eliminating all the clauses pertaining to people with disabilities and hereditary diseases and changing its name to the Maternal Body Protection Law. Shortly prior to this, the Prevention of Leprosy Law, which stipulated the compulsory institutionalization of patients with Hansen's disease, was abolished. Following the termination of both laws, patients with Hansen's disease who had been segregated for a long period of time and who had been forced to undergo sterilization and abortion brought legal actions against the state for discriminatory treatments and won a total victory in 2001.

On the other hand, activists of the disability rights movement organized a group in 1997 that demanded the Ministry of Health and Welfare apologize and compensate for forced sterilizations and hysterectomies conducted under the Eugenic Protection Law. The Ministry of Health and Welfare, however, responded that eugenic sterilization was legal when these operations were done and demanded evidence for the practice of forced hysterectomies on disabled women. Currently, disability rights activists are conducting fact-finding surveys among women with disabilities in order to investigate the realities of forced hysterectomies under the Eugenic Protection Law. As a result, some of these victims came out of the closet and began to talk about their experiences (Yūsei shujutsu ni shazai o motomeru kai 2003). Recently, a video film entitled *I Don't Want You to Forget* was made featuring Chizuko Sasaki, a woman with cerebral palsy who was forced at age twenty to undergo cobalt-beam irradiation at a hospital in Hiroshima.

I have described the history of the Eugenic Protection Law at length because I believe that these experiences form the undercurrent, or a kind of tradition, of Japanese feminist thought as regards current reproductive rights issues. Generally speaking, Japanese feminists have not been enthusiastic about utilizing new reproductive technologies for either fertility treatment or prenatal diagnosis, and some are explicitly critical of them. While a small number of feminist scholars assert that if there is "the right to control one's fertility by contraception and abortion," there should be as well "the right to use any available means to have children as one wants," they belong to a relative minority. Although the concept of "women's right to choose" or "women's right to control their own bodies" is considered to be of vital importance for feminism, the past experiences with the Eugenic Protection Law made many feminists sensitive to a possibility that this concept can be utilized conveniently by either state, market, medicine, or even women themselves in such a way as to legitimize choices that are discriminatory or exploitative of some people.

As regards prenatal screening in Japan, while ultrasonography is routinely used during normal pregnancy, other prenatal diagnostic techniques such as amniocentesis, chorionic villus sampling (CVS), alpha feto protein (AFP) testing, and the triple-marker test (maternal serum screening) are not used so frequently as in other developed countries. For instance, the number of triple-marker tests conducted in the United States is about 167 times that of Japan, and the frequency of amniocentesis in Germany is more than 10 times that of

Japan (Satō 1999, 52). However, there are medical professionals and corporation executives who aim at further advancing utilization of these technologies in Japanese society.

Although prenatal diagnostic technologies are regarded as important tools for managing pregnancy and ensuring fetal health and welfare, it is also true that they are used to detect fetal defects or abnormalities and that once some defect is found or suspected in the fetus, an abortion is chosen in many cases to terminate that pregnancy. The World Health Organization (WHO) states that the application of prenatal screening and subsequent abortion cannot be called "new eugenics" because there is no coercion to have tests and the "woman's right to choose" whether to keep that pregnancy or not is guaranteed (Wertz, Fletcher, and Berg 1993). However, the opinion of women's health activists in Japan is different. They are afraid that, just as women's right to abortion was used by the state to control the quantity of population in postwar Japan, the individual woman's "choice" is now used voluntarily to control the quality of human being to be born. One of them, Tomoko Yonezu, is a feminist activist with a disability who fought against the revision of the Eugenic Protection Law in both the 1970s and the 1980s, and she asserts that selective abortion after prenatal screening should not be considered a "woman's reproductive right." She writes:

> Abortion after prenatal screening is conducted, not because pregnancy itself is unwanted, but in expectation of having a baby. It is a deed to decide whether to welcome that child or not, depending on existence or nonexistence of defects. I think that a fetus is neither an independent life nor a part of woman's body. It is not the same as a person after birth but has a potentiality to be one. Just as discrimination against a living human being because of her or his attributes is wrong, so is discrimination against a fetus. . . . Notwithstanding the fact that it is the society that is unkind to people with disabilities that makes their lives difficult, proponents of prenatal diagnosis pretend there is no such liability and try to induce women to select their children, designating such selection a woman's "right" to be practiced at her own responsibility. That is exactly a new trend of eugenics and is nothing but an infringement of women's reproductive rights. (Yonezu 2002, 17–18)

Yonezu, however, does not support some disability rights activists' claim that selective abortion should be formally banned by law. She maintains that, for the purpose of preventing the normalization of prenatal screening and selective abortion, more information and support to make bearing and rearing a child with a disability easier have to be provided, while development and application of technologies for preselection should be placed under careful control. "If there exist conditions under which one can bring up a child with a disability in a manner not entirely different from that of an ordinary child," writes Yonezu, "then we will be able to choose not to choose our children" (Yonezu 2002, 21).

Presently in Japan, to conduct pre-implantation diagnosis (PID) of embryos is tightly restricted, not only for social reasons such as sex selection but also for medical reasons such as the detection of genetic diseases. In 2004 the Japan Association of Obstetrician-Gynecologists, however, changed its former stance and began to admit clinical application of PID in some cases. There is strong apprehension not only among feminists and disability rights advocates who oppose introduction of PID but also among the general public that liberalization of such techniques might open another door to the eugenic selection of people. I presume that at least some part of such skepticism of and caution against applying cutting-edge medical technology is related to reflections on our past experience with the Eugenic Protection Law.

As regards new techniques for assisting reproduction, ever since the birth of the first IVF child in Japan in 1983, fertility treatment has rapidly grown as a lucrative medical industry, and many fertility doctors are eager to try new technologies at an experimental stage on their patients. These treatments place high psychological, physical, economical, and social costs and risks on their core recipients, women. For those who eventually succeed in having their own children through assisted reproduction, the development of these technologies might be called a blessing. On the other hand, however, the net success rates of treatments are not high. There are a number of women (these women constitute a majority in number) who, once placed on the conveyer belt of fertility treatment, find it very difficult to get off from the endless cycle of various tests, artificial insemination, in vitro fertilization, and intracytoplasmic sperm injection. Doctors rarely listen to their complaints about the pains and various side effects of the treatment, and finally these women end up worn out both mentally and physically, still without having a child. New reproductive technologies also have brought about fragmentation of both the process of procreation and women's bodies, which are divided into modular parts such as ovum and uterus that can be donated, sold, or hired.

Doctors often justify the clinical application of experimental and painful techniques by asserting that they are merely trying hard to help infertile women or couples who desperately desire to have their own children, and that it is "women's right to self-determination" to resort to such treatments. For instance, as I mentioned at the beginning, presently in Japan, the use of surrogacy and some other techniques is prohibited by the guidelines of the medical professional association. A doctor, however, challenged this guideline by publicizing that he had successfully undertaken several cases of surrogate birth involving sisters. Recently, another doctor announced that he had carried out a pre-implantation diagnosis of embryos for a patient who already has two sons and strongly wants to bear a baby girl. Both of them claim that they support the women's right to choose in reproductive matters and that neither the medical association nor the public has any right to forbid women to use techniques when they are available.

But are they really assisting women's free choice? Surely we cannot deny the fact that there are women and their partners who sincerely and desperately hope to have their own children at any cost. Neither do I want to criticize infertile women undergoing long and painful treatments as victims of "false consciousness." Nevertheless, it is also often true that what one desires and chooses is shaped by what society wants her or him to want. In a society where deep-rooted ideologies such as "a woman who cannot bear a child is not a real woman" or "a marriage without children is a failure" still hold power, the ostentatious display of brand new reproductive technologies works to ignite and drive infertile persons' desire in the specific direction of wanting and purchasing such services. We have to notice that the "right to choose" of infertile women and couples is evoked only in so far as it contributes to justify the development and hasty clinical application to them of reproductive technologies still at an experimental stage. The fact that there is little professional or business interest in more legitimate but not so profitable research to find out and eliminate one by one the causes of infertility provides evidence for this speculation.

The development of new reproductive technologies seems to pose new dilemmas for women's right to choose. Although the concept of a woman's self-determination and autonomy over her body is an essential part of feminist thought, our experience with abortion under the Eugenic Protection Law teaches us that we must be careful and reflective about the context in which the "right to choose" is sanctioned and exercised. And I believe that such feelings of apprehension and cautiousness are not peculiar to Japanese feminists alone, because I know there are some American feminists, with or without disabilities, who have courageously questioned the primacy of the "right to choose" in the context of new reproductive technologies. For example, Ruth Hubbard calls prenatal screening "new eugenics" and warns that "the choice ideology that is part of the thinking of those of us who support abortion rights keeps many of us from acknowledging the one-sidedness of our 'choice' to assent to predictive testing" (Hubbard 2001, 4; see also Asch and Fine 1990, Saxton 1998, and Levine 2002). The current way in which the idea of individual autonomy and reproductive choice is evoked and used concerning new reproductive technologies such as prenatal diagnosis and fertility treatment seems to be dangerously incomplete, because there is not enough consideration for the effects of such technologies on others, including future generations, social systems, and women themselves. However difficult it might be, it is time for feminists with different social and historical backgrounds to share each other's experiences and begin straightforward discussion of the meaning of new reproductive technologies for women and their welfare.

Note

1. The number of forced sterilizations in Germany is based on testimonies by Klaus Dorner and Christine Teller in *Yūsei hogo-hō ga okashita tsumi*, 2003, ed. Yūsei shujutsu ni shazai o motomeru kai (Tokyo: Gendai shokan), 170 and 173.

References

Asahi Shinbun. 2001. Hikari no sono de nedayashi, May 8, p. 35.

Asch, Adrienne, and Michelle Fine. 1990. Shared Dreams: A Left Perspective on Disability Rights and Reproductive Rights. In *From Abortion to Reproductive Freedom: Transforming a Movement,* ed. Marlene Gerber Fried, 233–43. Boston: South End Press.

Hubbard, Ruth. 2001. Eugenics, Reproductive Technologies, and "Choice." *Gene Watch* 14, no. 1: 3–4.

Levine, Judith. 2002. What Human Genetic Modification Means for Women. *World Watch,* July/August, pp. 26–29.

Matsubara, Yōko. 2002. Botai hogo-hō no rekishiteki haikei. In *Botai hogo-hō to watashi-tachi,* ed. Yukiko Saitō, 35–48. Tokyo: Akashi shoten.

Satō, Kōdō. 1999. *Shusseizen shindan: Inochi no hinshitsu kanri eno keishō.* Tokyo: Yūhi-kaku.

Saxton, Marsha. 1998. Disability Rights and Selective Abortion. In *Abortion Wars: A Half Century of Struggle, 1950–2000,* ed. Rickie Solinger, 374–93. Berkeley and Los Angeles: University of California Press.

Tanaka, Mitsu. 1973. Matamata yūsei hogo-hō kaiaku nanoda! Shōgaisha mondai o chūshin ni. *Ribu News* 3:1–4.

Tsuge, Azumi, Yasutaka Ichinokawa, and Shuichi Katō. 1996. Yūsei hogo-hō o meguru saikin no doko. In *Seishoku gijutsu to jendā,* ed. Yumiko Ehara, 375–90. Tokyo: Keisō shobō.

Wertz, D. C., J. C. Fletcher, and K. Berg. 1995. *Guidelines on Ethical Issues in Medical Genetics and the Provision of Genetic Services.* Geneva: World Health Organization.

Yonezu, Tomoko. 2002. Shōgaisha to josei: Rendō-shī hokan-shiau sabetsu soshite kaihō. *Soshiren News* 204: 10–21.

Yūsei shujutsu ni shazai o motomeru kai, ed. 2003. *Yūsei hogo-hō ga okashita tsumi.* To-kyo: Gendai shokan.

16 Refusing Utopia's Bait: Research, Rationalizations, and Hans Jonas

William R. LaFleur

Mann kann auch in die Höhe fallen, *so wie in die Tiefe*
[One can just as easily *fall* into heights as into depths]

—Friedrich Hölderlin

Historical events and processes do not make clones of themselves. *Exact* replicas will not show up even in much later times—simply because each event and each historical process possesses its own particularities. Yet we scrutinize the past because, in spite of such particulars, some features, sequences, or reasoning processes tend to reappear. If that were not so, and if each event were presumed to be *totally* unique, our study of history would be stripped of much of its rationale.

Safeguards and Rationalizations.

Morally reprehensible events and processes such as the medical research of Unit 731 and the experiments carried out by Nazi-era physicians—that is, the two most salient examples scrutinized in this volume—are ones we study primarily because we wish to build strong safeguards against even milder forms of their reappearance in our world. Certain kinds of safeguards, the Nuremberg Code for example, have been brought into being in precisely that way (Annas and Grodin 1992). Bioethics as a field of study, even if arising later, was surely urged into existence in part because the Third Reich's atrocities in medicine remained in the public mind as being such a serious abuse of human beings that our societies did not wish to see it replicated (Jonsen 1998, 136ff.).

The question of critical importance today is whether our existing safeguards against new forms of unethical medical research are, in fact, sufficient. This is a question implicit in most, perhaps in all, of the essays in this volume. It may be the most important question we can ask, since "bulwarks," just by being built and by subsequently standing in the public eye, can produce a dangerous illusion of safety.[1] We already know that neither the Nuremberg Code nor the fact that early bioethicists had already discussed the ethics of using presumptively voluntary human subjects were sufficient to prevent the atrocious treatment of African-American men by American government officials in the infamous Tuskegee experiments, which lasted until 1972 (Jones 1993; Brandt 2000). Nor did these "safeguards" do anything to stop the U.S. government from subjecting thousands of its citizens to harmful radiation levels in Cold War experiments that lasted into the 1990s (Welsome 1999; Moreno 2001).

Based on the evidence to date, it seems fairly clear that the "safeguards" are not working as anticipated. And this is why it becomes especially important to scrutinize both how rationalizations for unethical behavior take shape and how specifically they may be operative in our own time. My hypothesis is that *rationalizations* work with maximum effect precisely *when* "safeguards" have been put in place and have come to be regarded as effective obstacles to carrying out ethically flawed plans and programs. The circumvention of bulwarks constitutes the raison d'être and the special genius of the rationalization.

Two Eugenic Heavens, One Eugenic Hell

Concerning eugenics, for instance, we have not yet figured out exactly how to apply to the present what we know about its history in the first half of the twentieth century. During that period within the West a rhetoric that had promised a virtual eugenic heaven on earth buckled under a demonstrated reality of terrestrial hell when it turned out that the eugenics of the Third Reich was targeting, sterilizing, and simply murdering persons and groups deemed biologically unfit.

The documentation is convincing. As graphically shown by Christine Rosen's *Preaching Eugenics: Religious Leaders and the American Eugenics Movement,* the hard sell given to eugenics policies in the United States during the early twentieth century combined messages about a rapidly "deteriorating state of human heredity" with others from some religious leaders that viewed "eugenics as a means for ushering in the Kingdom [of God]" (Rosen 2004, 7 and 126). And an optimism about eliminating everything that could pose an inheritable "problem" to this eugenic purification of the human gene pool was in no way limited to the discourse of the Germans. Charles B. Davenport, the first director of the Station for Experimental Evolution at Cold Spring Harbor on Long Island, wished he had a way to cleanse his own American "fatherland" of racial elements that were not Anglo-Saxon; in 1925 he bemoaned to a friend the fact that America had "no place to drive the Jews to" (Rosenberg 1997, 95–96). In 1923 Harry Laughlin, a director of Cold Spring Harbor's Eugenics Records Office, testified to the American Congress that people from Southern Europe are genetically prone to criminality. At a California "eugenics rally" in 1933 Laughlin praised the Nazi law designed to prevent the birth of persons with hereditary defects (Watson 1998, 191–92).

Adolf Hitler, of course, went much, much farther. He wanted to eliminate bad genes by liquidating the persons or, more precisely, the groups of persons presumed to be carrying them. Yet today, as we are in the midst of new conversations about genetics, there is something not a little sobering in realizing that it was really only during the late 1930s and 1940s that, because of growing awareness of the program of the Third Reich, eugenics programs in the Anglo-American world, in order to avoid association and embarrassment, were quietly dropped. For almost half a century the very word "eugenics" tagged a practice that many assumed would be incapable of ever finding rehabilitation.

Again, we see an oscillation between extremes. If eugenics was forced into association with a program seemingly designed in hell, its recent reemergence is, at least in the rhetoric of some, again starting to sound at times like the earlier promise of heaven on earth. In 1988 Joseph Fletcher, the American theologian who invented "situation ethics," already presaged the redemption of eugenics as an ideal that society would do well to pursue, even though, of course, it would now be voluntarily chosen rather than state-mandated. Fletcher's denigration of the way human beings have made their children throughout all time was articulated in his reference to the old way as "reproductive roulette," a hit-or-miss method that, tragically and now unnecessarily, lets bad genes get through.

And what about the past? Fletcher's *The Ethics of Genetic Control: Ending Reproductive Roulette* includes one and only one reference to the Third Reich: it flippantly dismisses what happened then as "cruelties" that "were neither genetic nor eugenic anyway" (Fletcher 1988, 88). Here, as in virtually all the work of this influential early American bioethicist, a self-serving amnesia about past medical atrocities was conjoined to a naive belief in America's unique capacity to bring unqualified progress to mankind and to do so especially through innovative and boldly executed medical research. Fletcher, a heady utopian, seemed incapable of seeing that his own promotion of preemptive eugenics was to be shoving medicine into a very dark place. And, showing that Fletcher's approach is alive and well, the author of a 1998 book advocating human cloning, one that also has next to nothing to say about the past, sanguinely concludes: Let's not "limit human reproductive liberty. Call me Joe Fletcher's clone" (Pence 1998, 175).

Elimination Theory

In *Leibsein als Aufgabe* Gernot Böhme reminds us that we should not try to discuss genetics without recognizing the role played historically by René Descartes (Böhme 2003, 171ff.) That observation is correct, and I would point out how that philosopher's vision of the future presaged where we are today in our discussions of eugenics. In the sixth portion of the *Discourse on Method,* we find Descartes writing as follows:

> For the mind is so dependent upon the humors and the condition of the organs of the body that if it is possible to find some way to make men in general wiser and more clever than they have been so far, I believe that it is in medicine that it should be sought. It is true that medicine at present contains little of such great value; but without intending to belittle it, I am sure that everyone, even among those who follow the profession, will admit that everything we know is almost nothing com-

pared with what remains to be discovered, and that we might rid ourselves of an infinity of maladies of body as well as of mind, and perhaps also the enfeeblement of old age, if we had sufficient understanding of the causes and of all the remedies which nature has provided. (Descartes 1950, 40)

Descartes was, as it were, already envisioning a day when the putative "aging gene" might be located and eliminated: the "enfeeblement of old age" would be no more. Moreover, his vision was blatantly utopian. We someday might, he wrote, "rid ourselves of an *infinity* of maladies of body as well as of mind."

Descartes's vision of science was one of pure potential—and a potential without attendant, unplanned, and unwanted side consequences. The "infinity of maladies" might be tackled and eliminated in a seriatim fashion. But Descartes seems not to have asked himself what we as humankind would *be* if the series of eliminations were ever to be brought to perfection—that is, to the *telos* where each and every defect had been expunged. His "theory of elimination," one that perhaps has been the preferred theory of much modern medical science, was uncomplex—and, as such, utopian. He did not ask, for instance, whether or not we can achieve the envisioned "eliminations" without along the way announcing or implying, in effect, that persons and groups of persons who "have" such maladies are *persons and groups of persons* whose very existence is one our world would do well to be without.

That is, the nasty-sounding consequence may be an unintentional one, but it is, nevertheless, a consequence—and one that itself is repugnant. You cannot, for instance, work to eliminate congenital deafness from the human species without implying, willy-nilly, that humankind would be much better off if all congenitally deaf persons simply did not exist. However good a case can be made for eliminating such deafness, we cannot simply ignore the fact that our societal intention of preventing certain kinds of persons from being born in the future implicitly conveys to similar persons—that is, those already living with such a disability—a message about their own nonexistence as the desideratum of others.

As evidenced in Shimazono's essay here and also in sustained research and writing by Masahiro Morioka (especially Morioka 2001), the community of Japanese persons with disabilities has been contesting energetically the notion of no-fault eugenics—and probably gaining more public attention than its counterparts in England and America.[2] Refusing to be taken by the larger society as a type of human whose very existence may soon become technologically preventable, Japanese with disabilities have been instrumental in making at least the use of *yūsei*, the word for "eugenics," and its compounds increasingly objectionable in their society. And this, ironically, has been occurring while "eugenics," now qualified as "positive" or as "liberal," has been making a comeback within the Anglo-American world. What, one may rightfully ask, is so different between current claims that we ought not burden society with the "costs of abnormality" (see Nelkin and Lindee 1995, 190) and von Weizsäcker's early assumptions about the *Rentenneurose* as persons who, costly to the larger society, had lost their right to live?

Flawed Physicians and No-Fault Science

In her chapter, Renée Fox tags "iatrogenesis as intrinsic to medicine and medical action in all of its forms"[3] and offers what she calls a "counter-intuitive" hypothesis. Is it possible that physicians find it more difficult to deal with the adverse consequences of their actions that are *not* caused by mistakes than those that are, because such outcomes confront them with situations inherent to medicine, things for which readily available means of explanation and rectification do not exist and that make the limitations in their control over doing harm so starkly apparent to them?

That is, unhappy outcomes are assumed to result from mistakes made by physicians. They are *human* errors. By contrast, it is assumed, science—that is, medical science in this case—will through this deflection be protected from being recognized as having had *within itself* a dynamic that could not avoid causing harm. Morality, and therefore also fault, is all packed into the later, "application" phase. Böhme traces this kind of convenient differentiation back to Bacon's *Novum organum,* where one can find "the rudiments of a distinction between neutral knowledge and morally responsible application—a distinction that has long served as a defense for science" (Böhme 1992, 4).

Although Böhme presents a strong case for why the epoch of Baconian science appears to be coming to an end,[4] its hold on the public consciousness remains sufficiently strong so that, in spite of detectable uneasiness about certain specific forms of medical research,[5] we can see this countered primarily by two things: first, claims that international competition requires the lifting of moratoriums on the very research about which the public expresses concern, and second, a rhetoric that employs remnants of the old Baconian equation of scientific progress with human progress. Both of these can serve the rationalization process. Both can justify kinds of research that sooner or later will start seeking for the cover of darkness, research the results of which may prove largely harmful and then later be explained as having consequences that had been "unforeseen."

We see the first of these—that is, international competition—as reason enough to justify the Japanese government's decision in 1997, despite deep and largely unabated public uneasiness, to legalize the notion of brain death and permit cadaveric organ transplantation. It is instructive to note that the Japanese decision to recognize brain death as death, after a moratorium of three decades, came not because the brain death concept itself finally had irrefutably been proven coherent—since, in fact, by 1998 it was beginning to seem *less* coherent than earlier (see Truog 1998, 24–40)—but because the Japanese Diet had been persuaded by the argument that nonacceptance of this concept made Japanese medical science appear to the outside world as incapable of keeping a competitive edge. This argument for moving "forward," based not on scientific proof but on national prestige in a competitive world, is central to an appeal for legalizing brain death made in a book by Dr. Jurō Wada, both famous and infamous in Japan for performing a questionable heart transplant there in 1968 (Wada 1998), and in an interview with him that I conducted in Tokyo on November 6, 1996.

The intense American debate about whether or not to proceed with stem-cell research showed the same feature, that is, its proponents including among their arguments the specter of losing out in international competition. Top-flight scientists doing research in this area would, we have been told, surely move away and do their work in countries without any moratoriums, and it then would be those countries, not the United States, that would harvest the technological, industrial, and economic benefits of what are certain to be breakthroughs in stem-cell research. In fact, because particular states within the United States can legislate much of their own way in these matters, not just international but also intranational competition surfaced strongly in this matter—with, for instance, California voting to legalize and support research in this area and in this way gain an "edge."

Although competition of this sort is not entirely new, the "globalization" push that has come to be so strong in our own times clearly intensifies it. Precisely because the rewards—prestige, prizes, and economic profit most especially —are now enormous, the deployment of the argument for meeting and beating the competition has all the marks of being the most potent "rationalization" of our age. Böhme sums it up accurately: "[A]rguments are bluntly presented from the perspective of economic and military competition. If we do not promote science and technological development intensively, we will fall behind in the international competition" (Böhme 1992, 8).

The Enduring Utopia

In his *New Atlantis* of 1627 Francis Bacon boldly sketched a future utopian world in which scientists assumed de facto political power and were bringing untold benefits to mankind. It would probably be impossible today to find anyone as sanguine as Bacon about such unalloyed benefits deriving from a full-throttle pursuit of science. There is an element of truth in the claim by Paul R. Gross and Norman Levitt in 1994 that some recent attacks on "Baconian science" have, in contrast to the critique offered by Böhme, been sweeping, lacking in nuance, and too ready to demonize the "West."

That said, even if they do not reach the full-blown scientific utopia of *New Atlantis,* Gross and Levitt by their own admission continue to maintain that science and science alone will "improve the prospects for human life." They write: "Let's raise a glass to Bacon! He wasn't much of a scientist or mathematician, but he made some shrewd guesses as to how our species might crawl out of the rut of ignorance. And here's to Baconian science—if that misattribution is to persist in our universities—Baconian in the sense of a rigorous adherence to the empirical and a faith that what we learn that way can improve the prospects for human life" (Gross and Levitt 1994, 178).

It was noted above that Joseph Fletcher, also an advocate of getting us out of "the rut of ignorance," advised us to abandon what had till now been the only way of producing progeny and to substitute for it a rational, scientific, and "foolproof" method. And Gregory Pence, with an eye toward what is offered by "liberal eugenics," deems Fletcher to have given us good advice.[6] The prospect of reaping unanticipated and bad consequences is moved off the shelf of what ought to be kept in view.

Amazingly, the utopian dream still has its advocates, sometimes in very visible places. Close scrutiny of the language used, for instance, by Gregory Stock, a bioethicist at UCLA, is warranted. In his book *Redesigning Humans: Our Inevitable Genetic Future*, Stock implicitly employs Frederick Jackson Turner's famous but overworked "frontier thesis" to give America, Stock hopes, the competitive edge in fashioning the world's eugenic future. In rhetoric not unlike that of the sermons and lectures analyzed by Rosen in *Preaching Eugenics*, Stock writes:

> A key aspect of human nature is our ability to manipulate the world. . . . We are now reaching the point where we may be able to transform ourselves into something "other." To turn away from germline selection and modification without even exploring them would be to deny our essential nature and perhaps our destiny. Ultimately, such a retreat might deaden the human spirit of exploration, taming and diminishing us. This seems particularly clear to the American psyche, influenced as it has been by the frontier. (Stock 2002, 172)[7]

Patent nonsense not infrequently, as here, goes jingoistic. Stock's progression merits scrutiny. "Human nature" is said to have a "key aspect" and that is "our ability to manipulate the world." And, although this is a universalized "essence" of humanity, Americans seem to have a special "destiny," one now inscribed in our national "psyche" for realizing and pursuing it. And to fail to do so—especially in biotechnology—would not only betray our *national* destiny but would even "deaden the human spirit."[8]

There are good reasons for skepticism vis-à-vis any claim that a nation has a special destiny to make dramatic changes in what it means to be human. *Cheerleaders for the Third Reich made such claims. And when the issue is eugenics the comparison is surely warranted.* Stock shows signs of being aware that what he wrote could invite the very kind of comparison suggested here. But he brushes that aside, writing: "Given Hitler's appalling foray into racial purification, European sensitivities are understandable, but they miss the bigger picture. . . . We have spent billions to unravel our biology, not out of idle curiosity, but in the hope of bettering our lives. We are not about to turn away from this" (Stock 2002, 13). In other words, we have already put a lot of money, billions in fact, into this project. And, since it is an "American destiny" thing, we cannot help it if hypersensitive Europeans—Germans, for instance—cannot or will not see its importance in America and the *certainty* of its positive outcome! It is almost as if Stock were making his position a classic instance of the observation made by Benno Müller-Hill in his paper here—namely, that "science lives in the present" and "its past does not interest scientists."

On Refusing the Bait—Jonas's Cautions

Utopias are not really benign. In a trenchant analysis, Paul Ricoeur has unearthed their agenda, writing,

> The scientists . . . have power for the sake of liberating creativity in a kind of chain reaction. This emphasis, which persists from Bacon to Saint-Simon, corroborates the claim of Mannheim's which at first seems paradoxical, that a utopia is not only a dream but a dream that wants to be realized. It directs itself towards reality; it shatters reality. The utopia's intention is surely to change things, and therefore we cannot say with Marx's eleventh thesis on Feuerbach that it is a way only of interpreting the world and not changing it. On the contrary, the thrust of utopia is to change reality. (Ricoeur 1986, 289)

Surely, although he expresses occasional ambivalence, Lee M. Silver, a Princeton biologist who authored *Remaking Eden,* is basically sanguine about the repro-genetics that, he thinks, will "inevitably" change our species by way of first producing a genetically improved variant of it, one he refers to as "GenRich humans" (Silver 1997). If implementation for the sake of *changing* reality is, as Ricoeur notes, the hallmark of utopians, then Silver too is such a utopian.

Hans Jonas (1903–93) deserves a special place among modern philosophers of science who have excavated and criticized the utopian agenda still only partially concealed in the writings of optimistic apologists for radical improvement of the human species. Jonas, largely because he has been cited by Leon Kass, has recently been castigated by some of Kass's critics—but in ways that suggest Jonas himself has not been read or, at least, has not been read carefully (e.g., Charo 2004).

It is, I suggest, telling that no major thinker or writer among those still expressing hope for some kind of utopia through biotechnology has directly addressed and countered what Jonas had to say. This is no doubt in part because Jonas was a very formidable thinker, and his arguments were tightly formulated. Up until now those who would be expected to disagree with the conclusions Jonas drew appear to have found it more expedient to ignore him—more precisely, to keep him so far on the periphery of the Anglo-American discourse about bioethics that he would not even be read.[9]

There may also be another reason for skirting him. Jonas's own mother was murdered in Auschwitz, and he had seen up close the horror of being among the vulnerable. The continuities are important in his career. A Jewish student of Martin Heidegger, Jonas saw his teacher slip into a mode of rationalizing that accommodated the agendas of the Third Reich. After escaping from Germany, he increasingly turned his attention to the philosophy of biology and bioethical topics. When, for example, in his important 1969 essay, "Philosophical Reflections on Experimenting with Human Subjects," he insisted upon a virtual *inversion* of practices by which the vulnerable were "obviously" the ones selected for experiments, it is important to realize that what he had himself seen in the Holocaust had taught him that the "vulnerable" should not be the subjects of medical experimentation. Those selected for such, he wrote, should be persons "where a maximum of identification, understanding, and spontaneity can be expected—that is, among the most highly motivated, the most highly educated, and the least 'captive' members of the community" (Jonas 1980). It is surely significant that Allan M. Brandt, in an important essay on racism and research, cites Jonas as having demonstrated precisely what had been criminally wrong in the Tuskegee syphilis experiment (Brandt 2000, 33).

But what about utopias and research?

First, it bears noting that Jonas, who himself had done extensive research on biology—as reflected in his 1966 book, *The Phenomenon of Life*—defended himself against any charge of being "anti-technology." Implicitly agreeing with Ricoeur that science has long been moving in the mode of a "chain reaction," Jonas insisted that "the 'technological imperative' is [in his own work] nowhere questioned, as it is indeed unquestionable in its anthropological primacy and integral to the human condition" (Jonas 1984, 203). It is obviously true in our era that "the technological drive takes care of itself" and is surely in no need of augmentation, especially via hype.

If *our* era has a need, it is for prudence. And this is why Jonas expressed his skepticism concerning the rationalizing ruse provided by utopian thinking about science and technology, especially when such thinking determines the decisions we make concerning medical and biotechnical ethics. While it was especially the unabashed utopianism of Ernst Bloch's book *Das Prinzip Hoffnung* that served as the text dismembered by Jonas's analysis (Jonas 1984, 194ff.), the author of a recent essay on Jonas rightly observes that Jonas was "puzzling [to] those readers who always ask if a writer is a rightist or a leftist," because that was difficult to discern (Hösle 2001, 32).

What Jonas found explicit in Bloch was something he found implicit in *all* utopian thinking—namely, a tilt toward valuing what humans will become in the future and a readiness to view that future development as the emergence at last of a *real* humanity. As a logical consequence, the humanity of both ourselves in the present and our ancestors in the past is seen as merely preparatory and, as such, inadequate, undesirable, and in need of being superseded. Jonas saw in such utopianism an "underlying ontology of the 'not yet' and the 'yet to come.'" And he described its flaw, one both fundamental and dangerous, as follows:

> The basic error of the ontology of "not yet" and its eschatological hope is repudiated by the plain truth—ground for neither jubilation nor dejection—that genuine man is already there and was there throughout known history; in his heights and his depths, his greatness and wretchedness, his bliss and his torment, his justice and his guilt—in short, in all the *ambiguity* that is inseparable from his humanity. Wishing to abolish this constitutive ambiguity is wishing to abolish man in his unfathomable freedom. In virtue of that freedom and the uniqueness of

each of its situations, man will indeed be always new and different from all before him, but never more "genuine." Never also exempt from the intrinsic perils, moral and other, that belongs to his genuineness. The really unambiguous man of utopia can only be the flattened, behaviorally conditioned homunculus of futuristic psychological engineering. This is today one of the things we have to *fear* of the future. *Hope* we should, quite contrary to the utopian hope, that in the future, too, every contentment will breed its discontent, every having its desire, every resting its unrest, every liberty its temptation—even every happiness its unhappiness. It is perhaps the only certainty we have about the human heart that it will not disappoint us in this expectation. But as regards the much-needed improvement of *conditions* for much or all of mankind, it is vitally necessary to *unhook the demands of justice, charity, and reason from the bait of utopia.* (Jonas 1984, 200–201)

I find it not unimportant that, in the same work within which Jonas levels cogent arguments against utopianism, he also makes a strong case for our generation's full responsibility to preserve humanity *as we have received and presently are it.* And, he argues, what it is our deepest responsibility to pass to future generations is *this* humanity in all its ambiguity—and clearly not some version of our species supposedly "improved" or ratcheted "upward" by eugenic bioengineering (Jonas 1984, 36–44).

Jonas upped the ante on so-called unintended consequences. Especially when something of crucial value is at stake, to pretend that such consequences may not show up, or that if they do, they will be deftly and safely handled, is not so much naïve as deceptive—to the individuals and the societies involved. And when we are tinkering with something such as the way we reproduce, we are, in fact, changing something basic to the way we have as humans always experienced our humanity. To *hope* for a satisfactory outcome or to express optimism about one will not suffice. Precisely because our proclivity (backed up by institutional pressures to beat the competition) is to be overly sanguine about outcomes, we need a corrective. We need strong reminders that consequences both unintended and unforeseen are the norm, not the exception. This is why Jonas insisted on our responsibility to imagine the *malum*—that is, unquestionably *bad* outcomes in projects, especially if those projects operate in a "chain reaction" in ways that will alter our way of being human. And in writing of our need to exercise what he called "the heuristics of fear," Jonas explained why such a heuristic could have a positive result, writing "it is an anticipated *distortion* of man that helps us to detect that in the normative conception of man which is to be preserved from it" (Jonas 1984, 26).[10]

I suggest that Hans Jonas invested so much of the time and energy of his final decades on bioethical questions precisely because, having witnessed within Germany the thought-trajectory that led to one kind of holocaust, he wished to articulate how we could detect the pattern of another if and when it would begin to take shape. It is why he indicated that loose talk about *improving* the species could lure us, in our naïveté, into incrementally and inadvertently destroying the species we not only have long been but also now have a duty to remain. He pointed out that we humans, simply by refusing to learn from history and with minds easily hooked on the "bait of utopia," could put not just what we have but *what we are* into a research trajectory that results in drastic, even tragic, changes. Recognizing that some research trajectories function almost like unstoppable chain-reactions and that humankind itself has begun to be the subject of technologies making changes at a very fast rate, Jonas challenged our generation to recognize that its prime duty is not to "improve" what we are as a species but to refuse—out of the highest ethical obligation—to put what we are at risk.

> For there is . . . an *unconditional duty* for mankind to exist, and it must not be confounded with the conditional duty of each and every man to exist. The right of the individual to commit suicide is morally arguable and must at least for particular circumstances be conceded; under no circumstances has mankind that right. Herewith we have found at last a *principle* that forbids certain technologically feasible "experiments," and of which that rule for decision making—to give the bad prognosis precedence over the good—was the pragmatic expression stated in advance. The ethical axiom, which validates the rules, is therefore as follows: Never must the existence or the essence of man as a whole be made a stake in the hazards of action. (Jonas 1984, 37)

Notes

1. Essays here by Winau and Frewer demonstrate how the establishment of "safeguards" can lead to a delusive sense of security.

2. In Japan the public appearances and books by Hirotada Ototake, born with neither arms nor legs, not only have done much to enhance the likelihood that persons with severe disabilities may no longer be hidden from public view but has also reinforced an awareness that even a very severe disability does not necessarily mean grave personal unhappiness or a "life" that either parents or society would have been wise to eliminate preemptively (Ototake 1998 and Ototake 2003).

3. This is another expression of what Tetsuo Yamaori, with a special skill for creating memorable metaphors, refers to in his essay here as both "a divine face and a demonic face" inevitably emerging within the world of medical research and application.

4. In English in Böhme 1992, 1–17, but in much more detail in German, Böhme 1993.

5. This is why, for instance, a public "uneasiness" about stem-cell research is not limited, in spite of what its proponents often claim, to persons opposed to abortion and intractably conservative on religious issues. See Shimazono in this volume. Note also that even Jürgen Habermas, in a clear departure from his earlier disregard of such matters, has recently urged reengagement with questions about the nature of human beings (Habermas 2002 and 2003).

6. In her chapter in this volume, Miho Ogino shows how, from within a feminist position, the kind of agenda laid out in Fletcher would appear, in any final analysis, to consist of *bad* advice.

7. The reappearance of the term "human nature" is instructive, in discourse such as this and its flagrant self-contradiction. The argument is: Our "choice" to follow the

path laid out by Stock is "inevitable" because it is our fixed "human nature" to alter an infinitely malleable human nature.

8. It is worth recalling what Fox and Swazey wrote concerning what they found disturbing in the ethos of American transplantation and artificial organ pioneers: "This ethos includes a classically American frontier outlook: heroic, pioneering, adventurous, optimistic, and determined" (Fox and Swazey, 1992, 199). See also LaFleur 2003a, 100–105, for other uses of the "frontier" metaphor to justify research that appeared to being going "too far."

9. This is certainly much less true in Germany and, at least in comparison with the Anglophone societies, less true in Japan as well. In 2003 the German government issued a special stamp to commemorate the centenary of Jonas's birth.

10. Although—typically—unmentioned, Jonas's concept of "heuristic fear" would seem to be included in what Pence targets as "knee-jerk condemnations arising out of fear and ignorance" (Pence 1998, 2). "Knee-jerk" scarcely applies to Jonas's carefully considered and articulated concepts. See LaFleur 2003b.

References

Annas, George J., and Michael A. Grodin. 1992. *The Nazi Doctors and the Nuremberg Code: Human Rights in Human Experimentation.* New York: Oxford University Press.

Böhme, Gernot. 1992. *Coping With Science.* Boulder, Colo.: Westview.

———. 1993. *Am Ende des Baconschen Zeitalters: Studien zur Wissenschaftsentwicklung.* Frankfurt: Suhrkamp.

———. 2003. *Leibsein als Aufgabe: Leibphilosophie in pragmatischer Hinsicht.* Zug: Die Graue Edition.

Brandt, Allan M. 2000. Racism and Research: The Case of the Tuskegee Syphilis Experiment. In *Tuskegee's Truths: Rethinking the Tuskegee Syphilis Study,* ed. Susan M. Reverby. Chapel Hill: University of North Carolina Press.

Charo, R. Alta. 2004. Passing on the Right: Conservative Bioethics Is Closer than It Appears. *Journal of Law, Medicine, and Ethics* 32, no. 2: 307–14.

Descartes, René. [1637] 1950. *Discourse on Method.* Trans. Laurence J. Lafleur. Indianapolis: Bobbs-Merrill.

Fletcher, Joseph. 1988. *The Ethics of Genetic Control: Ending Reproductive Roulette.* Buffalo, N.Y.: Prometheus Books.

Fox, Renée, and Judith P. Swazey. 1992. *Spare Parts: Organ Replacement in American Society.* New York: Oxford University Press.

Gross, Paul R., and Norman Levitt. 1994. *Higher Superstition: The Academic Left and Its Quarrels with Science.* Baltimore: Johns Hopkins University Press.

Habermas, Jürgen. 2002. *Die Zukunft der menschlichen Natur: Auf dem Weg zu einer liberalen Eugenik?* Frankfurt: Suhrkamp.

———. 2003. *The Future of Human Nature.* Cambridge: Polity.

Hösle, Vittorio. 2001. Ontology and Ethics in Hans Jonas. *Graduate Faculty Philosophy Journal [The New School]* 23, no. 1: 31–50.

Jonas, Hans. 1966. *The Phenomenon of Life: Towards a Philosophical Biology.* New York: Harper and Row.

———. 1980. *Philosophical Essays: From Ancient Creed to Technological Man.* Chicago: University of Chicago Press. Reprint.

———. 1984. *The Imperative of Responsibility: In Search of an Ethics for the Technological Age.* Chicago: University of Chicago Press.

Jones, James H. 1993. *Bad Blood: The Tuskegee Syphilis Experiment.* New York: Free Press.

Jonsen, Albert R. 1998. *The Birth of Bioethics.* New York: Oxford University Press.

LaFleur, William R. 2003a. Transplanting the Transplant: Japanese Sensitivity to American Medicine as an American Mission. *Society and Medicine: Essays in Honor of Renée C. Fox,* ed. Carla M. Messikomer, Judith P. Swazey, and Allen Glicksman, 87–107. New Brunswick, N.J.: Transaction Publications.

———. 2003b. Philosophy and Fear: Hans Jonas and the Japanese Debate about the Ethics of Organ Transplantation. In *Technology and Cultural Values: On the Edge of the Third Millennium,* ed. Peter D. Hershock et al., 158–75. Honolulu: University of Hawai'i Press.

Moreno, Jonathan D. 2001. *Undue Risk: Secret State Experiments on Humans.* New York: Routledge.

Morioka, Masahiro. 2001. *Seimeigaku ni nani ga dekiru ka? Nōshi, fueminizumu, yūsei shisō.* Tokyo: Keisō shobō.

Nelkin, Dorothy, and M. Susan Lindee. 1995. *The DNA Mystique: The Gene as a Cultural Icon.* New York: W. H. Freeman.

Ototake, Hirotada. 1998. *Gotai fumanzoku.* Tokyo: Kōdansha.

———. 2003. *Ototake repōto—'03 Han.* Tokyo: Kōdansha.

Pence, Gregory E. 1998. *Who's Afraid of Human Cloning?* Oxford: Rowman and Littlefield.

Ricoeur, Paul. 1986. *Lectures on Ideology and Utopia.* Ed. George H. Taylor. New York: Columbia University Press.

Rosen, Christine. 2004. *Preaching Eugenics: Religious Leaders and the American Eugenics Movement.* Oxford: Oxford University Press.

Rosenberg, Charles E. 1997. *No Other Gods: On Science and American Social Thought.* Baltimore: Johns Hopkins University Press.

Silver, Lee M. 1997. *Remaking Eden: How Genetic Engineering and Cloning Will Transform the American Family.* New York: Avon Books.

Stock, Gregory. 2002. *Redesigning Humans: Our Inevitable Genetic Future.* New York: Houghton Mifflin.

Truog, Robert D. 1998. Is It Time to Abandon Brain Death? In *The Ethics of Organ Transplants: The Current Debate,* ed. Arthur L. Caplan and Daniel H. Coelho. New York: Prometheus Books. Originally published in 1997.

Wada, Jurō. [1992] 1998. *Nōshi to shinzō ishoku: Are kara 25 nen.* Tokyo: Kanki shuppan.

Watson, James D. 1998. Afterword. In *Murderous Science: Elimination by Scientific Selection of Jews, Gypsies, and Others in Germany, 1933–1945,* by Benno Müller-Hill; trans. G. R. Fraser. Woodbury, N.Y.: Cold Spring Harbor Laboratory Press.

Welsome, Eileen. 1999. *The Plutonium Files: America's Secret Medical Experiments in the Cold War.* New York: Random House.

Williams, Peter, and David Wallace. 1989. *Unit 731: The Japanese Army's Secret of Secrets.* London: Hodder and Stoughten.

Contributors

Gernot Böhme is founder and Director of the Institut für Praxis der Philosophie and prior to that was Professor of Philosophy at the Technical University of Darmstadt. His studies of mathematics, physics, and philosophy were at the Max-Planck-Institute for Research in the Conditions of Life in the Scientific-Technical World in Starnberg, whose directors were C. F. von Weizsäcker and Jürgen Habermas. The primary foci of his research are classical philosophy, Plato, Kant, the Sociology of Science, Philosophical Anthropology, Aesthetics, Ethics, Goethe, and Theories of Time. He is author and editor of more than forty works in German, including *Leibsein als Aufgabe: Leibphilosophie in pragmatischer Hinsicht*. Among Böhme's publications in English are *Coping with Science* and *Ethics in Context: The Art of Dealing with Serious Questions*. He contributes regularly to Europe's public media, held the distinguished Jan-Tinbergen-Professorship at the University of Rotterdam in 1985–1986, and received the Denkbar-Award for *Obliques Denken* in 2002.

Arthur L. Caplan is the Emmanuel and Robert Hart Professor of Bioethics, Chair of the Department of Medical Ethics, and Director of the Center for Bioethics at the University of Pennsylvania in Philadelphia. He served on President Clinton's Advisory Committee on Gulf War Illnesses. Caplan is author or editor of twenty-five books and over five hundred papers—on the ethics of medical experimentation, IVF, organ transplantation, and the costs of health care. His edited works include *When Medicine Went Mad: Bioethics and the Holocaust; Health, Disease and Illness; The Case of Terri Schiavo: Ethics at the End of Life* and among the books he has authored are *Due Consideration: Controversy in the Age of Medical Miracle; Am I My Brother's Keeper? The Ethical Frontiers of Biomedicine; If I Were a Rich Man Could I Buy a Pancreas?* and *Smart Mice, Not So Smart People*.

Frederick R. Dickinson is Associate Professor of Japanese History at the University of Pennsylvania. Born in Tokyo and raised in Kanazawa and Kyoto, Japan, he holds an M. A. and Ph.D. in History from Yale University and an M. A. in International Politics from Kyoto University. He is author of *War and National Reinvention: Japan in the Great War, 1914–1919* and "Dai-ichiji taisengo no Nihon no kōsō: Nihon ni okeru Uirusonshugi no juyō," in *Nijū seiki Higashi Ajia no chitsujo keisei to Nihon*, edited by Yukio Itō and Minoru Kawada. Dickinson has received grants from the Japanese Ministry of Education, the Fulbright Commission, and the Japan Foundation. He was a National Fellow at the Hoover Institution, Stanford University (2000–2001) and has held visiting professorships at Swarthmore College, Katholieke Universiteit Leuven in Belgium, and Kyoto University. His current research focuses on Japanese political and cultural reconstruction following the Great War, 1919–1931.

Renée C. Fox, a sociologist of medicine, is the Annenberg Professor Emerita of the Social Sciences and a Senior Fellow at the Center for Bioethics at the University of Pennsylvania. She is also a Research Associate at Queen Elizabeth House at the University of Oxford. Among her books are *Experiment Perilous: Physicians and Patients Facing the Unknown* and *The Sociology of Medicine: A Participant Observer's View. The Courage to Fail: A Social View of Organ Transplants and Dialysis* and *Spare Parts: Organ Replacement in American Society* were both coauthored with Judith P. Swazey. A Fellow of the American Association for the Advancement of Science and of the American Academy of Arts and Sciences, Fox holds nine honorary degrees, is a recipient of the Centennial Medal from the Graduate School of Arts and Sciences of Harvard University, and been named a Chevalier of the Order of Leopold II by the government of Belgium.

Andreas Frewer, a Professor at the Institute for History, Ethics, and Philosophy of Medicine at Hanover Medical School since 2002, studied medicine, philosophy, and the history of medicine in Munich, Erlangen, Oxford, Jerusalem, and Berlin. His Ph.D. is from the Free University of Berlin, and he has a Masters in Bioethics from the University of Leuven. He earlier held a position at the University of Göttingen and served as temporary director of the Institute for History and Ethics of Medicine at the Goethe-University in Frankfurt. Among his publications are the books *Medizin und Moral in Weimarer Republik und Nationalsozialismus: Die Zeitschrift "Ethik" unter Emil Abderhalden* and *Bibliotheca Sudhoffiana,* as well as several publications on euthanasia, on research ethics, and on the historical and ethical aspects of medicine. He is editor of the series *Culture of Medicine* (21 vols.) and a member of the Academy for Ethics in Medicine and of the Editorial Board of *Theoretical Medicine and Bioethics.*

G. Cameron Hurst III is Professor of Japanese and Korean Studies at the University of Pennsylvania and Director of its Center for East Asian Studies. Educated at Stanford, the University of Hawaiʻi, and Columbia University, he was a professor at the University of Kansas before joining the Penn faculty. Fluent in Korean and Japanese, he has focused his research as a historian on premodern Japan. He has held teaching and administrative positions in Hiroshima, Kyoto, Seoul, and Hong Kong. He is author of *Insei: Abdicated Sovereigns in the Politics of Late Heian Japan, 1086–1185,* co-translator of Yukichi Fukuzawa's *Outline of a Theory of Civilization,* and co-author of *Samurai Painters.* His *Armed Martial Arts of Japan* is the first of a two-volume work. Hurst wrote many of the entries on premodern history in the *Kodansha Encyclopedia of Japan* and regularly contributes essays, especially on politics and society, to American and East Asian newspapers.

Yoshihiko Komatsu is a Professor at Tokyo University of Marine Science and Technology. Born in Tokyo, he did graduate work and research for his Ph.D. in the Division of the Natural Sciences at the University of Tokyo. The areas of Komatsu's concentration are the History of Science and Bioethics. Important among his published works is a research article, "Kurōdo Berunāru no seimei-kan no rekishiteki kyōi," in a collection of essays in Japanese on Claude Bernard, a French physiologist of the nineteenth century. Komatsu has examined the right to autonomous decision making in bioethics from both historical and philosophical points of view—first in *Shisō*, Japan's premier journal of philosophy, and then in a 2004 book. His widely hailed 1996 book on death, brain death, and organ transplantation is entitled *Shi wa kyōmei suru: Nōshi, zōki ishoku no fukami e*. Another book, *Tasogare no tetsugaku: Nōshi zōki ishoku, genpatsu, daiokishin*, was published in 2000, on a range of social, industrial, and bioethical problems.

William R. LaFleur is the E. Dale Saunders Professor in Japanese Studies at the University of Pennsylvania. Having a Ph.D. from the University of Chicago, he taught at Princeton University and the University of California–Los Angeles before joining the Penn faculty. Although his earlier research and books dealt with medieval Japan, during the past two decades he has focused more on modern Japan, especially the relationships among religion, philosophy, and ethics there. His *Liquid Life: Abortion and Buddhism in Japan* was widely noticed. A Senior Fellow at Penn's Center for Bioethics, he has lectured in various venues on Japanese topics and comparative issues in medical ethics. His work has been translated into German, Russian, and Japanese. A book in process compares bioethics in the United States and Japan. A recipient of numerous fellowships, he was awarded the Watsuji Tetsurō Culture Prize for scholarship published in Japanese.

Susan Lindee is Professor of the History and Sociology of Science at the University of Pennsylvania. She is author of *Suffering Made Real: American Science and the Survivors at Hiroshima*, which explores the Atomic Bomb Casualty Commission–sponsored and funded scientific efforts to decipher the biological effects of radiation. Her most recent work, *Moments of Truth in Genomic Medicine*, places the history of genetic disease in a Cold War context. With the late Dorothy Nelkin, she published *The DNA Mystique: The Gene as a Cultural Icon*. Her review in *Science* of James Watson's latest work expressed profound skepticism about his ideas and elicited positive responses from scientists around the world. Her contribution to the present volume is part of a larger study for which she was awarded a Guggenheim Fellowship; it deals with the relationship between war and science in the United States from 1914 to the present and has "Knowledge to Heal, Knowledge to Injure" as its working title.

Jonathan D. Moreno is the David and Lyn Silfen University Professor at the University of Pennsylvania. He is a member of the Board on Health Sciences

Policy of the Institute of Medicine (National Academy of Sciences) and a past president of the American Society for Bioethics and Humanities. Moreno co-chaired the National Academy of Sciences Committee on Guidelines for Human Embryonic Stem Cell Research and is a Fellow of the Hastings Center, a Fellow of the New York Academy of Medicine, and an adjunct scholar at the Center for American Progress. His multiple books include *Deciding Together: Bioethics and Moral Consensus; Undue Risk: Secret State Experiments on Humans,* nominated for the Los Angeles Times Book Prize and a Virginia Literary Award; *In the Wake of Terror: Medicine and Morality in a Time of Crisis; Is There an Ethicist in the House? On the Cutting Edge of Bioethics;* and *Mind Wars: Brain Research and National Defense.*

Benno Müller-Hill studied chemistry in Freiburg and Munich and worked as a research fellow in the laboratory of James Watson at Harvard University. He isolated the Lac Repressor Protein with Walter Gilbert. Until 1998 he was Professor at the Genetics Institute of University of Köln. His main areas of research in the field of genetics have been protein-DNA interaction and gene control. He published *The Lac Operon: A Short History of a Genetic Paradigm,* as well as *Tödliche Wissenschaft,* a history of human genetics during Germany's Nazi period and a work credited with exposing the collusion between eugenic programs and racist politics during that period. Translated into English as *Murderous Science: Elimination by Scientific Selection of Jews, Gypsies, and Others in Germany, 1933–1945,* its paperback edition includes an afterword by James D. Watson. Müller-Hill is an elected member of the Academia Europaea, an Honorary Fellow of the Hebrew University of Jerusalem, and *Doctor Honoris Causa* of the Israel Institute of Technology (Technion) in Haifa.

Miho Ogino is Professor of Japanese Studies in the Faculty of Letters at the Graduate School of Osaka University. The areas of her research are the history of women's bodies and gender. She published *Seishoku no seijigaku: Feminizumu to bāsu kontororu* (The politics of reproduction: Feminism and birth control), followed by *Chūzetsu ronsō to Amerika shakai: Shintai o meguru sensō* (The abortion controversy and American society: A war over bodies) and *Jendāka sareru shintai* (Gendering the body). Ogino authored numerous articles on these topics and the politics of reproduction in both Japan and the Western world. One published in English is "Abortion and Women's Reproductive Rights: The State of Japanese Women, 1945–1991," in *Women of Japan and Korea,* edited by Joyce Gelb and Marian Leif Palley (1994). She contributed to the Life and Death Studies project at the University of Tokyo and is currently working on both the politics of the family planning movement in post–World War II Japan and feminist views on reproductive technologies.

Susumu Shimazono, Professor in the Department of Religious Studies of the University of Tokyo, has published widely on modern and contemporary religious movements, especially those of Japan. He is author of nine books in Japanese, one in Korean, and one in English entitled *From Salvation to Spirituality: Popular Religious Movements in Modern Japan* (2004). Although Shimazono's works focus mainly on empirical and historical research on Japan, his interest in comparative perspectives is keen. He has been invited to teach at the University of Chicago, at Ecole des Hautes Etudes en Science Sociales, and at Eberhardt Karls Universität in Tübingen. His interest in bioethics, and especially in the relationship between religion, medicine, and ethics, is reflected in his directorship of a multiyear project on Death and Life Studies at the University of Tokyo and his 2006 book, *Inochi no hajimari no seimei rinri*. He also serves on the Japanese Prime Minister's Research Council in Bioethics.

Kei-ichi Tsuneishi is Professor of the History of Science at Kanagawa University in Japan. A student of both physics and history, in 1981 he published *Kieta saikin senbutai*, the first major work of research on the infamous 731 Unit. He continued research on Japan's wartime use of human subjects and published books such as *Igakushatachi no soshiki hanzai*, a work showing physicians engaged in what was tantamount to institutionalized murder. He has begun research on the Japanese materials seized by the American army after the end of World War II and now kept on microfilm in the Library of Congress. Tsuneishi has also been leading the grass-roots movement in Japan to identify the bones discovered in 1989 on the Tokyo site where the Japanese army's medical college had been during World War II. By putting together the results of this archeological find, what is already known about Unit 731, and the materials he is researching in Washington, D.C., Tsuneishi expects to provide a comprehensive account of this horrendous wartime medical research.

Rolf Winau was, until his sudden death while this book was in preparation, Professor of the History of Medicine and Chair of that department at the Charité Berlin. He studied history, literature, philosophy, and medicine, gaining his Ph.D. at the University of Freiburg and his medical doctorate at the University of Mainz. Winau was the founding director of the Center for Humanities and Health Sciences at the Charité. He served as president of the German Society for the History of Medicine, Science, and Technology and also of the Association for the History of Medcine. Among his many publications are books such as *Versuche mit Menschen* (with H. Helmchen), a study of experiments on human subjects, and *Versuche mit Menschen: Historische Entwicklung und ethischer Diskurs*, an examination of the historical development and ethical discourse of the same topic.

Tetsuo Yamaori recently retired as Director-General of the International Research Center for Japanese Studies, located in Kyoto. Born in San Francisco, he has made the comparison of cultures, religions, and ethical systems the major focus of his research and writing. Specializing early in the study of Indian philosophy, he served as Professor at the National Museum of Japanese History, as Dean of the Graduate School of Kyoto University of Art and Design, and as

President of Hakuhō Women's College. Known widely within both Japan's academic world and the general public as an authority on religion, philosophy, and ethics, Yamaori presents his views on public affairs frequently in national newspapers and television. Among his numerous books are *Rei to niku* (The spirit and the flesh), *Rinshi no shisō* (Critical questions about facing death), *Nihonjin no shūkyō kankaku* (The religious sensibility of the Japanese), and, in English, *Wandering Spirit and Temporary Corpses: Studies in the History of Japanese Religious Tradition*. He received the Watsuji Tetsurō Culture Prize and the NHK Broadcast Cultural Award.

Index